MCAT Reasoning

CARS and Science

blueprint

2nd Edition Acknowledgments
Reviewers: Elizabeth Flagge and Mackenzie Perkins
Editors: Sumedha Attanti, Amanda Koch PhD. Paul Forn, Brian McGrew, and Lauren White
Copywriters: Aislinn McCormack, Zoe Mikel-Stites, and Emily Soto
Cover Design: Becca Roth and Lona Ryan

Special thanks to all of the writers, editors, and reviewers involved in prior editions

Printed in the United States of America

First Printing, 2022

ISBN 978-1-944935-33-7

Blueprint Education Subsidiary Holdings LLC
6080 Center Drive
Suite 520
Los Angeles, CA 90045

MCAT is a registered trademark of the American Association of Medical Colleges (AAMC). The AAMC has neither reviewed nor endorsed this work in any way.

Second Edition

This page left intentionally blank.

This page left intentionally blank.

STOP! READ ME FIRST!

Welcome and congratulations on taking this important step in your MCAT prep process!

The book you're holding is one of Blueprint's six MCAT review books, and contains concise content review with a specific focus on the science that you need for MCAT success. To get the most out of this book, we'd like to draw your attention to some distinctive aspects of our book set and their role in MCAT prep.

First and foremost, **books are not enough** for MCAT prep. Realistic practice is absolutely essential, and should include both MCAT-targeted practice questions and an ample number of full-length practice exams that simulate the MCAT itself.

Second, **our books reflect our experience**. Our book editing team is made up of a combination of people: they represent people who have been in your shoes and have excelled on the MCAT, people who are truly experts in MCAT style critical thinking and reasoning, and people who are experienced tutors and instructors with a focus on MCAT prep (not to mention a few skilled copywriters and communicators to keep us on our toes!). This makes our books unlike many other MCAT review products, which provide a dry, factual overview of scientific knowledge without MCAT-specific context. Our books recognize that the **MCAT is primarily a test of thinking**—and more specifically, a test that reflects how the American Association of Medical Colleges encourages future physicians to think. The "MCAT Strategy" sidebars throughout the book call out specific points to be aware of as you study, and in general, our approach to presenting science is informed by how science is tested on the MCAT—that is, in a way that draws upon passages, builds connections across subject areas, and prioritizes an understanding of fundamental principles. In a nutshell, it's our hope that by studying with these books, you can benefit from our team's unparalleled MCAT expertise.

Third, after completing a chapter, we urge you to test your knowledge with all of the online practice materials that were included with your Blueprint course: our Learning Modules, Qbank, End of Chapter Quizzes, and of course our Practice Tests.

We wish you the best of luck on your MCAT journey,

The Blueprint MCAT Team

This page left intentionally blank.

TABLE OF CONTENTS

This page left intentionally blank.

MCAT Basics

0. Introduction

Throughout your MCAT prep journey, you'll be engaging in regular, realistic MCAT practice and analyzing the results of that practice. Therefore, the first step in this process is to become familiar with what the MCAT *is* (a source of surprisingly many misconceptions) and what the experience of taking the MCAT is like.

> **MCAT STRATEGY >>>**
>
> Used to our books having MCAT strategy sidebars? You won't see them in this Reasoning book, as the entirety of the text is strategy focused! For key takeaways, refer to the Must-Knows at the end of each chapter.

1. What's on the MCAT?

The MCAT has four sections: three science sections and one verbal reasoning-based section, called Critical Analysis and Reasoning Skills, or CARS for short. The sections, in the order that you will encounter them, are:

> Chemical and Physical Foundations of Biological Systems, often shortened to Chem/Phys or C/P
> Critical Analysis and Reasoning Skills (CARS)
> Biological and Biochemical Foundations of Living Systems, shortened to Bio/Biochem or B/B
> Psychological, Social, and Biological Foundations of Behavior, abbreviated Psych/Soc or P/S

Each science section consists of 59 questions, while the CARS section is slightly shorter with 53 questions.

The majority of questions on the MCAT are associated with a **passage**, which is a piece of writing intended to be used as a reference for at least some of the associated questions. Passages predominate in the science sections, with 10 passages and 44 associated questions per section, and only 15 **discretes**, or non-passage-associated questions. In CARS, there are nine passages per section, and all questions are passage-associated.

Science passages can vary in length, but usually fall in the range of 100-400 words. They can contain one or multiple figures and tables. Question sets in these sections alternate between passage-associated and discrete sets. **CARS passages** are structured similarly to the reading comprehension passages you may have encountered previously on standardized exams. Specifically, they lack figures and are typically closer to 500-600 words.

With the exception of CARS, which requires no outside content knowledge, each of the MCAT sections requires a familiarity with several different subject areas. The subject area coverage in each section: consists of the following breakdown:

SECTION	BREAKDOWN
Chemical and Physical Foundations	30% general chemistry, 25% physics, 25% biochemistry, 15% organic chemistry, and 5% biology
Biological and Biochemical Foundations	65% biology, 25% biochemistry, 5% organic chemistry, and 5% general chemistry
Psychological, Social, and Biological Foundations of Behavior	65% psychology, 30% sociology, and 5% biology

Figure 1. Breakdown of MCAT sections

A key takeaway is that Chem/Phys, for instance, is not just limited to chemistry and physics. A common theme across MCAT science sections is that passages are nearly always focused on some biological, biochemical, or physiological phenomenon, even if the test-makers then use that passage to ask physics- or general chemistry-based questions. Additionally, keep in mind that some variation, typically ±5%, can happen across examinations with regard to those percentages.

Combining the above percentages for all three science sections, we can see that biology is the most heavily-tested subject, as well as the only subject that appears in all three sections. On the other end of the spectrum, organic chemistry is the most lightly tested.

Finally, it's worth noting that no section contains fewer than three subjects. This is important, because it gets at the heart of a fundamental truth about how the MCAT is designed: the MCAT test-makers love **integrating multiple subject areas**. For example, the test-makers could ask a chemistry question that also requires knowledge of a biochemistry topic, or a question about an organic separatory technique that also presupposes knowledge of biomolecules.

The AAMC (American Association of Medical Colleges—or, in simple terms, the test-writers) classifies questions in two key ways: by content category and reasoning skill. The content categories are essentially topic-based categories that can be found in the official **content outline** provided by the AAMC (search online for "AAMC What's On the MCAT Exam" and you will find links to this PDF), and they range from 1A to 10A. Categories 1A through 3B refer to the Bio/Biochem section, categories 4A through 5E refer to Chem/Phys, and categories 6A through 10A classify questions that appear in the Psych/Soc section. On one hand, we don't recommend that you spend much time agonizing over these categories, because they can confuse more than they help. Specifically, because each science section integrates content from multiple subjects, it can feel like there's a lot of overlap. However, most courses and textbooks teach science content by *subject* and not by exam *section*, so the content categories are helpful in seeing, for example, exactly which section or sections a particular topic might appear on.

The other system of AAMC classification is by **reasoning skill**. The AAMC emphasizes the importance of a number of scientific inquiry and critical reasoning skills, and to that end, they've defined four core skills for science and three for CARS. Starting with science, the first reasoning skill is **Knowledge of Scientific Concepts and Principles**. Most students will find this to be the simplest skill, because it focuses on recognition and recall of the science concepts that you'll learn throughout your prep. In other words, these are the (relatively) simple science questions that you'll occasionally encounter. Skill 2 is **Scientific Reasoning and Problem-solving**, and these questions get a bit more complex, as they ask you to reason about scientific principles or analyze scientific predictions or explanations. Skill 3 is **Reasoning and Design about the Execution of Research**, and Skill 4 is **Data-based Statistical Reasoning**. These aren't necessarily more *difficult* than the other skills, but they are more specific.

2. MCAT Timing, Scoring, and Exam Day

As mentioned in Section 1, the science sections each consist of 59 questions, and you'll be given 95 minutes to finish each one. This boils down to about 1.5 minutes per question - although you need to factor in time to read the passages, too. The CARS section has only 53 questions and one fewer passage. Correspondingly its time allotment is lower: exactly 90 minutes. Some simple math tells us that nine passages in 90 minutes works out to exactly 10 minutes per passage. There are breaks between each section: a 10-minute break between the Chem/Phys and CARS section, a 30-minute break (for a quick lunch) between the CARS section and Bio/Biochem, and finally another 10-minute break between Bio/Biochem and Psych/Soc. It is not mandatory that you take the entire time of the breaks, although doing so can help provide a much-needed mental refresh.

Structure of the MCAT

	Minutes	Number of questions
Examinee agreement	8	
Tutorial	10	
Chemical and Physical Foundations of Biological Systems	95	59
Break	10	
Critical Analysis and Reasoning Skills	90	53
Extended break	30	
Biological and Biochemical Foundations of Living Systems	95	59
Break	10	
Psychological, Social and Biological Foundations of Behavior	95	59
Void question	5	
Satisfaction survey	5	

Figure 2. Time allowance breakdown of the MCAT

The above time constraints apply to students who are taking the MCAT under standard testing conditions. In certain cases, test-takers may qualify for testing **accommodations**. This most commonly applies in cases of impairments or medical conditions, for example sensory impairments and learning disabilities. While the AAMC provides a wide range of accommodations to students who qualify, the most common are timing accommodations, which can provide the test-taker with extra time per section or extended break times. Since qualifying for accommodations is a rigorous process that involves, among other steps, an evaluation by a qualified professional it's approval is not a guarantee by any means, even if you have received testing accommodations in the past. The AAMC is the arbiter of all requests for accommodations, so we recommend visiting the AAMC's website as soon as possible if you believe that you might qualify for accommodations. Since the process takes time, the earlier you can get the ball rolling, the better.

Moving on to a question at the top of every student's mind, how is the MCAT scored? On one hand, the answer is simple: a scaled score is assigned for each section from **118** to **132**, and the four scaled scores sum to a range between **472** and **528**. The median score is 500, so if you receive a score greater than 500, you've done better than 50% of test-takers, and vice versa. For reference, in the 2021-22 application cycle, the mean MCAT score of applicants to medical school (as distinct from test-takers, because not all test-takers apply) was around 506, and the mean MCAT score of *matriculants* (that is, people who applied to medical school, were accepted, and enrolled) was between 511 and 512. That said, it's important to note that what counts as a "good" MCAT score varies significantly depending on your goals, which may be one specific program, U.S. MD schools in general, DO schools, Canadian schools, or some other option. For this reason, we recommend researching the programs you plan to apply to so you can understand the score range you'll need to aim for to give yourself a solid chance.

Each scaled score can be converted to a **percentile score**. Percentile scores are common across standardized exams in general, and they refer simply to the percent of students who scored lower than you did. If your score falls in the 65th percentile, then you performed as well or better than 65% of test-takers. One final note about scores: unlike some exams, you will not receive your MCAT score immediately after finishing the exam. Instead, should you choose to have the exam scored, you'll receive it about 30 to 35 days after your exam day. The AAMC publicizes exact score release dates, so if you know when you'll be taking the exam, you can also look up when your scores will be released. Meanwhile, if you haven't registered for the exam yet, we recommend doing so as soon as possible unless you have a very extended timeline (for example, if you plan to spend the next six months prepping). Registering as early as possible is important, since seats do fill up, and you'll want to take your exam in a location as convenient to you as possible.

3. Basics of MCAT Prep

There are three core elements of MCAT prep: (1) a study plan, (2) content and reasoning-related review materials, and (3) practice materials. Blueprint offers abundant resources in all three domains, including a freely accessible study plan tool, a comprehensive online MCAT course, and a broad range of practice materials including a half-length diagnostic examination and 10 realistic practice Full Length MCAT exams. If you are a Blueprint course student, we would recommend using your online materials to acquaint yourself with the details of what the course offers. In this section, we will focus on some key points and frequent questions about MCAT prep in general.

The first point to make regarding your **study plan** is just how useful it can be to take advantage of others' accumulated expertise on MCAT prep in this regard. It's hard enough to actually *study* for the MCAT, but trying to figure out from scratch *how* to do so is exponentially more difficult. It's also important to create a realistic study plan. This is an area where it's hard to make 100% across-the-board generalizations, because people's MCAT prep timelines can vary widely (anywhere from three to six months is common), the time people have available for MCAT prep can be dramatically different (some students balance MCAT prep with full-time school and/or work commitments, others take time off to devote entirely to MCAT prep), and students can be at very different stages with regard to how long it has been since they completed their science coursework. That said, the AAMC has recommended that students spend about 300 hours preparing for the exam. That equates to roughly 20 hours per week, or a half-time job, over the course of three months. Some variation is certainly possible, but this is a useful benchmark to keep in mind. Once you start studying, if you find that you have unexpectedly little time available for MCAT prep or that MCAT prep is taking you longer than expected, it may be worth considering changing your exam date.

Let's now turn to content and reasoning-related **review materials**. The core takeaway here is that you need both content knowledge and reasoning skills to succeed, and MCAT success depends on applying them *together*, not in isolation. The reason for this is that the MCAT is all about integration of concepts. Many questions (especially those related to a passage) draw upon multiple science topics, and similarly most questions require *both* an understanding of some content information *and* a subset of reasoning skills. The integration of content and reasoning skills is a hallmark of the Blueprint approach to MCAT prep, informed by hands-on experience with thousands of students, and being aware of this idea at the beginning of your MCAT prep process will help you study most effectively.

Last but not least, **practice materials** are vital. Realistic MCAT practice should start at the *beginning* of your MCAT prep process, and for this purpose, we recommend our half-length diagnostic exam. The diagnostic exam is a test that is structured exactly like a full-length MCAT, except each section is half as long. For this reason, we sometimes refer to it as the "half-length diag" - half-length because, at this point, it serves two key purposes. First, it's scored, so it provides you with a score baseline, or initial sense of where you're at and how much you'll need to improve. Second, and arguably more importantly, *it gives you an early sense of what the MCAT exam is like*. We can't emphasize this enough: your MCAT study process will be *massively* more effective if you understand the test that you're studying for. Then, after the diagnostic, practice materials (including both realistic Full Length tests and shorter, more content-focused review questions) should be a regular part of your study schedule.

Taking practice materials, including realistic Full Length exams, is good, but the real magic comes from careful review. It should take at least as much time to review an exam as it did to take it. This might sound like overkill, but we're entirely serious. During the review process, we recommend:

> Analyzing both the questions you got right (especially those you were unsure of) and those you got wrong, to build a more comprehensive picture of your strengths and weaknesses at any given point in time.

> Focusing on the *reasoning* each question requires, above and beyond the content knowledge. In other words, what cognitive steps were required to solve the problems? If you didn't know some relevant science information, how would knowing that content have changed your process? Was there an alternate way of solving the problem that you could have used, even without the knowledge involved?

> Creating and using a tool we call the Lessons Learned Journal, or LLJ. An LLJ is just that - a document, whether on paper or in a spreadsheet or Word document, where you can list the lessons you learn from the passages, questions, and even content modules that you complete. Every student's LLJ can be slightly different, but the core principles are:

    — It should be easily searchable, or at least structured in a way that makes it easy to see which question or questions correspond to each "lesson" you identify.

    — Lessons should be written in concise, understandable terms that you'd comprehend even if paging through the journal in a few spare minutes. They should hit a sweet spot of usefulness in between the extremes of specificity and generality. For example, a good lesson might be something like "In ΔG problems, always make sure to convert the units for ΔH and ΔS to be the same." This is specific to a certain set of problems, but not limited to a *single* problem.

    — Lessons should correspond to *action points*. Integrating this with the previous point, we can see why "In ΔG problems, always make sure to convert the units for ΔH and ΔS to be the same" is a good lesson: in addition to hitting the sweet spot in terms of generalizability, it *gives you something to do* the next time you take a test. In comparison, some less good lessons could include "I'm so stupid - I've got to get this right!" (too general, demoralizing, no action points) or, alternatively, an entire essay about some content topic (too specific, no action points).

4. The MCAT Testing Experience

Next, let's switch gears to discuss what it's like to take the MCAT itself. This material will be relevant in the run-up to the exam, so you may want to bookmark it for then. We're including it here because it's also valuable to have a sense of what you're preparing for.

First off, expect the testing experience to **start early**, and last for **most of the day**. You'll want to arrive at your testing center at about 7:30 am. If you expect time delays with traffic or public transportation, give yourself additional wiggle room. For this reason, it can be useful to scout out the testing center sometime in the week or so before the exam. By doing so, you can familiarize yourself with the route, where to park, what the building looks like, and any surprises like road work or other predictable sources of delays and congestion.

You will need to bring several **items** with you to the testing center. The first, and most essential, is your government-issued photo ID. You *must* have this to take the MCAT. Most students bring a driver's license or passport, but any current, English-language, government-issued photo ID with an accompanying signature is acceptable. However, a student ID will *not* work. Additionally, you'll also want to bring a bottle of water and food for your breaks.

The **check-in process** can take a while, especially if others are in front of you, so don't be surprised if you find yourself waiting to be checked in. You might consider bringing a book to occupy yourself while you wait, or plan on taking that time to do some breathing or meditation exercises and get in the best mental state possible right before the test. What we do *not* recommend is taking that time to repeatedly and nervously rehearse pieces of rote content knowledge. By the time you're at the testing center itself, it's time to take a leap of faith and trust in all of the work you've already put in. On a similar note, we recommend taking the day before the test off from any sort of MCAT prep. Instead of reviewing amino acids, do something nice for yourself, and try to reconnect with who you are outside of the often-overwhelming process of MCAT prep. The one caveat here is that sometimes students feel like *not* studying might be an additional source of anxiety. If the only way to calm your racing mind is to review your chart of amino acids a few more times or do a few short, *easy* practice problems, that might be OK, but we really do suggest minimizing your last-minute studying as much as possible. Being rested and at peak focus is much more important than one last day of studying.

When you enter the testing center, you'll be given a check-in number and told to wait. Once your number is called, you'll verify your identity, sit for a picture, have your palms scanned, and hand over your photo ID. If you brought your phone, or any other electronic devices, they will be sealed in a small plastic bag, which will then be unsealed at the end of the exam. During your check-in, you may also be asked to remove certain accessories, such as wristwatches or hair pins. These can be stored, along with food and anything else you've brought, in an onsite locker provided for you. The check-in process shouldn't take more than a few minutes after your number is called. Once you're checked in, a proctor will walk you through a short security screening: you'll show them your ID, turn out your pockets, and repeat the palm scan. You'll repeat this security check anytime you leave the test room, such as on a break. After the security check is finished, you'll be given a booklet to take notes in, consisting of several laminated pages of grid paper, and an accompanying marker. These are wet erase pages, which is different from the *dry* erase that you might be more accustomed to, and this means you won't be able to erase your notes during the test.

With your check-in and security processes finished, it's time to enter the **test room**. You'll be escorted to your computer, carrying your ID, locker key, and dry erase booklet and marker. There will also be noise-cancelling headphones at the computer, if you wish to use them, and most centers will provide foam earbuds upon request. The proctor will start your exam, which will begin with the user agreement and tutorial. During the exam, if you ever need to get a proctor's attention, raise your hand and a proctor will come to your computer. You may need to call them over if your marker isn't working, if you run out of note-taking space and need another wet-erase booklet, or if any other unforeseen issue arises. The proctors will also walk the room periodically, so try not to be distracted if you hear someone moving behind you.

Unlike many standardized exams, everyone in the test rooms will start their exams, end their exams, and take their breaks at different times, rather than there being a single start and end time for everyone. This means that, when you are finished and ready to leave, you will need to call the proctor over to escort you out, rather than waiting for time to be called for everyone. You are allowed to leave during the section itself, such as if a bathroom emergency arises, but if at all possible try to wait until the scheduled breaks, as your time will continue to tick down if you leave in the middle of the exam. When you reach the end of the section and are ready to finish, raise your hand and the proctor will come. If you have any time left over at this point, you'll be required to end the section early, rather than adding that time to your scheduled break. For that reason, it's typically in your best interest to go back and review any difficult passages or flagged questions if you reach the end of the section with time to spare.

The MCAT is a long exam, more than **seven hours** if you take the entirety of each section and break, and it's natural to begin to fatigue as you progress through the test. This is part of why it's important to incorporate *realistic* Full Length practice into your study routine. Managing that fatigue is an essential skill, and can make a dramatic difference in your final performance. The most important contributor to your endurance will be your energy level, and for that you need food and water. Try to eat something for breakfast, even if the nervousness makes you lose your appetite, and eat and drink at least a little bit during each break, especially your longer lunch break. During your breaks, try to stand, stretch, and walk as well, because moving your body can make a huge contribution to revitalizing your mind. If you find yourself zoning out or feeling tired during a section, take 15 to 20 seconds to stop, breathe, and then refocus your attention on the passage or question that you're tackling. Refocusing can also be helpful if you find yourself feeling overwhelmed at a particularly challenging point of the test. Don't be afraid to do this once or twice on each section. Maintaining an acute and focused mind is worth more than the few seconds you'll lose doing so.

When you're finished with the exam, you'll be presented with the final **score/void screen**. At this point, you can choose to submit your exam, in which case it will be scored, or void it, which will erase it from your record, as if you had never taken it. Although virtually everyone at least thinks about voiding your exam, we don't generally recommend doing so. It's generally only advisable to void your exam if something went catastrophically wrong. If you've prepared thoroughly, but the examination still seemed difficult to you, it will seem difficult to other test-takers too. The scaled nature of the MCAT means that your score will account for that fact—so just being taken aback by questions or even entire passages, and maybe having to rush more than you did in practice sessions, should *not* automatically count as a reason to void. Likewise, it's not a good idea to void just because you don't feel good about your performance. That post-MCAT anxiety is completely normal, and happens to most students—even those who wind up receiving a top-percentile score! If you void your score, you will need to reschedule and retake the exam; if you score your exam, the worst thing that could happen is that you don't get the score you were hoping for, in which case you might choose to retake the exam anyway and then highlight your improvements on your application. Therefore, our general advice is to score your exam, even if you feel stressed about your score at the end of the test.

Once you've completed the score/void page, and done a short survey at the end of the exam, call over the proctor. They will check you out and certify your exam. Collect any items you may have brought with you, walk outside, and enjoy being done with the MCAT. You worked hard and earned that feeling of accomplishment, and if all goes well, you will never have to think about the MCAT again.

5. Basics of Medical School Admissions

The MCAT is a test with a purpose: getting into medical school. With that in mind, we'd like to cover some basics of the medical school application process. Depending on your personal timetable, some of this may already be very familiar to you, because it's entirely possible to arrange things such that the MCAT is one of the last items to finalize before submitting applications. This may also be mostly new to you, since it's equally possible to take the MCAT well before seriously thinking about the details of the application process. However, most students who take the MCAT are somewhere in between those two extremes.

The majority of medical schools in the United States are allopathic medical schools, or schools that award an MD. Most allopathic medical schools utilize a common application administered by the Americal Medical College Application System (AMCAS). The **AMCAS general application** typically opens in the first week of May, which means you can start entering your information into the application, even though you can't submit your application until June. The general application consists of your biographical and academic information, including your transcripts, a section for important experiences and accomplishments, such as academic awards or volunteer experience, and your personal statement. The AAMC has specific style guidelines for how certain information must be entered, so be sure to check the instructions posted on the AAMC website before beginning.

The **personal statement**, consisting of a maximum of 5300 characters, is your best chance to communicate directly to admissions committees who you are, why you want to be a physician, and why they should want you to be their student. If you're an MD/PhD applicant, there will be three personal statements, two of which focus on your research experience and pursuit of the physician-scientist pathway. For all that GPA and MCAT scores are at the top of pre-meds' minds when thinking about their odds of being accepted at various schools, and rightly so, the personal statement really is the focal point of your application. Every year, students with fantastic MCAT scores and high GPAs are rejected, and students with not-so-amazing statistics are admitted. Personal statements therefore play a huge role in tipping the odds in your favor. Spend time reflecting on what you want to say, revise it multiple times, and seek the input of others in crafting it. The personal statement is your chance to advocate for yourself beyond the numbers and unite your experiences into a cohesive narrative.

For your application to be verified, you will also be required to submit **letters of recommendation** and a set of official **transcripts** from any undergraduate or graduate programs you have attended. The verification of transcripts takes several weeks from the date of receipt, so be sure to have your college submit them as early as possible. It's okay if you're still taking classes, as you can update your application after it has been submitted.

You'll be required to submit multiple letters of recommendation. Recommendation letters can be written by physicians, professors, or others who know you and can speak to your aptitude and qualifications. Additionally, it's possible for your college's premedical advising committee to compose a committee letter, which can take the place of another letter of recommendation. Some institutions also manage the process of gathering recommendation letters and assembling them into a letter packet, which fulfills the requirement for recommendation letters completely. We recommend looking into the letter writer requirements specified by each program you intend to apply to, as some require a letter from a non-science professor, some require a letter from a non-academic individual, and some require or recommend a letter from a clinician. Therefore, to have your bases completely covered, you may end up requesting five or six letters in total. You should contact the people you wish to write your letters several months in advance of the actual application process, to give them time to prepare. Let them know your preferred timeline, giving them at minimum two to three weeks to craft your letter, although it's okay to give your letter writers polite reminders if the deadline is approaching. In addition to leaving enough leeway in terms of time, when approaching people for a letter, a useful tip is to ask them whether they would be able to write a *positive* letter for you. The details will vary depending on who you're asking for a letter, and how familiar he or she is with the process, but it's generally considered to be good form to make it as easy and seamless as possible for your recommender to write you a letter—so keep this in mind, and tailor your approach to specific recommenders accordingly. Fortunately, letters of recommendation can be submitted electronically, and AMCAS has useful information on their website to facilitate this process.

On your application, you will also have an opportunity to select which medical schools you wish to receive your application, and you can come back to your application after submitting to send your application to more programs. AMCAS opens to submissions in the first week of June, giving you at least one month to prepare your application before submitting it. While the application deadline for most allopathic medical schools is usually in the late fall or

December, submitting your application as early as possible is really in your best interest. First, AMCAS verification of your application can take weeks, and even longer if you submit later when the number of applications to be processed has piled up. More importantly, most programs have rolling admissions processes, which means that they begin offering interviews and acceptances and filling up seats as early as the fall. For this reason, you improve your chances the earlier you can submit your application, with June and potentially early July being your surest bets. If you're wondering where your MCAT fits into this timeline, you *can* submit your AMCAS application before you've taken your MCAT or received your scores, as long as you can enter your testing date in the application when you submit. That way, AMCAS can begin verifying your application while you're busy taking your MCAT.

After your application has been submitted, it will be sent to the medical colleges you wish to apply to, which will begin evaluating your application once your MCAT scores are in. Since the medical school admissions process is extremely competitive, most students apply to a relatively high number of schools, typically between 10 and 20 (although the specific "best" number of schools to apply to varies from person to person), with a mix of both relatively competitive and relatively "safer" schools.

After your application and transcripts have been submitted and verified, you will begin receiving secondary applications from medical schools. The first secondaries generally begin arriving in the middle of July. Each secondary is different, although most will ask for additional short essays with specific prompts, such as why you want to attend a particular medical school. Once a medical school has received your completed secondary application, they will begin considering you for a potential interview. Being notified for an interview can take weeks or months, so there is little to do but sit back and wait.

An offer of acceptance to a school will always be preceded by an in-person **interview**. Each school typically only interviews a small portion of their applicants, so don't be surprised if not every school you applied to offers you an interview. Interview offers can be extended as early as August and as late as February or March, so the timing can be unpredictable. A medical college interview is typically a day-long experience, during which you'll be given presentations about the school and curriculum, a tour of the campus, and sit for individual interviews with current students, faculty, and physicians. Some, but not all, medical schools incorporate MMIs, or multiple mini-interviews, into the process. MMIs are conducted at thematically distinct stations and involve scenarios ranging from more traditional interview topics to ethical dilemmas and even teamwork-based exercises. Regardless of the details, a major part of medical schools' goal in interviews is to get a sense for the person behind the application. As such, interviews are often less about giving a correct set of answers, and more about projecting an impression of who you are as well-rounded future physician.

Once an interview has been completed, you can generally expect to hear back from the school within four to six weeks, although some schools may take longer. Note that offers of acceptance are not given until October 15th at the earliest. Once you've started to receive offers of **admission**, you can hold onto these offers without making any decisions until April. If you were placed on any waitlists, it's around this time that you'll hear back with acceptance offers from programs where you were taken off their waitlist.

While most American medical colleges are allopathic and follow the admissions process we described above, a smaller number are osteopathic, meaning they confer a Doctorate of Osteopathy, or DO, to graduating physicians instead of a Doctorate of Medicine, or MD. Practically speaking, this difference is not very important in clinical settings, since, as of 2020, physicians with MDs and DOs train in the same residency programs and undergo the same licensing requirements. Nonetheless, there is still a tendency for DOs to be relatively over-represented in specialties like family medicine and primary care, and under-represented in competitive surgical specialties and academic medicine.

Students may consider applying to osteopathic schools due to their historical differences from allopathic schools, their location, or because they tend to be less competitive than allopathic schools. This final factor, competitiveness, is a very real reason why many students apply to DO schools. However, it's somewhat of a sensitive point for DO admissions committees, and if you *do* wind up applying to DO schools, be prepared ahead of time to discuss your motivations for doing so in a way that is more informative and specific than "your school would be a good fit for me because its average MCAT scores and GPAs are lower." As you can imagine, that doesn't give the best impression. The application system used by osteopathic schools, the AACOMAS, utilizes a similar timeline, though applying early is not as essential as in the AMCAS. Additionally, the AACOMAS requires at least one letter of recommendation from a physician, which they highly prefer to be a letter from an osteopathic physician. This echoes the point made above about how osteopathic schools generally want a sense of why you specifically want to become an *osteopathic* physician.

Students interested in application to medical colleges in Texas will have to fill out the TMDSAS application, as most Texan medical colleges do not participate in nationwide common applications. Canadian medical colleges in most provinces do not use a general common application, so any applications must be submitted to colleges individually. Their admissions requirements also tend to be highly institution-specific, and may involve very strict MCAT cut-offs, especially for CARS. Medical colleges in Ontario have their own regional application system called OMSAS. Due to all this complexity, if you're considering applying to Canadian medical schools, it's highly advisable to do research in advance about your options.

No matter which avenues of application you pursue, there are certain universal guidelines that can help maximize any student's chances of success in this competitive process. Apply early, and prepare your application, letters, and test scores (if possible) even earlier. Revise your personal statement and secondary essays multiple times, and have someone else give you feedback on them as well. However, the specifics of each student's strengths and weaknesses are unique and often hard to discern, so consider reaching out to a pre-medical advising service. Some undergraduate institutions offer these services through advisory committees, but Blueprint also offers admissions consulting and can help you navigate the admissions process from start to finish.

6. Must-Knows

> MCAT structure:
  - Chemical and Physical Foundations (59 questions, 95 minutes): 30% general chemistry, 25% physics, 25% biochemistry, 15% organic chemistry, and 5% biology.
  - CARS (53 questions, 90 minutes): nine passages on humanities and social sciences topics.
  - Biological and Biochemical Foundations (59 questions, 95 minutes): 65% biology, 25% biochemistry, 5% organic chemistry, and 5% general chemistry.
  - Psychological, Social, and Biological Foundations of Behavior (59 questions, 95 minutes): 65% psychology, 30% sociology, and 5% biology.
> MCAT Score: 118-132 per section; 472-528 total; median score: 500
> Key components of MCAT prep:
  - Study plan.
  - Review materials.
  - Practice materials.
  - Lessons Learned Journal.
> MCAT testing experience:
  - Starts early (plan on arriving around 7:30).
  - Can take roughly 7.5 hours with all breaks.
  - Plan ahead in terms of route to the testing center, food and beverages, etc.
  - Don't void the test unless something truly catastrophic and exceptional happens.
> Key concepts regarding admissions:
  - AMCAS application (opens in May, can be submitted in June).
  - Application requires transcripts, letters of recommendation, and personal statement in addition to MCAT.
  - Initial application is followed by secondaries, interviews, and acceptance.

Applied Practice

The best MCAT practice is realistic, with detailed analytics to help you assess where things went wrong. For those reasons, we recommend completing practice questions in an online setting that simulates the real MCAT interface, and using the analytics provided to help you decide how to best move your studies forward.

CARS does not require knowledge of specific subject areas, but it does require development of strong test-taking skills. To ensure you are honing those skills as you work through this book, we suggest you go online after wrapping up each chapter and generate a Qbank Practice Set of 2-3 CARS passages to practice and review. While not every chapter of this book is directly applicable to CARS, regular CARS practice is key to test day success.

As a further supplement, given the importance of active learning for effective studying, we also suggest that you consult the Must-Knows at the end of each chapter of this Reasoning text as a basis for creating a study sheet. This is not a sheet to memorize in the more traditional sense of content memorization, but rather a quick reference of the most important strategies for you to refer to during and after practice in your early prep. Frequently revisiting the most important strategies for the MCAT - in both CARS and the Sciences - will help you continue to improve your performance.

This page left intentionally blank.

This page left intentionally blank.

How to Read a CARS Passage

0. Introduction

The **Critical Analysis and Reading Skills** (CARS) section is a vitally important section of the exam, so preparation for it is an integral component of MCAT prep. In this chapter, we discuss how to read CARS passages effectively, starting with a review of the basic reading strategies and reasoning skills needed to tackle these passages, before moving on to cover multiple additional tips.

Before getting into the nitty-gritty details, we need to acknowledge a core truth about the MCAT: there's no such thing as a single "right" way to succeed on this exam. Everyone's brain is a little different, and there's no reason you should feel forced to rigidly adhere to a discrete series of strategic steps, at least without adapting them to work optimally for your own brain. However, the many different "right ways" of succeeding have certain features in common. With that in mind, our strategy is to present the framework that we've seen work best for the MCAT, and then discuss techniques for troubleshooting and adapting these techniques in order to find *your* best approach.

1. Core Reading Strategies

Three tools are at your disposal when working through the CARS section: (1) the pen and whiteboard, (2) the on-screen highlighter, and (3) your eyes.

You'll be provided with a **wet-erase pen** and a **whiteboard** to take notes during your MCAT. The whiteboard is wet-erase, meaning that unlike with dry erase boards, you won't accidentally erase it by smearing your hand across it. However, we do *not* recommend taking notes on your whiteboard on the CARS section. There's two big reasons behind this advice. First, note-taking can be time-consuming and inefficient, especially with wet-erase markers. Second, prioritizing note-taking can divert your attention away from synthesizing main ideas. For extremely complex passages you may choose to jot down a few words that summarize the main idea, but for most passages it is best to capture main ideas using your on-screen highlighter.

The goal of **highlighting** is to capture main ideas and to create an outline of the passage you can refer back to. In other words, highlighting is like adding post-it notes that capture the most salient points, which will help you find pertinent information when you need it. We recommend stopping at the end of each paragraph to reflect on the purpose and key ideas of that paragraph, and then using the highlighter tool to identify a select number of words that will serve as a visual reminder of those key ideas, without necessarily fully describing them in detail. Many students' first instinct with highlighting is to highlight as they read along. Doing so can help you focus, the retroactive method we've described is far more efficient for a test like the MCAT. In particular, **retroactively highlighting** makes you take a moment to synthesize what you've just read, enabling you to process the material more deeply than if you highlight in a way that tracks the initial movement of your eyes across the screen. Even without consciously summarizing the paragraph, this kind of deeper engagement helps to build awareness of the structure of the passage and how each paragraph fits into the larger argument, or main idea, of the passage. Nonetheless, highlighting is not mandatory. Some students find highlighting to be not especially useful, in which case it's completely acceptable to use the highlighting tool minimally or not at all.

The third tool you have access to is your **eyes**. In other words, the highlighting tool and wet-erase board may be valuable, but they're no substitute for reading, paying attention to, and making sense of the passage. In particular, the most important goal while reading is to capture main ideas. This means maintaining a relentless focus on what the author *means* as you read. A useful technique to do so is rephrasing the ideas that the author presents in your own words, which can involve simplifying the language to get at the heart of the idea. Eventually, this process should happen fluidly as you are reading, although as you're getting started—and especially if you run into a sentence or paragraph that's particularly dense—it's OK to take a few seconds to pause and think through what the author is saying. While reading, reflect on the main ideas of each paragraph, and identify words and short phrases you can highlight to capture those main ideas. Keep in mind that everything in the passage—every argument, every example, every opinion—always relates to the **main argument** of the passage. Furthermore, questions in the CARS section draw upon main ideas, both explicitly and implicitly. Taking the time to effectively read and understand the passages is the first step to acing these questions.

Although it may seem tempting to **skim** the passage, or even to skip over it entirely and go straight to the questions, doing so is generally inefficient. It doesn't ultimately wind up saving time, and it doesn't reliably lead to a performance benefit. The one important exception to this guidance is that skimming can be useful if you're low on time near the end of the CARS section. One option in such a situation is to skim through the text at a more rapid pace than normal, or, in a real time crunch, to read the first and last sentences of each paragraph. If at all possible, it's best to read the first paragraph fully, as the first paragraph often introduces the passage thesis or at least provides a basic sense of what the author is concerned with. Reading the first paragraph, and then the first and last sentences of the other paragraphs, will help you get the overall gist of what's in the passage and then immediately move on to the questions. The caveat to skimming when low on time is that you'll need to return to the passage as you answer questions since you didn't invest much time in the passage itself.

Let's put these techniques into practice by working through two paragraphs of a practice passage. First, read through each paragraph without highlighting. At the end of the paragraph, stop and reflect, asking what the author's key opinions or arguments are. Then, with that in mind, we'll show how to reflect that reasoning through highlighting.

Often hailed as the greatest example of experimental filmmaking, *Un Chien Andalou* was an attempt to fuse the aesthetics of surrealism with the arational modes of an analysis brought into vogue by Freudian psychoanalysis. Allegedly springing from a conversation between the director and Salvador Dali in which they each related random images they'd seen in dreams, the film presents a series of largely disjointed images and events with little logic connecting them. The director's stated goal was to ensure that the film would in no way be susceptible to any rational understanding and that "[n]othing, in the film, symbolizes anything."

Despite aggressive efforts to craft a film that stood in opposition to the tastes and style of the film scene in Paris at the time (efforts that led the director to fill his pockets with rocks on the day of the premiere, fearing he would need to throw them at the audience to defend himself), *Andalou* was greeted with a strongly positive reception. Dali's reaction to the positive reception was marked disappointment. The film's director was quoted at the time as saying, "What can I do about the people who adore all that is new, even when it goes against their deepest convictions, or about the insincere, corrupt press, and the inane herd that saw beauty or poetry in something which was basically no more than a desperate impassioned call for murder?"

In the first paragraph, we encounter the intent of the film's director, or what he was trying to achieve by making *Un Chien Andalou*. Specifically, the director wanted to synthesize the aesthetics of surrealism with arational modes popularized by Freudian psychoanalysis so that it wouldn't be susceptible to any kind of rational understanding. We can highlight those short phrases to capture these insights. It's often tempting to highlight proper nouns, like Dali's name, or the name of the film itself. However, if you're generally able to find names in the passage quickly, then don't bother. We want to highlight sparingly so that it really stands out. Sample highlighting for this paragraph is shown below:

> Often hailed as the greatest example of experimental filmmaking, *Un Chien Andalou* was an attempt to fuse the aesthetics of surrealism with the arational modes of an analysis brought into vogue by Freudian psychoanalysis. Allegedly springing from a conversation between the director and Salvador Dali in which they each related random images they'd seen in dreams, the film presents a series of largely disjointed images and events with little logic connecting them. The director's stated goal was to ensure that the film would in no way be susceptible to any rational understanding and that "[n]othing, in the film, symbolizes anything."

Next, let's return to the second paragraph, where we're given more insight into the director's goals. We learn about what he was trying to achieve by making the movie, and then we hear about the reaction from the public. An important contrast emerges between what the director and Dali were attempting to achieve (a desperate impassioned call for murder, a film opposite to the current film scene) and how the audience actually reacted (positively). We want to capture this contrast with our highlighting. The director's use of the phrase "inane herd" to describe how he felt about the audience of the time is particularly vivid, making it an excellent section to highlight. It is precisely the kind of opinionated expression that we should make note of, both to understand the logic of the passage as a whole and to prepare for related questions. Sample highlighting is below:

> Despite aggressive efforts to craft a film that stood in opposition to the tastes and style of the film scene in Paris at the time (efforts that led the director to fill his pockets with rocks on the day of the premiere, fearing he would need to throw them at the audience to defend himself), *Andalou* was greeted with a strongly positive reception. Dali's reaction to the positive reception was marked disappointment. The film's director was quoted at the time as saying, "What can I do about the people who adore all that is new, even when it goes against their deepest convictions, or about the insincere, corrupt press, and the inane herd that saw beauty or poetry in something which was basically no more than a desperate impassioned call for murder?"

From here, we would continue reading each paragraph, stopping to highlight the core opinions, contrasts, and cause-and-effect relationships that capture main ideas before moving on to the questions.

2. Reading Comprehension Fundamentals

The CARS passages on the MCAT contain academic, college-level writing, often on topics that you may never have heard of before. When faced with abstract academic writing about obscure topics it's all too easy to panic. However, the ultimate metric of the difficulty of a passage is the percentage of questions that you answer correctly. Sometimes dense, difficult passages are associated with surprisingly easy questions, and vice versa. Keeping this fact in mind can help you stay motivated while reading abstract, challenging passages and force you to stay alert during seemingly easy ones.

With difficult passages, the key is **taking it a sentence at a time**. Within each paragraph, within each sentence, try to pare away the complicated language until you've understood the basic meaning. Consider the following example, drawn from the beginning of a passage:

> To say that the jury determines the facts and the judge determines the law is, it goes without saying, a radical oversimplification that obfuscates the near-totally deterministic effect that extra-legal sociological considerations and rigid legal formalisms have on the actual process of supposed justice-seeking that occurs daily in our nation's courtrooms.

The first phrase we see reads "the jury determines the facts and the judge determines the law." This part isn't too complicated; it describes how the legal system works. Next, the sentence says that this is an "oversimplification." Now we understand that this divide between the jury and the facts, versus the judge and the law is *too simple*.

Next, we read that this "obfuscates the near-totally deterministic effect." Here, the language gets much more complicated. Even if we don't understand exactly what this phrase means, we can identify that it likely has a negative connotation, if only because it comes right after "oversimplification". In other words, this "radical oversimplification" isn't good. The use of the word "obfuscates" here is a good example of how to handle difficult vocabulary on the MCAT. Although CARS passages can contain challenging vocabulary, the core purpose of this section is not to be a vocab test. Therefore, when you encounter vocabulary that you don't understand, the best thing to do is infer what you can from contextual clues like tone, and then *move on*.

Next, we reach the phrase "extra-legal sociological considerations and rigid legal formalisms" that have a "near-totally deterministic effect." It might not be clear what "extra-legal" means, but we can focus on "sociological," since we know what sociology is. More specifically, sociology isn't the same thing as the law, so the author is essentially pivoting to say that we need to focus on something beyond the narrow scope of the law. Just as a note, if we consult a dictionary—which of course is not an option when taking the test—we will learn that "extra-legal" means something that is outside of the law's authority or not regulated by the law. In other words, this is the same meaning of "extra" as a prefix that is used in science, in words like "extracellular," which means "outside of the cell." However, the point here is that you didn't actually have to know that; even just processing this phrase as "sociological considerations" is enough to draw our attention to sociology as distinct from the law.

At this point, we've recognized that the author thinks that it's an oversimplification to say that the jury deals with facts and the judge determines the law, and that other things like sociology matter. More specifically, sociology and legal formalisms have some kind of effect on the "process of supposed justice-seeking that occurs daily..." Thus, the author is transitioning to talk about finding justice in courtrooms. We might even pick up on the sarcastic tone of "supposed justice-seeking," which hints that the author thinks that justice-seeking is *supposed* to occur but actually doesn't. Thus, we can roughly summarize this sentence as saying, "okay, so the whole jury-finds-facts and judge-determines-law idea is too simple, there's sociology stuff that matters, and this is important in our courtrooms." That level of understanding, while far more basic than the original sentence, is the core of what's needed to keep moving through the passage.

If you find yourself totally lost, don't fret. CARS passages are often repetitive! In particular, a confusing or convoluted sentence may be followed by a simpler sentence that recaps the sentiment from the prior sentence. Furthermore, it's helpful to pay careful attention to the context of a difficult sentence within a passage, because that can give us important clues about how that sentence fits into the main idea of the passage. Along those lines, we can also watch for the author's **tone**. Adjectives and adverbs tell you what the author thinks about a given noun or idea, and verb choice can show you the overall thrust of the author's opinion. Consider a simple example: (1) *The red car failed to brake in time and contacted the rear of the blue car* versus (2) *The driver of the red car was negligent and didn't use his brakes, smashing into the blue car*. Sentence (1) reads more neutrally, framing things in terms of "cars," rather than "drivers," and using factual phrases like "contacted the rear of the blue car." Sentence (2), in contrast, is both more vivid and more personal, using words like "smashing" to create a more dramatic picture in our heads, "negligent" to place blame on the driver of the red car, and "didn't use his brakes" to frame the action in terms of the agency of the driver. In other words, sentence (2) is much more negative towards the driver of the red car, and finds that driver to be at fault on a personal level.

Take another example: *Historians of ancient Rome present three stories about the end of Emperor Trajan's rule, starting with an emphasis on the outsized importance of the economic motives behind his Parthian campaign.* If we encounter this at the beginning of a passage, it's clearly a signal that the passage will deal with the history of ancient Rome. However, the author's choice to use the word "stories" signals that the author probably doesn't agree with what historians of ancient Rome have to say, in that the author presents these as "stories" as opposed to objective, factual accounts. Something as simple as detecting the author's opinions can be instrumental in correctly answering CARS questions.

A useful exercise for solidifying this point is to read the well-known poem "Jabberwocky" by Lewis Carroll, the author of *Alice in Wonderland*. It's full of nonsense words, but it contains numerous, vivid indicators of tone.

'Twas brillig, and the slithy toves
Did gyre and gimble in the wabe:
All mimsy were the borogoves,
And the mome raths outgrabe.

"Beware the Jabberwock, my son!
The jaws that bite, the claws that catch!
Beware the Jubjub bird, and shun
The frumious Bandersnatch!"

He took his vorpal sword in hand;
Long time the manxome foe he sought—
So rested he by the Tumtum tree
And stood awhile in thought.

And, as in uffish thought he stood,
The Jabberwock, with eyes of flame,
Came whiffling through the tulgey wood,
And burbled as it came!

One, two! One, two! And through and through
The vorpal blade went snicker-snack!
He left it dead, and with its head
He went galumphing back.

"And hast thou slain the Jabberwock?
Come to my arms, my beamish boy!
O frabjous day! Callooh! Callay!"
He chortled in his joy.

'Twas brillig, and the slithy toves
Did gyre and gimble in the wabe:
All mimsy were the borogoves,
And the mome raths outgrabe.

Nonsense words account for the majority of this poem, but we can get a decent idea of what's going on just by focusing on the basic actions and analyzing the tone. For example, in the fifth stanza, the word "galumphing" describes the character's movement after having successfully killed the Jabberwock, suggesting that it's a kind of triumphant, positive, energetic sort of movement. Similarly, here, "beamish," "frabjous," and "callay," are all nonsense words, but given that the poem then immediately states that he "chortled in his joy," we can see the strongly positive tone of all of those adjectives. Of course, the MCAT won't have literal nonsense words on it (even though it may feel like it at times!). Nonetheless, focusing on the overall tone and context of a passage can help us make sense of even the most nonsensical MCAT passages.

Another key to understanding MCAT passages is paying close attention to **pronouns**. A single 500-to 600-word passage can be awash with various opinions, perspectives, and contrasting schools of thought, and authors can use pronouns to refer back to things in a way that makes it easy to lose the thread of the discussion.

As you read, whenever you see pronouns, make sure you understand what noun it refers to back to. Options can include people, names, ideas, or schools of thought. In addition to pronouns like *he, she, it,* or *they,* be on the lookout for the demonstrative pronouns *this, that, these,* and *those.* Passage authors constantly say things like "this theory" or "that view," and if you start to zone out, you'll miss the key connections being made by those pronouns. This is especially common when transitioning from one paragraph to the next. Let's examine two quick paragraphs to illustrate this.

> To say that the jury determines the facts and the judge determines the law is, it goes without saying, a radical over-simplification that obfuscates the near-totally deterministic effect that extra-legal sociological considerations and rigid legal formalisms have on the actual process of supposed justice-seeking that occurs daily in our nation's courtrooms. These two concerns are treated with depth and subtlety in Johnson's latest contribution to the Critical Legal Studies movement. In her monograph, "Practical Considerations in Courtroom-Based Fact Determination," we see a thoroughgoing deconstruction of the distinction between findings of fact and findings of law. Legal formalisms and the manipulations thereof are considered briefly before Johnson moves on to a summary of the past decade's sociological findings on the operation of courts at the city and county level, where the overwhelming majority of citizens will rarely find their lives intersecting with the legal system, if at all.

> This summary then serves as a springboard for Johnson's larger analysis, which deftly moves between statistical analysis and values-based logical argumentation before ending in a line that has been repeatedly quoted in law review journals: "Would that facts mattered. Would that it were so." For all that this work has earned Johnson any number of new adherents, it is not without its flaws nor does it lack for critics happy to discuss those flaws at length.

Since we've already discussed the opening sentence, we don't need to repeat that discussion here. Instead, let's focus on the pronouns, starting with the second sentence. The second sentence begins with "these two concerns," and we should take a moment to make sure we understand what "these" refers to. Here, it's referring back to "sociological considerations" and "legal formalisms." Connecting demonstrative pronouns with their antecedents is necessary in order to know *exactly* what concept the author is referring to.

The next sentence uses the pronoun "her," which is a reference back to Johnson. Moving to the second paragraph, we see the classic AAMC strategy of beginning a paragraph with the word "this". Here, the demonstrative "this" refers back to Johnson's summary of sociology. Later in the paragraph, we see the pronouns "this" and "it," which refer back to the monograph that Johnson wrote. This constant double-checking to make sure you understand what you've read will certainly take time at first, but it should become second nature by the time you take your MCAT. Try to get in the habit of connecting the various ideas within and between paragraphs to ensure you'll understand the author's main idea well enough to answer the questions.

3. Pay Attention!

It's a fact of life that some CARS passages on the MCAT will be boring. Very boring. This is not a *unique* feature of the premed experience, but CARS presents us with a paradoxical situation. The pressure of the exam means we're totally amped up, but we start zoning out when we see a passage about 17th century French philosophy. Ideally, the goal is to cultivate the ability to get into the swing of things with the passage. After all, every passage—no matter how dry it seems at first—has an audience and is making an argument, and we can leverage that fact to channel at least enough interest to be able to read the passage effectively and to follow its main idea. However, that can be easier said than done. Especially in the initial stages of studying CARS, it's worth acknowledging that some passages will feel profoundly boring, which underscores the need to develop strategies to cope with them.

To succeed, you'll have to learn to build your stamina and sustain **focus**. To do so, try starting small by focusing on individual sentences. Even if the whole passage is a snooze-fest, getting through a single sentence and understanding it as best you can is a realistic goal. Focusing on concrete tasks, like identifying the subject and verb of the sentence, can also help you stay engaged. Once you can reliably keep yourself focused on one sentence after the other, it's time to start building your focus up to the paragraph level. You can motivate yourself by viewing each paragraph as a separate task on your to-do list, or by reframing what you're reading in ways that make sense to you, as if you were teaching it to someone else. Instead of a dense wall of text, imagine you're listening to an audiobook or a speech. Hear the text in your head as you read and try to picture actually listening to a person at a podium enthralling the audience with their brilliance on the topic of fourth-century Etruscan pottery. Alternatively, tell yourself a story about why you're reading this paragraph, this passage. Pretend someone you want to impress is totally into the topic, so you want to learn about it, too. Or read the passage as if your best friend is saying the passage out loud, as this will unconsciously help you focus better.

During practice, see how long you can last until your mind starts drifting off. When that happens, what are you thinking about? Are there any distractions that affect you? Start making note of these things, and see if you can extend the duration of time until you begin to lose focus. Before you take practice tests, write down a to-do list of all the things you have to take care of or that are stressing you out. By jotting these down in a physical list, you're allowing your mind to free yourself of these worries, letting you leave stress and distractions at the door.

There's a notorious saying "fake it til' you make it," which can certainly apply to maintaining your focus on dry or dense CARS passages. Try to maintain a curious attitude when studying CARS to ward off frustration, and understand that some passages may be *designed* to be overly complicated or poorly organized. CARS is meant to test how well you operate in gray areas where the right answer cannot be calculated using a simple algorithm. That said, it's best practice to treat boring practice passages as if they are just as important and high-stakes as passages on your real MCAT. As much as possible, do your best not to become bored or frustrated by a passage, otherwise your reading speed and comprehension may be affected.

Now, in addition to building up your focus a little bit at a time, or using little cognitive tricks like "fake it til' you make it," you should be attentive to your own **physiology**. Many people find it helpful to begin an exercise routine, as even short bouts of exercise have been shown to improve mental acuity and focus, both in the moment and longer-term. This doesn't have to be an intense running program, though. For instance, you can try yoga, lifting weights, swimming, or something completely different. If you're unable to or not interested in exercise, consider starting a simple meditation practice for the mindfulness benefits.

Your ability to control your mental focus will be significantly impacted by how comfortable and relaxed your body is. During a practice test, if you find your mind wandering and find yourself getting bored, irritable, and distractible, especially near the end of the section, you may need to get in the habit of taking a little micro-break after the fourth or fifth passage. A micro-break is simple: it provides a very brief chance to reset your body and mind to help you regain focus for the remainder of the section. Simply put down your pen and close your eyes after you've completed the fourth or fifth passage. Sit up straight. Put your feet flat on the ground. Close your eyes. Take a long slow breath in while clenching up one muscle at a time, then exhale while relaxing the muscle. Do this three times: for your feet, your hands, and for your face. We also encourage you to explore other guided relaxation techniques to give yourself that much-needed mental refresh at the midpoint of the CARS section.

4. Study Strategies for CARS

Preparing for the CARS section of the MCAT is a marathon, not a sprint. That is, you need to work at it a bit every single day for weeks or months. Although each student ultimately finds an individualized strategy for analyzing passages, the overall approach to prepping for the CARS section has important underlying principles that will benefit everyone.

First and most importantly, cramming is not a viable option for the CARS section. Instead, **consistent practice** is key. Every single day you can, work your way through one or two practice passages. As you move along in your prep, step it up to doing regular timed practice, and eventually full timed sections. Although timing is certainly an important part of success on the CARS section, we would also advise you not to worry about timing too early. Your first goal is to find your own optimal method for success in understanding the passage and tackling the questions. After finding the approach that works best for you, it's time to focus more seriously on optimizing timing.

Early on, good resources to use include your course CARS passages, as well as the AAMC CARS Question Packs and Official Guide CARS passages. Once you have a handle on passages and have done plenty of untimed work, you can move to full timed sections using section tests and full length exams. Another important thing to keep in mind early in your prep is the value of being experimental. You don't want to simply pick an approach and stick with it if it's not working for you. If you feel that your CARS performance has flatlined and you don't know what to do, try something different! **Troubleshoot** your approach to passages and questions, and figure out how to use the highlighting tool, and maybe even the wet erase board from time to time, to your advantage.

Even more important than endless hours of practice is that high-quality practice involves **reflection**. That is, it's important to look back and ask yourself *why* you did what you did and *why* you got a question right or wrong. If you answer a question incorrectly, ask yourself specifically what went wrong. Did you misread or misinterpret the question? Did you eliminate the right answer choice too quickly? This process of painstaking review is time-consuming and not very exciting. It's understandable, then, why we often fail to do it. There's always more science to learn, more practice questions to answer, and more exciting things than MCAT prep to be doing. And yet if you want to master the CARS section, we've got to keep pushing ourselves, asking "why" over and over while reviewing our work. After all, the best way to minimize future mistakes is to learn from the ones you've already made.

We recommend identifying at least **three trends each week** that indicate clear areas for improvement, and setting specific goals to tackle those areas. For example, say your performance analytics indicate that you're rushing on passages toward the end of the section, or that you're missing strengthen/weaken questions. For your next practice session, you should work on one of these areas at a time, and then at the *next* practice session, revisit the goals you set to evaluate your improvement. This will help you overcome frustrating plateaus in your CARS performance, especially if you're aiming for a high score.

A helpful technique for this kind of reflective practice is **prediction**. That is, instead of looking backwards and just asking why something was right or wrong, the goal is to look forward and make predictions that help us deepen our analysis. For example, we can start with predicting passages. After reading the first paragraph, stop and ask yourself what's coming up. What is the author doing here? Where is she going with this? What opinions are likely to emerge? What contrasts? After you've made your predictions, read the second paragraph. Did you get what you were expecting? Stop and make new predictions again. Regularly doing this over time will help your ability to follow passages improve significantly.

After reaching a certain level of familiarity with predicting passages, practice **predicting the questions**. That is, after reading a full passage, stop and make notes on questions you expect to see. Imagine the AAMC has recruited you to write the questions for the passage, and see how close you can get to the questions that actually show up. If you get good at this, you can get to a point where you can, while still reading, recognize that a certain sentence or phrase might be exactly the kind of thing that the AAMC is likely to ask about, meaning that it's crucial to pay attention to. Realizing that there really *is* a finite amount of material and ways in which the questions can be asked will also help boost your confidence.

Next, practice **predicting the answer choices**. After reading the passage and a related question, stop before reading the choices. You can even cover them up with your hand on the screen! Then try to imagine what the right answer might say. Students who become skillful at this kind of prediction can often zero in on the right answer, with minimal distraction from the wrong answers. Each of these approaches to prediction can help keep you focused and thinking on a deeper, "why" level, which can dramatically improve your score.

There's a final point we should address in our first chapter on CARS prep, because it's a question that comes up often: what about **outside reading**? The idea that you can improve on the MCAT by practicing reading books, newspapers, and dense articles every day is a common one. To some extent, it *is* true that reading a good, difficult text every single day will make you a stronger reader, and all things being equal, stronger readers tend to do better on the MCAT. That said, for the purposes of MCAT prep, we do recommend specifically focusing on CARS passages. The real MCAT isn't a magazine, newspaper, or nonfiction book, so even the best-written texts in the world won't build up those MCAT muscles in the same way—and time is usually at a premium when it comes to MCAT prep. As such, an exception to this generalization can be if you have a long time to prep, perhaps six months or more. In such circumstances, you could consider doing some of the most difficult outside reading there is: philosophy. After working through, and critically engaging with, a few hundred pages of philosophy text, the MCAT will feel like a cakewalk by comparison.

5. Must-Knows

> Tools at your disposal for the CARS section:
  - Wet-erase pen and whiteboard: cumbersome and typically best used only for the most difficult, complex passages.
  - Highlighting: use to create an outline of main ideas while reading the passage.
  - Eyes: pay attention!
> Reading comprehension tips:
  - Take it one sentence at a time.
  - Pay attention to tone.
  - Understand what pronouns refer to.
> Tips for studying CARS:
  - Practice to build stamina and attention.
  - Explore how physiology (exercise, meditation, sleep, etc.) affect focus.
  - Routine practice.
  - Troubleshoot and reflect upon your practice materials.
  - Practice predicting passage transitions and questions as you read.

Applied Practice

The best MCAT practice is realistic, with detailed analytics to help you assess where things went wrong. For those reasons, we recommend completing practice questions in an online setting that simulates the real MCAT interface, and using the analytics provided to help you decide how to best move your studies forward.

CARS does not require knowledge of specific subject areas, but it does require development of strong test-taking skills. To ensure you are honing those skills as you work through this book, we suggest you go online after wrapping up each chapter and generate a Qbank Practice Set of 2-3 CARS passages to practice and review. While not every chapter of this book is directly applicable to CARS, regular CARS practice is key to test day success.

As a further supplement, given the importance of active learning for effective studying, we also suggest that you consult the Must-Knows at the end of each chapter of this Reasoning text as a basis for creating a study sheet. This is not a sheet to memorize in the more traditional sense of content memorization, but rather a quick reference of the most important strategies for you to refer to during and after practice in your early prep. Frequently revisiting the most important strategies for the MCAT - in both CARS and the Sciences - will help you continue to improve your performance.

This page left intentionally blank.

Pacing in CARS

CHAPTER

3

0. Introduction

Pacing is a major contributor to MCAT success, both on the science sections and on the CARS section. For some students, pacing winds up being one of the major challenges that they wrestle with throughout their test prep process. For others, pacing is one of several factors to optimize. Regardless of where you stand personally, when it comes to pacing it can only be beneficial to review the key components of successful time management.

1. CARS Pacing and Time Management

Your initial reaction to the topic of time management might be to look for *tricks*: clever ways to take shortcuts or to manage the clock. However, the core of effective time management for the CARS section is about being fully mentally committed to each passage. That's because the CARS section is ultimately about transforming a bunch of words on a screen into coherent messages, so that you can critically evaluate the evidence and the strength of the author's arguments. Therefore, the fundamental techniques for promoting focus and cultivating attention that we discussed in Chapter 2 also apply in the context of pacing.

Section	Questions	Time
Chemical and Physical Foundations of Biological Systems	59	95 min
Critical Analysis and Reasoning Skills	53	90 min
Biological and Biochemical Foundations of Living Systems	59	95 min
Psychological, Social, and Biological Foundations of Behavior	59	95 min

Table 1. Timing of MCAT sections

On the CARS section, you'll have 90 minutes to complete nine passages, each associated with five to seven questions, or 53 questions total. This means that you have 10 minutes to complete each passage and its five to seven questions. Of course, this value will be an *average*, because some passages will naturally take longer than others. We recommend aiming for **nine minutes on each passage**, with a roughly equal division between time spent on the passage and time spent on questions. This pace will also provide a buffer of five to ten minutes at the end, which will give you a little breathing room on the day of your test.

As we mentioned, it usually works best to divide your time as evenly as possible between the passage and questions, although this isn't necessarily a one-size-fits-all rule. An alternative approach is to digest the passage very thoroughly, spending most of the allotted time on reading the passage, and then picking off questions one by one without looking back. The problem with this approach is that CARS is fundamentally about analysis, not memorization, and you'll be better equipped to answer the questions correctly if you balance your time by focusing on the big picture as you read while also giving yourself time to go back to the passage for details and evidence in order to answer questions. It's not that reading thoroughly is a problem; rather, the problem can be having too little time while answering questions to effectively problem-solve. Since you earn points based on correct answers, it makes sense that you will spend a good amount of time thinking through the questions and selecting the most appropriate responses.

On the other end of the spectrum, it can also be tempting to breeze through the passage or even to skip it entirely and go straight to the questions. After all, you can always go back to the passage, right? This works fine for questions requiring simple fact recollection, but those aren't the kinds of questions that are asked in the CARS section. These questions require you to synthesize information across an entire passage and derive main ideas, and there's no shortcut to doing so. If you spend nearly all of your time on the questions, there's a good chance you'll be going back and re-reading more than you need to, and this approach may end up taking more time, as well as increasing the risk of wrong answers.

Rather than obsessing over the clock, which can exacerbate test anxiety, we suggest **checking the timer roughly every other passage**. This way, you'll have plenty of time in the beginning to modulate your pacing without the clock sneaking up on you at the very end, while at the same allowing you to focus your attention on the passage at hand. Consider toggling the timer to the hidden position during MCAT practice, and compare that to your performance when the timer isn't hidden. This can be helpful to some people, and you never know until you try! This is also true of any other approach you might take to CARS. The best way to convince yourself that a given approach is effective is to try it out yourself and see whether the evidence suggests that it is effective for *you*.

2. Avoiding CARS Pitfalls

Doing the right thing is sometimes about avoiding the wrong things, so let's discuss some pitfalls that eat away at the clock. The number-one time-sink on CARS passages is **note-taking**. For CARS, taking notes generally doesn't make much sense. A major reason for this is that we're not really concerned with memorizing or regurgitating details. In the rare case it's necessary, you can always go back to the passage later to remind yourself of any small detail. Furthermore, jotting down information verbatim diverts your attention away from processing main ideas and making important connections. It also just takes time, and a LOT of it, especially given that you'll only have access to a wet-erase board for notes. As if that wasn't enough, taking notes on the wet-erase board sets you up for a disjointed experience when answering questions, since your attention and literal gaze will have to shift back and forth between the question you're answering, your handwritten notes, and the passage itself. In general, taking notes on CARS passages, either on details within the passage or even on main ideas, will divert attention and time away from the passage itself without yielding much tangible benefit.

Instead use of the **highlighter** function is much better suited to CARS passages. A pitfall here is over-highlighting, or highlighting ineffectively. A well-highlighted passage should serve as a roadmap, or outline, of its main ideas. Avoid highlighting entire sentences or 20 different parts of the passage, as neither will make for a particularly effective roadmap from a glance. Rather, as you read through each paragraph, choose just a few key words or phrases to serve as reminders of the paragraph's purpose and its overall connection to the passage's main idea. Not only will effective highlighting yield a nice skeletal outline of the passage, but it also helps make reading a more physical, active process, and reduces the tendency to drift off.

Another strategy that isn't particularly logical is **skipping questions or entire passages at a time**. Wherever you are in your CARS practice, the ultimate goal should be to try to complete all or as many passages as possible within the allotted time. Therefore, skipping around carries more risks than it does benefits. First of all, it takes time to evaluate whether a passage is one you think you should skip. On a basic level, the actual process of skipping around takes time, and it can result in accidentally leaving questions blank. Then, navigating back to unanswered questions requires you to get back in the mental framework of that passage, which increases the chance of error, as well as the amount of time you're spending on passages. Furthermore, it's very difficult to assess whether a passage truly *is* hard, both because a dense-looking passage might have easy questions, and because students often over-rely on the passage *topic* as an indicator of how difficult the passage will be. Another point that often gets lost in this conversation is that, by telling yourself certain passages are hard, or that you're not very good at a particular type of passage, you may be setting up a self-fulfilling prophecy or mental roadblock that can hold you back from what you're capable of. It also makes it more difficult to keep track of your pacing. We recommend going passage by passage, question by question, during MCAT practice. Of course, if you have extra time it's always a good idea to go back and check answers you're not confident in, but in that initial pass-through, tackling questions in order is the way to go.

When taking any test, it can be extremely easy to **lose focus**, and find your attention drifting off to random topics, or things going on in your everyday life. This is something we're all predisposed to, but avoiding or minimizing such distractions is also a skill at which we can improve. Drifting off and losing focus means we have to re-read parts of a passage, which is an inefficient use of time. In fact, this is an issue underlying many students' perceptions of themselves as "slow readers." In many cases, being a "slow reader" doesn't mean actually processing each sentence unusually slowly, but instead reflects a pattern of getting stuck reading and re-reading the same sentence or paragraph over and over. The best protection against a wandering mind is anything that will keep you laser-focused on the passage.

In connection with maintaining focus, keep in mind that it is not always necessary to understand every single word or phrase or even sentence of a passage. In fact, some passages—especially dense philosophy passages or those with convoluted opinions and arguments—are designed to be difficult for *any* reader to fully comprehend without taking significantly more time than is reasonable for a CARS passage. If you don't feel confident in your understanding of a given sentence or paragraph after a careful read-through, it might be that you don't *need* to really understand it comprehensively, and that your time is better spent **moving on** rather than reading the same sentence or sentences over and over again, which is unlikely to reveal new insights. It's quite possible that the meaning of a difficult section might become clear upon reading later paragraphs or the questions associated with the passage, or reading the passage might not even be necessary to answer the questions at all.

Active reading strategies tend to be effective for maintaining focus. Try to figure out why the author thinks the topic of a passage is interesting or important enough to talk about. Even if the topic doesn't immediately seem relatable or compelling, the author must have had a reason to write about it! For example, the author might be waxing philosophical about Socrates's early theories, but perhaps at the same time throwing shade at Plato. Alternatively, you might notice that the author is weirdly enthused about an obscure form of art involving plants. Your job is to figure out what the author is *really* trying to say, and why.

Active reading can also be **task-oriented**. The next time you have an opportunity to review a CARS passage, ask yourself questions as you read about the purpose of each sentence and paragraph, or about the author's motivations. The goal is to ask these questions in such a way that you can set incremental goals for yourself. For example, what words do you need to highlight in this paragraph to remind yourself of what's being discussed, or what its main idea is? Another useful technique is to review a CARS passage as if you were teaching it to someone else. Ask yourself: What should that person focus on? What parts are details supporting a broader argument? Furthermore, our brains are especially good at encoding text that is emotionally salient. For example, if an author claimed that pineapple doesn't belong on pizza, you might be either highly offended or deeply enthusiastic, depending on your personal pizza preferences, and therefore you'll be really interested in what evidence the author has to back that claim. You'll probably also be highly engaged with that passage, and, as a result, have greater retention of its content. It's extremely unlikely that you'll encounter a discussion of pizza toppings in the CARS section, but the point holds that, if you can connect with a passage, or with the author, *even a little bit*, that'll help you maintain focus and do well in the CARS section.

Additionally, sometimes your brain needs a little time to **rest**. We previously discussed the strategy of taking a microbreak halfway through the section, but it's also possible to give your brain designated five-second breaks at the beginning of a passage to clear your mind of old concepts, rather than having it wander off onto other thoughts in the middle of a passage.

3. CARS Passages

Reading CARS passages is about **efficiency** as much as it is about thorough analysis and reasoning. Normally, we want to read a CARS passage in approximately four to five minutes, which gives us enough time to read through the passage and gather our thoughts before moving on to the questions. Most CARS passages will be between 500 and 600 words in length, and since the average reading speed is about 200 words per minute, you may be able to read a CARS passage in as little as three minutes. Therefore, four to five minutes gives you some buffer room. You can demonstrate this to yourself by timing how long it takes you to read a CARS passage. There's a good chance you *can* read a CARS passage efficiently in isolation, although you may be surpassing your time budget if you find yourself re-reading, getting distracted, or navigating through questions non-strategically.

Let's take a look at a CARS passage together. First, we'll discuss how to read CARS passages thoroughly but efficiently, and then compare this method to skimming when you're running low on time. There are a few things you can be doing to read a CARS passage efficiently. First, we're going to be **task-oriented**: we're actively reading to identify **main ideas**, as well as the author's **perspective**. We're also looking for terms to **highlight** that capture these ideas. Read through the passage below with these goals in mind, and then we'll discuss the passage in more depth.

> The camera extends, and is modeled after, the eye. Does this make the eye a tool, or the camera an organ? Is the distinction meaningful? Flusser's characterization of the camera as a form of intelligence might have raised eyebrows in the 20th century, since, surrounded by cameras, many people had long since reinscribed the boundaries of intelligence more narrowly around the brain—perhaps, as we have seen, in order to safeguard the category of the uniquely human. Calling the brain the seat of intelligence, and the eye therefore a mere peripheral, is a flawed strategy, though. After all, we are not merely brains in biological vats. Even if we were to adopt a neurocentric attitude, modern neuroscientists typically refer to the retina as an outpost of the brain, as it is largely made out of neurons and performs a great deal of information processing before sending encoded visual signals along the optic nerve.

> Do cameras also process information nontrivially? It is remarkable that Flusser was so explicit in describing the camera as having a program and software when he was writing his philosophy of photography in 1983, given that the first real digital camera was not made until 1988. Maybe it took a philosopher's squint to notice the programming inherent in the grinding and configuration of lenses, the creation of a frame and field of view, the timing of the shutter, the details of chemical emulsions and film processing. Maybe, also, Flusser was writing about programming in a wider, more sociological sense.

Be this as it may, for today's cameras, this is no longer a metaphor. The camera in your phone is indeed powered by software, amounting at a minimum to millions of lines of code. Much of this code performs support functions peripheral to the actual imaging, but some of it makes explicit the nonlinear summing-up of photons into color components that used to be physically computed by the film emulsion. Other code does things like removing noise in near-constant areas, sharpening edges, and filling in defective pixels with plausible surrounding color, not unlike the way our retinas hallucinate away the blood vessels at the back of the eye that would otherwise mar our visual field. The images we see can only be beautiful or realistic because they have been heavily processed, either by neural machinery or by code, operating below our threshold of consciousness. In the case of software, this processing relies on norms and aesthetic judgments on the part of software engineers, so they are also unacknowledged collaborators in the image-making. There is no such thing as a natural image; perhaps, too, there is nothing especially artificial about the camera.

The flexibility of code allows us to make cameras that do much more than producing images that can pass for natural. Researchers like those at the Massachusetts Institute of Technology Media Lab's Camera Culture group have developed software-enabled nontraditional cameras (many of which still use ordinary hardware) that can sense depth, see around corners, or see through skin. Abe Davis and collaborators have even developed a computational camera that can "see" sound, by decoding the tiny vibrations of houseplant leaves and potato chip bags. So, Flusser was, perhaps, even more right than he realized in asserting that cameras follow programs, and that their software has progressively become more important than their hardware. Cameras are "thinking machines."

Adapted from Aguera, B (2017). "Art in the Age of Machine Intelligence." Arts, 6(4) under CC BY 3.0.

The first paragraph starts out somewhat medically related—the author claims the camera is modeled after the eye—and then says something about how cameras may be organs, and eyes may be tools. This latter part simply enhances that first point about the relationship between cameras and the eye, so we should highlight this phrase. Then the author introduces Flusser, whose name we may want to remember in case it comes up in a question later. More important is this new idea we're introduced to, that the camera may be a form of intelligence. We can highlight the word "intelligence" to capture this idea. This paragraph then introduces a point of contention: is intelligence "uniquely human"? Is the brain alone the seat of intelligence, or does the eye, or the camera, play a role too? The author seems to think the latter.

We're just one paragraph in, yet we've already been exposed to several differing viewpoints, including the author's own. Let's review the terms we chose to highlight and reflect on the main idea here. This passage will clearly focus on the camera, and builds up the argument that the camera is, controversially, linked to intelligence. Most of the rest of this paragraph is supporting text - it's still important, and it's still highly relevant to the author's major arguments, but we can always come back to the passage when asked about supporting details.

Now let's consider a situation where we're really crunched for time. Say, we have two passages to complete in 10 minutes. While this isn't much time, it's enough to spend some on the passage, which we know is actually a more efficient strategy than jumping straight to the questions and having to navigate back through the passage haphazardly. In such a situation, you may need to rely on skimming techniques to gather the major ideas of the passage before working through the questions. With this approach, read the first and last sentences of each paragraph, and, with CARS passages in particular, focus on the introduction and conclusion. The author will generally introduce the major premise or thesis of the passage in the first paragraph, and end by synthesizing their arguments in a decisive conclusion at the end of the final paragraph. Let's examine that in the last paragraph of this essay, this time only reading the first and last sentences.

"The flexibility of code allows us to make cameras that do much more than producing images that can pass for natural." And then, "Cameras are 'thinking machines.'" So we cut out a lot of information from this paragraph, and what we're left with is a statement about how much cameras are capable of, thanks to coding, and finally the author concludes that cameras are intelligent, thinking machines. In fact, this lines up perfectly well with the author's views as they are presented in the introductory paragraph. What we're missing here is the evidence. If you read these sentences in isolation, it's going to require a lot more convincing to believe that cameras are "thinking machines," at least in the absence of any supporting information. We can assume that this or the prior paragraph discusses coding and natural images, so we would want to return to this part of the passage if we encountered questions related to these ideas.

Ideally, we'd want to read each paragraph in its entirety, but skimming when you're really pressed for time can give you an outline of the author's main premises and where they're located so you can return to the relevant parts of the passage later if needed. When skimming it's okay to highlight, but since you'll be reading from the passage selectively, it's not necessary to highlight as much as you normally would. Note that from just those four words alone at the end—"Cameras are thinking machines"—we obtain what appears to be the author's thesis. Maybe we got lucky this time, but the conclusion paragraph is the author's last chance to make a closing argument, so it tends to be rich in conclusive arguments and testable material.

4. CARS Questions

After reading through a passage, we recommend proceeding through its associated questions in order, and selecting an answer choice before moving on from each question, since there are no penalties for guessing. Based on just what we've read, let's see how we fare on this question:

> Which of the following best describes the author's primary argument?
>
> A. Cameras have become progressively more complex in recent years.
> B. Philosophers are still struggling to properly describe cameras.
> C. There are strong parallels between cameras, computers, and the human brain.
> D. Cameras are programmed in the same manner as computers.

Our goal here is not only to get the right answer, but to do so as efficiently as possible. There are four answer choices, but before we address those, what would we say is the author's primary argument? The author seems focused on convincing us that cameras aren't just series of lenses with some internal circuitry; rather, they're intelligent, as described by the phrase "thinking machines." For a question as general as this, we probably won't need to return to the passage for specifics, which will save us some time. Therefore, we are looking for an answer choice that most closely relates to this idea.

Choice A says that cameras have become more complex in recent years. This *may* be true, but if anything, a statement like that would likely be used to reinforce the author's real argument, that cameras process information in ways analogous to the brain. In fact, we haven't even encountered any information about cameras becoming more advanced in the introductory or conclusion paragraphs, so it'd be surprising if this were really the author's main point.

Choice B says philosophers don't totally know how to describe cameras. Whether or not this is true, or the author believes this, it doesn't really align with the author's thesis.

Choice C says that cameras parallel computers and the human brain. This is the moment where we transform from feeling lukewarm about the first two answer choices to that incredibly satisfying feeling of finding an answer choice that's a perfect fit. So far, this best captures what we've considered the main idea of this passage.

Let's examine choice D just briefly to be thorough, although on test day you should move on to the next question once you believe you've selected the correct response. Choice D again relates cameras to computers, but, like our earlier answer choices, this is information that might be supportive of the author's main argument, but not the primary thesis itself. In addition, it's somewhat of an extreme answer choice, as it's unlikely that cameras are programmed in the *exact* same manner as computers are. Therefore, we can be pretty confident that choice C is correct.

Now let's tackle a separate question where we could benefit from returning to the passage:

> According to the passage, which of the following was true prior to the 21st century?
>
> A. Flusser's philosophy of cameras was held in higher esteem than that of his peers.
> B. Cameras were less common and people were less familiar with them.
> C. The idea of non-human intelligence was more contentious.
> D. Digital cameras were adopted more slowly than non-digital cameras.

Ideally, we would go through each answer choice in succession, but our goal here is to model a highly time-efficient approach. Recall that the passage described events of the 20th century in the first paragraph, so we'll want to go back to that part of the passage. If we had skimmed, numbers are pretty easy to identify within a passage, so we could likely still navigate to this section. According to the passage, Flusser made some provocative statements about the camera being a form of intelligence, at a time when everyone else considered the brain the hub of intelligence, adhering to the notion that intelligence is "uniquely human."

We can easily eliminate choice A, as "raised eyebrows" doesn't exactly translate to a raised esteem - in fact, probably the opposite. We can also eliminate choice B, as the passage quite literally claims that people at the time were "surrounded by cameras." Choice C says that non-human intelligence was a controversial idea, which is a promising answer choice since the author claimed that people at the time were desperate to safeguard the concept of intelligence as being uniquely human. Let's look at choice D briefly, too. This is another poor answer choice, as it's not stated by the passage, so choice C must be correct.

We moved through these questions pretty quickly, which is great! That will often be the case when you understand the passage, especially the author's opinion. However, there will be times when you feel stuck between multiple tempting answers on a CARS question. When this happens, you risk wasting a lot of time debating between answer choices, which both takes up time and increases the risk of being drawn to making logical leaps and speculations that lead to an answer choice that doesn't clearly follow from the passage information.

To combat this tendency, try to stay conscious of how much time you're spending on each question relative to the other questions on the test. If you catch yourself wavering between answer choices for longer than normal, say for 20 or 30 seconds, then choose the answer choice that best matches your original gut instinct. Then flag the question, and move on. Your gut instinct can be more reliable than you think, particularly when it points you to the answer choice that most closely matches the main idea and the author's tone.

If you're running short on time, these methods can help you efficiently maximize the number of questions you answer correctly. Of course, the best approach is time management prophylaxis. In other words, keep tabs on your pacing as you go along so that the clock doesn't sneak up on you. But if it does, now you have a few strategies up your sleeve that you can employ in the nick of time.

5. Pacing Through Practice

As we've discussed, practice is key to MCAT prep in general, and for the CARS section in particular. By practicing with new passages on a regular basis, you'll become more comfortable with expecting the unexpected, and processing new information analytically, no matter if it's about Egyptian obelisks or punk rock sub-genres.

Using CARS passages for practice is really the best way to familiarize yourself with the right pacing for the MCAT. **Passage practice** can be timed or untimed, each with a different purpose. During **untimed practice**, the goal should be to focus solely on your performance. Ask yourself questions like: Are you understanding the passage correctly? Are you able to interpret and answer the questions? What areas can you improve upon? This is ideal when practicing with one or more passages at a time, followed by review of these passages. **Timed practice** has another purpose: to master the passage, but under a time crunch. In other words, once you've optimized your performance, can you become more efficient and still achieve the same score? Ideally your full-length MCAT practice should be timed, giving you an opportunity to simulate the real MCAT, and timed practice can also be used on individual passages or sets of passages as you fine-tune your pacing strategy.

When you're first getting started, work through untimed CARS passages, and don't worry about how long it's taking you. Once you're getting 70-80% of questions right, then you can consider the clock: time how long it takes you to work through the passage and still achieve a good score. Then see if you can do another passage while reducing the time by 30 seconds to a minute. Then see if you can cut your time down by another 30 seconds to a minute, and so forth until you're hitting your goal time. You can also decouple the passage from its questions and just focus on one issue at a time: first, just see how long it takes you to read a passage, but always complete its questions in as much time as you need to test your understanding of the passage. If you start missing more questions, you might be reading too fast! Then see how long it's taking you to answer questions. You might find that you're more efficient with questions when you have a better understanding of the passage, which means that your investment in the passage text is paying off. Then, by treating your timed full-length practice as a true simulation of the real MCAT, nothing should feel completely new on the day of your exam, and you'll be as ready as you'll ever be.

As you practice, you'll become more adept at estimating how long you've spent on a passage, and more importantly, whether you're on track with your **pacing**. While this may seem like a daunting task, finding the right pace with which to proceed through CARS passages is a skill that can be practiced and learned. Although we've discussed various pacing-related skills and techniques, you should absolutely troubleshoot these methods, as they can be tailored to your own experience. For example, if you spend a lot of time trying to remember where to go back and find information at specific locations within a passage, a highlighted outline might serve you well. In contrast, if you constantly feel rushed towards the end of the section, minding the clock and using skimming techniques as needed may benefit you more.

In addition to these benefits, practice has another advantage: **analysis**. If you're spending eight hours on a given practice exam, you may as well use your results to troubleshoot your strengths and areas for improvement. A thorough review will help you unveil patterns in the types of questions or passages that you find particularly challenging, and it can also help guide your next steps in improving your pacing. For example, if you find that you're missing questions predominantly in later passages, it could be because you're rushing toward the end of that section, or because the clock is contributing to feelings of test anxiety. Take advantage of the analytics available to you so that you're setting and meeting specific goals each time you take a practice test.

Passage practice is also an excellent way to build up endurance for an eight-hour exam. Starting off, complete passages in manageable chunks of two or three to build your familiarity with CARS passages. From there you can build up to entire section tests and full-length MCAT exams in no time. As you begin doing this, you may find it helpful to give yourself a short, five-second break between passages to clear your mind of old concepts and reset your CARS brain. While regular passage practice is important, working through multiple passages in timed sets and in one sitting will best simulate and prepare you for the real MCAT.

6. Must-Knows

> Key to pacing on CARS: full mental commitment to each passage, not tricks.
> Some timing-related pitfalls to be aware of:
  - Checking the timer too often or too rarely (we recommend once every couple passage).
  - Spending too much time note-taking.
  - Skipping questions or entire passages.
  - Losing focus.
> Strategies to improve pacing:
  - Cultivate awareness of your timing.
  - Utilize active reading strategies (identifying main ideas, perspectives, etc. and using highlighter tool to create outline).
  - Make reading CARS passages into a task-oriented activity.
  - Focus on emotionally salient points.
  - Move through questions in order.
  - Utilize a mix of untimed and timed practice to hone your pacing skills.
  - Carefully analyze how and where you encounter pacing problems in order to improve.

Applied Practice

The best MCAT practice is realistic, with detailed analytics to help you assess where things went wrong. For those reasons, we recommend completing practice questions in an online setting that simulates the real MCAT interface, and using the analytics provided to help you decide how to best move your studies forward.

CARS does not require knowledge of specific subject areas, but it does require development of strong test-taking skills. To ensure you are honing those skills as you work through this book, we suggest you go online after wrapping up each chapter and generate a Qbank Practice Set of 2-3 CARS passages to practice and review. While not every chapter of this book is directly applicable to CARS, regular CARS practice is key to test day success.

As a further supplement, given the importance of active learning for effective studying, we also suggest that you consult the Must-Knows at the end of each chapter of this Reasoning text as a basis for creating a study sheet. This is not a sheet to memorize in the more traditional sense of content memorization, but rather a quick reference of the most important strategies for you to refer to during and after practice in your early prep. Frequently revisiting the most important strategies for the MCAT - in both CARS and the Sciences - will help you continue to improve your performance.

This page left intentionally blank.

This page left intentionally blank.

Opinions in CARS Passages

0. Introduction

Whether you're a science major more comfortable with memorizing chemical formulas and calculating torque than reading art history, or one of the thousands of humanities and social sciences majors that matriculate to medical school, or somewhere in between, there's always room for further developing and refining your CARS skills. One of the foundational aspects of success on the CARS section is attending carefully and accurately to authors' opinions.

1. Identifying Opinions in CARS Passages

CARS questions will frequently ask about the author's **perspective**, either directly or in contrast with other perspectives discussed in the passage. Therefore, our first goal is to identify and distinguish between opinion-based versus fact-based statements. **Facts** are verifiable statements rooted in an objective truth. Facts can be proven, or disproven, with evidence. For example: The earth revolves around the sun. Slugs have four noses. It's impossible to breathe and swallow at the same time. In contrast, **opinions** are non-verifiable, subjective judgments like: it's a good thing that the earth revolves around the sun, or four noses is a lot of noses, or trying to breathe and swallow at the same time is a silly endeavor.

Opinionated statements often contain **qualifiers**, like "may," "might," "probably," "suggests," "should," and "very." These statements can also be identified by the presence of **adjectives** indicating value judgements, such as "terrible," "bad," "beautiful," and so on. Sometimes comparisons can even hold opinions, so look out for words or phrases that signify them, like "worse/worst," "better/best," "favorite," "inferior," and even "similar" or "the same as." Such cues will help you pick up on the author's attitude and overall position. Remember that the author is or was a real person with real emotions and attitudes and opinions. They wrote their passage on a topic they care or cared deeply about, so their text is bound to be full of those feelings. We just need to be reading carefully and critically. After each paragraph, see if you can gauge the mood of the writer. After all, you'll be asked to put yourself in the author's shoes while answering questions such as, "Which of the following statements would the author most likely agree or disagree with?" An important factor here is that opinionated statements can be packed with emotion, but they don't have to be. In fact, they're often a bit more subtle in MCAT passages.

When dealing with these sneaky passages, it's critical to distinguish fact from opinion. For a given claim, you can ask yourself, "Is this a claim that can be demonstrated to be true? Can it be observed and verified?" If yes, it's probably a fact. If no, you're probably dealing with an opinion. Statements aren't always so clear-cut though. Opinions can also be embedded within a factual statement. For example, "The man thought his handlebar mustache was rather tasteful" is technically a fact if the man quite literally did experience that thought, but whether or not his mustache is objectively tasteful is an opinion that's up for debate. These expressions often are used by the author to present someone else's argument or an opinion. In these cases, we know what this other person or group of people think but not necessarily what the author believes.

For example, a passage might state: "The researcher posits that annual screening is the best approach to cervical cancer prevention." If the researcher did literally posit or state this belief, the statement as a whole is a fact. But, more importantly, whether annual screenings are indeed the best approach to cervical cancer prevention remains the researcher's opinion, even if it's a popular belief. Contrast this with the factual statement: "Annual screenings reduce cervical cancer incidence by 10%." This is an unbiased, verifiable fact. Still, though, even this piece of evidence doesn't change the fact that whether annual screenings are the best approach is up for debate. Maybe it's expensive or there are other preventive approaches that are just as effective. And even if every single clinician agreed that these screenings were the absolute best approach, we're still dealing with an opinion until it's backed up by verifiable, factual evidence.

Next, consider the statement: "Michelangelo is thought by many to be the greatest artist of all time." Similarly phrased statements are common in CARS passages. Note here that the author states what many other people believe or think but does not reveal his or her own personal beliefs. Commonly, the author will present one or more positions only to counter them later in the passage, using wording like "It is thought by many…" or "Some would say…" or "According to some…" On the other hand, if the author states directly and matter-of-factly that "Michelangelo was the greatest artist of all time," then that would be the author's own opinion. If, instead, this sentence said, "Michelangelo ate more gelato than did any of the contemporary artists of his time," technically this would be a factual statement. In theory, we could go back and measure the exact gelato consumption of Michelangelo and all of his contemporaries to try to verify the truth of this statement.

Having taken the first step to identify opinionated claims, the next step is to analyze them in the context of the passage. This means asking questions like:

> What does this tell me about what the author believes?
> Why might the author believe this?
> Is this consistent with the passage as a whole?
> How does this contribute to the author's agenda and the main arguments of the passage?
> Based on this, what other ideas might the author support, and what other positions is the author likely to disagree with?

In addition to the author's opinion, we need to address *your* opinion. The MCAT view on **personal opinions** in CARS is that they don't belong. In other words, you should always answer questions based on what the passage says, not your opinions or outside knowledge. But it's harder than it sounds. Sometimes your opinions can seep in around the edges, even if you're trying to keep an open mind. And it's not just about agreeing or disagreeing with the author, or someone the author refers to. Sometimes, your opinion may just be that something is *boring*. On one hand, that's legitimate. Everyone has their own preferences, and no one can force you to like art history or economics or whatever. On the other hand, as we've discussed, that can negatively impact your performance by diminishing your ability to focus, so be sure to engage active reading techniques to combat this tendency.

The opposite danger also exists. If you encounter a passage on a topic you like or are knowledgeable about, your initial reaction might be excitement: CARS passages can be on anything but this one actually matches your interests! This is risky because if you feel strongly about a topic, or have outside knowledge about it, you may inadvertently bring your own opinions to the table. When you do that, some devious wrong answer choices can start to look really appealing. This can be a particular danger on passages about population health or medicine, since many pre-med students have strong points of view on these topics. In such a situation, step back and focus on the words on the screen, not your own insights into the topic, and be alert for perspectives that might seem surprising.

2. Identifying Opinions in Practice

Let's practice identifying opinions in CARS passages by examining a sample passage together:

According to the Declaration of Helsinki, research studies should 1) be approved by an independent research ethics committee (REC) and 2) seek informed consent (IC) from the participants. These principles have in turn been addressed by the International Committee of Medical Journal Editors (ICMJE) and the Committee on Publication Ethics (COPE). Both groups publish core requirements for editing and reporting research findings. For example, the ICMJE states that "the requirement for informed consent should be included in the journal's instructions for authors. When informed consent has been obtained, it should be indicated in the published article." The COPE code of conduct asks editors to ensure that reports of clinical trials cite compliance with the Declaration of Helsinki (DoH), good clinical practice, and other relevant guidelines on safeguarding participants. Editors are encouraged by the ICMJE and COPE to apply and distribute these guidelines.

However, empirical data from several studies throughout the last two decades suggest insufficient reporting of ethics review approvals and informed consent procedures in peer-reviewed articles and meta-analyses. Weil and colleagues demonstrated that only 52% of the articles in pediatric journals reported ethical approval, and one in seven studies had not undergone REC review.

Insufficient reporting of ethical issues can negatively affect how trustworthy the public judges the biomedical research community to be. Public trust in the research community requires evidence that the community has qualities such as competence and goodwill which merit that trust. Insufficient reporting of ethical issues may not only give the impression to the public but also to the research community itself that the ethical quality of research is judged far less important than its scientific validity. However, designing a study demands both critical reflection on relevant methodological aspects (e.g., randomization and blinding to minimize the influence of confounding biases) and on ethical issues (e.g., fair selection of, minimizing risks for, and obtaining valid informed consent from trial participants). Furthermore, ideal scientific design sometimes needs to be compromised for ethical reasons.

The better-established requirement to report standard methodological aspects, such as eligibility criteria, blinding, and randomization procedures, has two main consequences. First, as a direct consequence, it helps editors, reviewers, and readers assess the reliability and validity of the research. Second, as an indirect consequence, it signals to future authors the importance of critical reflection on methodological quality in the design and conduct of a study. Likewise, editorial policies should require reporting of pertinent ethical considerations for the following reasons: A) to allow editors, reviewers and readers to assess the ethical quality of the research; B) to foster the design and conduct of future studies that meet appropriate standards of ethical research; C) to raise the visibility of ethical research and thereby maintain public trust; and D) to facilitate a discussion and scientific evaluation of current standards and variations in real-life research ethics.

Statements such as "the study was approved by the local institutional review board (IRB)" or "informed consent was obtained from all study participants" are too general to meet the criteria for, and aims of, reporting ethical issues. These platitudes are especially lacking when the research involves patients with disorders that impair decision-making capacity, such as Alzheimer's disease and schizophrenia, and in studying interventions that pose ethical concerns.

Passage adapted from Strech, D., Metz, C., & Kahrass, H. (2014). Do Editorial Policies Support Ethical Research? A Thematic Text Analysis of Author Instructions in Psychiatry Journals. Research Ethics Forum Ethics and Governance of Biomedical Research, 125-134 under CC BY.

This passage is an ethics passage that, at first glance, may appear to be strictly factual but is rich in opinionated adjectives and statements. Consider the first paragraph. We're looking for any words or phrases that suggest an opinion or bias. The first sentence says, "according to the Declaration of Helsinki, research studies *should* do" certain things. The qualifier "should" tells us what the creators of the Declaration think are the basic criteria research studies must meet for publishing. But what does the passage's author think of these requirements? We have no idea at this point. This first paragraph basically outlines the requirement guidelines for publication that various ethics committees have established, including review by an ethics committee and informed consent.

Paragraph two begins with the linkage word "however," transitioning to a contrasting idea from those in the first paragraph. The author states that data *suggest* that fulfillment of these criteria has been *insufficient*, which is an opinion, as what one person considers insufficient might differ from the next person's definition. Opinions tend not to stand by themselves without some kind of support, and that's certainly the case here. The author backs up their statement with facts, stating that only 52% of pediatric journal articles reported ethics approval, and one in seven hadn't been reviewed by an independent research ethics committee. Notice, though, that even these factual statements have been modified with words that signify the author's opinion. For example, the word "only" in the phrase "only 52% of articles in pediatric journals reported ethical approval" tells us that the author believes that 52% is a low value.

Moving on to paragraph three, the author's purpose here is to persuade us that such insufficient reporting is bad in terms of public opinion of the biomedical research community. This is clearly an opinion, as the value words "insufficient" and "negatively" tell us that the author personally thinks this is a problem. The author says midway through this paragraph that inadequate ethics reporting *may* give people the idea that researchers believe ethical standards aren't as important as the science itself. There are actually a few layered opinions embedded in this statement. The first is the idea that ethical standards aren't as important as the science. However, the author doesn't believe this. Rather, the author believes that if researchers don't follow certain ethics guidelines and reporting procedures, then the public may begin to mistakenly think it.

The author then shifts, using the transition word "however" again, to bridge these two seemingly conflicting needs, emphasizing the necessity of sound scientific methods as well as ethical considerations in research. The author even goes so far as to claim that scientific methods sometimes need to be compromised in light of ethical considerations. Take note of the moderating word "sometimes" used in this latter sentence, and notice the lack of any qualifiers in the prior one: both of these choices reveal opinions. We know that these are the author's beliefs (pretty critical ones in the context of the entire passage, in fact) because the author directly states them, rather than framing them as others' beliefs.

Expanding upon the contrast between reporting scientific methods versus ethics issues, paragraph four opens by discussing the benefits, according to the author, of reporting scientific methods. First, reporting methods help others determine whether a research study is reliable and valid. Second, other researchers may be more inclined to use sound and rigorous methods in future studies. These are opinionated claims that together tell us more generally that the author thinks reporting scientific methods is a really good idea! Where do you think the author is going with this? Let's make a prediction by considering what we've seen earlier in the passage. We know from paragraphs two and three that the author thinks ethics reporting in scientific papers has been lacking. However, the author argues that the reporting of scientific methods has been fairly strong, so it would be logical to predict that the author would argue that the reporting of ethical considerations should be treated as rigorously as methodological reporting.

This is indeed what happens, beginning with the linkage word "likewise." The author states that journals *should* require ethics issues to be reported, and that qualifier "should" is a big clue that this is an opinionated argument asserting one of the author's major positions. Here, this statement is followed by four reasons in support of this position, and it's up to you to decide whether this support is actually persuasive.

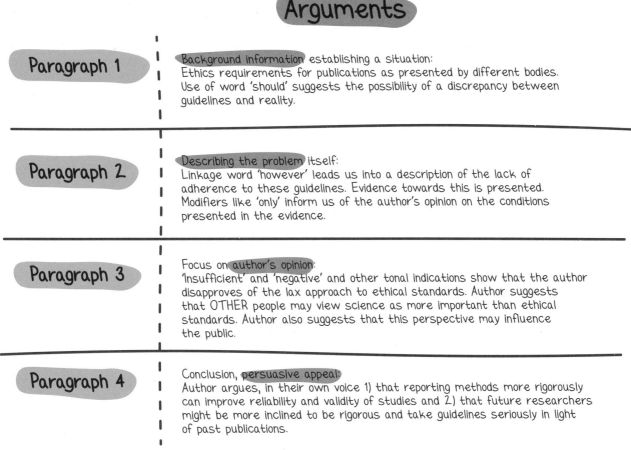

Figure 1. Paragraph outline of passage on pages 41-42, *Do Editorial Policies Support Ethical Research? A Thematic Text Analysis of Author Instructions in Psychiatry Journals*

Based on what we know about the author's perspective, we can infer that the author is clearly knowledgeable about publishing scientific articles in the biomedical research sphere and is invested in responsible ethics reporting, so this person is almost certainly involved with the biomedical research community in some way. Thus, it's not surprising that such a person would be motivated to improve publishing standards, not only to better the scientific literature but also the quality of scientific research and study design. We want to avoid extrapolating too far beyond the text in any attempt to predict the author's position on other issues. For example, if we were presented with a question about various study designs for theoretical experiments, we might predict that the author would favor a study design that compromises scientific methods somewhat in order to accommodate ethical considerations. However, it would be too extreme to conclude that the author would pursue a perfectly ethical study with poor scientific methods.

In the final paragraph, the author criticizes journal articles that simply state the study was approved by an ethics review board or that informed consent was obtained, arguing that such statements are "too general." Furthermore, the author calls these statements "platitudes" that are "especially lacking" in studies with particular ethical concerns. Such word choice indicates the author's strong, negative attitude towards such statements. We shouldn't be too surprised to find such forceful claims in the conclusion, as conclusion paragraphs are the author's last chance to make his or her position crystal clear. If the author presents multiple perspectives within a passage, it should become clear by the conclusion where he or she stands.

We've taken quite a journey through this passage. A few points are particularly worth emphasizing. First, don't be fooled if a passage seems technical or factual at first. The author most likely still has opinions, and there's even a good chance they might be pretty strong, as they are in this case. This is normally true, even if those opinions are cloaked by technical language, field-specific jargon, or a series of factual statements that the author uses to support their opinions. In the CARS section, you will *never* get a passage that just presents a bunch of facts, followed by simple questions about those facts. Therefore, you should always be on the lookout for opinions. Even if the author doesn't have strong opinions or remains neutral, it's virtually certain that one or more other individuals in the passage are opinionated.

This passage is also interesting from the point of view of managing your own emotional reaction. Many of you might have had an overall neutral reaction, and that's more than OK. As future clinicians and/or biomedical researchers, though, some of you might actually feel pretty strongly about issues of medical ethics and reporting. There's nothing at all wrong with that, but an intense gut-level engagement can also be a warning sign to step back and focus only on what the *author* is bringing to the table in the passage. Alternatively, this passage might have seemed dense and dull, perhaps because your interest in medicine is purely clinical and action-oriented, or because research isn't really your thing. Those are also totally legitimate perspectives. Likewise, though, getting bored can be a problem, so as we've discussed, try to boost your emotional engagement by connecting the topic to something that you are interested in.

3. Opinion Questions

CARS passages are littered with **opinions**, and CARS questions just love to ask about them. Think about it: does it require greater critical reasoning to recall a fact stated by the author or to get into the author's mind and truly understand his or her perspective? We discuss CARS questions more specifically in Chapters 6 and 7, but it's worth previewing these issues early on in your CARS journey.

CARS questions test three fundamental **skill categories**. The first category, *Foundations of Comprehension*, contains questions that assess your ability to understand the basic components of the passage and to make inferences about the author's tone, word choice, or point of view. For example, you might be asked about the author's response or attitude toward something discussed in the passage.

Returning to the passage on medical ethics presented above, suppose we were asked how the author feels about reporting scientific methodology in journal articles. Is the author skeptical of its value to the scientific community? Is the author critical because it detracts from the reporting of ethical issues? Is the author neutral? Is the author just plain accepting of it? Or is the author fully supportive of methods reporting while also arguing that a similar approach ought to be applied to ethics reporting? Note that adjectives like "accepting" and "supportive" both strike a positive tone, but "supportive" is a better fit here. We might also be asked how the author feels about particular information or opinions that were mentioned in the passage. These questions could look something like: what does the author think of the study by Weil et al. that showed almost half of the articles in pediatric journals did not report ethics approval? The passage used this study as support for the claim that ethics reporting has been insufficient in the last 20 years, and, furthermore, the passage doesn't offer any direct criticism of it. Thus, we can conclude that the author very likely believes this study to be legitimate.

The second category of CARS questions is *Reasoning Within the Text*. These questions will ask you to dive a little deeper, integrating separate parts of the passage to evaluate the author's arguments, claims, and biases. This is particularly relevant for opinions within CARS passages because, by interpreting them, you'll be better able to assess how credible the author is and what's objective versus what isn't.

For example, suppose we are given the following MCAT question: the author most likely believes that statements such as "informed consent was obtained from all study participants…" are "especially lacking when the research involves patients with disorders that impair decision-making capacity" because… This is referring to the statements made in the conclusion paragraph, but it requires us to integrate information from elsewhere in the passage. For one, we know that the author thinks the research community needs to step up its game when it comes to reporting ethical considerations in research studies. That point is made clear in paragraphs three and four. But why should this be especially important for studies involving patients with impaired decision-making? Let's look closely at the conclusion with those opinions from earlier paragraphs in mind. The author specifies that ethics reporting is especially relevant when ethical issues are raised in a study, and the author also feels that informed consent should be *valid* informed consent. Therefore, it makes sense that the author would argue that we should take special precautions when considering how to obtain informed consent from participants with impaired decision-making. Thus, by understanding the author's beliefs and motivations, we can more readily deconstruct an author's arguments and find the best answer choice. A Reasoning Within the Text question could also ask us about the author's probable identity, which is ultimately a question that really gets at how the author's point of view and biases shape his or her arguments. This requires us to draw upon information throughout the passage. The author is clearly knowledgeable about publishing practices within the biomedical research community and seems highly invested in improving such practices. Thus, the author is likely someone closely tied to biomedical research in some capacity and probably has some experience writing or reviewing scientific publications.

Reasoning Beyond the Text questions form the third category of CARS questions, and these are arguably among the toughest of the three question groups. These questions go a step further from Reasoning Within the Text questions, requiring you to apply the passage text to new situations outside of the text or to take new information and interpret it in light of the passage. Such questions are presented in one of two ways. The first way will ask you to identify how the author would feel about some new idea or piece of information. The second way will give you new information and then ask how that affects your interpretation of the passage. Thus, the common thread of Reasoning Beyond the Text questions is their inclusion of new information, either in the question stem or the answer choices.

For example, we might be asked: what statement might the author of this passage agree or disagree with? Here, the "new" information will be found in the answer choices, which will contain statements that weren't present in the passage. As we search for our answer, however, we should be careful not to extrapolate too far beyond what is evident from the text. For example, the author would likely agree that some aspects of study design may need to be compromised to accommodate ethical concerns, but completely neglecting methodological considerations to avoid any ethical issues would be too extreme of a position. Alternatively, a different question might give us a new piece of information (e.g., 30% of studies involving dementia patients do not report approval by an ethics review board), and then we might be asked how that would affect the argument made in the conclusion paragraph. We could also be told that many pediatricians feel that reporting approval by an ethics review board is cumbersome and unnecessary, and be asked how the author would feel about such a belief. These types of questions require us to apply passage information beyond the text, so it's critical to gain a solid understanding of the author's beliefs and perspective as you read through CARS passages.

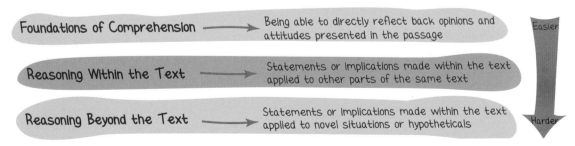

Figure 2. The three CARS question types

4. Multiple Points of View

CARS passages are generally written to persuade their readers of some **viewpoint**. The thesis is less often a fact like, "Capitalism is an economic system that prioritizes private ownership," but more often an opinion such as, "Free market capitalism is good for the economy," or "Capitalism exacerbates economic disparities." Alternatively, the author may choose to maintain a more balanced, objective stance on an issue while presenting others' views, such as "There are several different positions on the value of capitalism as an economic system." Opinions on any given subject will likely vary throughout society, so essays that take differing viewpoints into account are more likely to win over their readership or at least give their readers something to think about. For example, if you're critical of capitalism for one particular reason, or prefer a specific alternative to capitalism, you're unlikely to agree with an essay that simply lists the benefits of capitalism. But if the author acknowledges and addresses your viewpoints, you might be persuaded to change beliefs or find that your original beliefs are actually compatible with the premise of the author's argument.

This is not the only reason that a CARS passage might expose you to **multiple viewpoints**. There are many reasons why using different viewpoints can be useful to an author. For example, an economist may wish to provide nuance to a particular argument by incorporating a diverse array of competing ideas, or perhaps a sociologist wants to summarize the controversy around his or her position by presenting all the prevailing theories. The author might even choose to begin with the evidence for a variety of ideas, examining each individual position until arriving at an evidence-backed conclusion drawn from the patterns and similarities that held these ideas together. Such an approach is considered a bottom-up approach. This is in contrast to the common top-down approach, which begins with a thesis followed by pieces of evidence that provide support to the thesis. Most often, though, multiple points of view will be offered in opposition to the author's main argument, giving the author an opportunity to predict and swiftly defeat each potential counterpoint.

CARS passages with multiple viewpoints won't always follow the same organizational structure, so it's important to recognize which and whose argument is being presented at each step of the way rather than trying to memorize structural formulas. For example, you might encounter a passage where the author's opinion is introduced at the beginning, followed by one or more counterpoints in successive paragraphs, and returning full circle to the author's position by the end. Another option is that the author might begin with the opposing argument, or arguments, followed by the author's position on the stated issue. Still another option would be for the author to present an issue in a more objective fashion, noting the various positions on this issue to add nuance, discussing their pros and cons, and then narrowing down or refining these views to illuminate the author's position in the debate. Sometimes, the author will voice an opinion on select topics within the passage while the author's opinion on other topics is left ambiguous. Whether the author incorporates one or more opinions, the author's main argument should become clear by the end, even if that opinion is "we need more research to answer this question with total certainty!"

Different complementary viewpoints

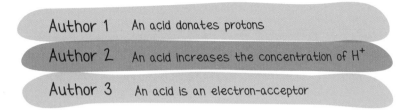

Different contradictory viewpoints

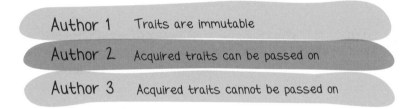

Figure 3. Multiple subtly different viewpoints

The relationships among multiple points of view may be complex and not necessarily clear-cut, and CARS questions love to test your understanding of them. Sometimes you'll even be asked what a supporter of one idea in the passage might think about another idea in the passage. Identifying viewpoints within a passage is vital here, and the process starts with recognizing opinion statements, as we discussed earlier. Often such arguments will introduce more nuance than simply black-and-white, "good versus bad" type debates. Likewise, the differences between two dissimilar viewpoints may be subtle. For example, one might argue not that "capitalism is good," but rather that "capitalism can be good when regulated appropriately," and the difference between the two competing viewpoints might be over what level and types of regulation would be appropriate.

Sometimes differing viewpoints will be blindingly obvious. The author may be describing the debate between two theories, positions, or scientists, with each discussed in separate paragraphs. At other times, it's less clear. For example, the author might cite multiple individuals who have views that are identical, complete opposites, or somewhere in the middle, and it's these subtle differences that tend to be highly testable on the CARS section. A *temporal* contrast might also be made between perspectives held at different points in time, such as how today's society views capitalism versus how capitalism was viewed 100 years ago. Furthermore, the proponents of a particular viewpoint might not be explicitly stated. In some cases, the author will identify the names of particular economic theorists or distinguish between capitalists versus socialists, but at other times, the author may refer to a more widely-held view with language like, "some believe," "it is thought that," or "a common belief is that," none of which indicate whether the author agrees with the view in question. Although more often than not in these cases, the author is preparing to either counter or refine that commonly-held view, but we should never assume this is the case with a given passage. The only way to know whether the author agrees is to look for the author's own assertions.

As we touched on earlier, two viewpoints in a CARS passage might be in direct opposition to one another, or they might be compatible and in agreement with each other, or somewhere in between. For example, two economists might be cited as being in support of capitalism but for different reasons. These two economists might support the same position, but the author might cite each with a different purpose in mind. If the author quotes one or more individuals, we have to decide on a case-by-case basis whether or not they agree with each other or with the passage thesis. The latter point (whether a given viewpoint is consistent with the author's) is particularly important. Does the author simply present others' viewpoints objectively? Does the author disagree or agree with certain perspectives, or do they try to find common ground? Is someone's perspective given as evidence in support of the author's thesis? It's important to distinguish the author's position from others' beliefs in the passage. To get that coveted top score, you need to identify the precise relationships between these views and really get at why the author chose to include each viewpoint.

For these reasons, it's critical to recognize **shifts in ideas**. For example, is the author comparing two different things? What language does the author use when shifting from one idea to another? If the language is negative when shifting to a second idea, the author probably disagrees with it. If it's positive, the opposite is likely true. The highlighter tool can be very helpful for keeping track of these differing viewpoints, especially when you're just starting out.

Transition words can tell you a lot about how an author shifts from one viewpoint to another. Contrasting transition words, like "however," "but," "in contrast," "on the contrary," "on the other hand," "nevertheless," or "despite," are good indicators that a differing viewpoint is being introduced. The words "likewise," "similarly," or "in the same manner" might be used to make a comparison between similar positions or pieces of support that reinforce the same position. If the author wants to expand on a given position with support, he or she might use words such as "furthermore," "also," "besides," or ordinal words like "first," "next," or "finally." An example in support of a position might begin with phrases like, "to illustrate," "to demonstrate," "specifically," "for instance," or "for example." The author might clarify a position by using phrases like, "that is to say," "in other words," "to clarify," or "to put it another way." You might also see words that highlight cause-and-effect relationships, which might be "because," "so," "consequently," "therefore," "thus," or "for this reason." Recognizing these words isn't a foolproof guarantee of an author's reasoning, but they can certainly be used to map out the various viewpoints and elements of support used within a passage. These transitions are important for understanding a passage and for correctly answering CARS questions, which frequently ask about the beliefs within the passage, the relationships between views, and the examples used to support each position.

5. Multiple Points of View in Practice

Keeping in mind that our job on the MCAT isn't to determine which position is "more right" or "more wrong" but rather to identify and analyze those positions, let's examine a CARS passage that discusses several positions on the topic of brain death in medicine:

Recent advances in science and medicine, including ventilator breathing and tube feeding, can maintain a body in the absence of conscious brain activity indefinitely. This raises the question: when does death truly occur? Many groups use the neurological standard of brain death: total brain failure (TBF) is identified in comatose, ventilator-dependent patients with no capacity to spontaneously breathe or otherwise exhibit signs of life. There are two popular positions regarding the neurological standard of death. Position One rejects brain death as a valid indication of true "death" of a patient, while Position Two accepts this standard as valid.

There is a third position which distinguishes the death of the "organism" from the death of the "person." Philosopher John Lizza states that life-supporting technology has interfered with the process by which death creates a corpse. He states that the person's remains "take the form of an artificially sustained, living organism devoid of the capacity for consciousness." However, due to the ethical difficulty of distinguishing the loss of personhood versus a "consciousness-compromising" condition, in which a patient can move, wake up, and groan when in pain, it is preferable to focus on the first two positions.

To those who support Position One, death can be hidden with a ventilator once a patient loses brain function and spontaneous breath. Loss of breath, once an indication of death, is now obscured by a ventilator. There is no reliable "second window" to evaluate for the death of a comatose, ventilator-dependent patient. In 1974, the Harvard Committee declared that an "irreversible coma" should be synonymous with death. Hans Jonas dissented, stating that the border between life and death is unclear. He cites "sufficient grounds" to suspect this artificially supported state may still be one of life. Jonas poses, "the only course … is to lean over backward toward the side of possible life."

Further, a 1998 article by Shewmon in *Neurology* notes that age, etiology, and somatic integrity of a person's body determines survival past brain death. He argues that integrated bodily functions persist after brain death, including wound healing, waste elimination, and regulation of body temperature. Shewmon studied hundreds of brain-dead patients surviving past one week's time. However, critics of the study cited faulty data, inappropriate TBF diagnoses, and the rarity of cases with survival past brain death. In fact, the majority of patients enter asystole, or "flat-line," shortly after brain function ceases.

Position Two retorts that TBF is indicative of death as it ceases organismic work, the drive of an organism to work as a whole to interact with its environment. Work is defined as an organism's receptivity to stimuli and environmental signals, ability to act to selectively obtain what it needs, and the basic felt need of the organism to act as it must to stay alive. Although individual tissues, cells, and organ systems can persist long after brain functioning ceases, the organism loses its openness to the surrounding world with TBF. From this viewpoint, Position Two poses that clinical judgment may be used to declare death due to an absence of the work of the organism to interact with the outside world, a characteristic that defines all living things.

Adapted from The President's Council on Bioethics (2009). Chapter Four: The Philosophical Debate. Controversies in the Determination of Death. Washington, DC: The President's Council on Bioethics under CC BY.

The initial paragraph gives us some background science information, then poses a critical question: when does death actually occur? This is followed by several positions, which are highlighted quite explicitly. Everything in this paragraph points back to that central question of when death occurs. It's easy to imagine how this could be a contentious topic. Now let's dissect this paragraph for opinions. The author says that "many groups use...total brain failure" to define death. The author refers vaguely to "many groups," which doesn't tell us much about who these groups are, let alone what the author thinks about this definition of death. All we know for certain is that this is a common definition, as it's a "standard" adopted by "many groups." More interestingly, we're told that there are two "popular" opinions on this: one that doesn't think that brain death defines death and one that does. Note the subordinating conjunction "while" in that paragraph's last sentence establishes a contrast between these positions. Again, the author hasn't revealed his or her views on this issue, either by asserting his or her stance or by using positive or negative value words to describe these positions.

From this paragraph alone, we get a pretty good map of the passage ahead of us. This passage is going to flesh out the two positions (yes or no) on whether brain death should be used to define death. It's clear what's coming next — most likely a discussion of Positions One and Two, and at some point, the author may share their own perspective. At other times, however, the direction in which the passage is headed might be hard to predict. In this case, we're thrown for a loop because paragraph two introduces a third position, which says that an "organism" dying is not the same thing as the death of one's "personhood." This position is supported by a philosopher, John Lizza, who says a person's remains may linger long after that person has lost the capacity for consciousness and thus the body may still be around long after the "person" has passed. Therefore, we can distinguish between these two "deaths" as two separate things.

What does the author think about this? So far the author has avoided using value words, tending to stick with the objective stance of an observer. That is, until the last sentence of paragraph two. Here the author pivots with the contrast word "however," explaining why the author is choosing not to focus on this position for the passage. The author states the "ethical difficulty" of identifying when one truly has lost personhood versus when one's consciousness has just been "compromised." In other words, who is to say when a ventilator-dependent, comatose individual has truly lost "personhood"? Now we have an author opinion to work with! Isn't it interesting that the author chose to put "consciousness-compromising" in quotation marks? What this suggests is that Lizza meant something specific by a "consciousness-compromising condition," and the author wanted to retain that original meaning. So, the author doesn't say that this position is fundamentally flawed, or that this view is unimportant, or that John Lizza is completely wrong (although the author doesn't deny this either). All we know is that the author wants to avoid this ethical quandary, so we move onto Positions One and Two.

Paragraphs three and four return to Position One, which posits that brain death does not define true death. The initial phrase "to those who support position one" is kind of like a "to whom it may concern" address, introducing a counterpoint to Position One. However, we transition half-way through paragraph three to those supporting Position One, who "dissent" or disagree with this argument. Hans Jonas tends to err on the conservative side of the life versus death debate, preferring to assume one is alive when in the gray middle area.

Shewmon also agrees with Position One, arguing that one can technically "survive" and perform biological functions after brain death. The rest of this text here is all largely used in support of that one idea. But then the author transitions yet again! Fortunately, the contrast word "however" and the mention of "critics" signal this shift. These critics disagree sharply with Shewmon's work and, by extension, the premise of his argument. According to these critics, Shewmon had bad data, bad diagnoses, and few examples, and in fact, most patients don't really survive after brain death. So we're given a ton of useful information in paragraphs three and four, but it's important to distinguish between opposing perspectives (in this case, those that support Position One and those that do not).

Let's turn to the last paragraph to learn more about Position Two, according to which brain death is an indication of true death. This is best captured by the third sentence of this paragraph, which states that the loss of bodily functions may occur long after brain death and the loss of one's drive to interact with the world. Verbs like "retort," just like "dissent," indicate a contrast. On the MCAT, you should immediately notice transition or contrast words, but don't necessarily highlight them. Instead, highlight the terms that capture the general main ideas of each paragraph, like that this paragraph focuses on Position Two, which posits that "death" ought to be defined as an "absence of the work of the organism to interact with the outside world."

To recap, let's look at the big-picture structure before we dive into the individual layers. The passage opens with a question (when does death really occur?) and continues to discuss two positions on the issue. Then we take a quick detour in which the author explains why we should ignore a third position for the sake of the argument. Our goal here is to get a sense of the overall structure of the passage so we can better understand the relationships between these viewpoints. In paragraphs three and four, the author outlines the support for Position One, bookended by some critiques of this view, and finally, the author concludes with Position Two. We frequently saw transition or contrast words indicating a shift from one viewpoint to another, and we even encountered more than one person in support of the same position. Note that, in most cases, value statements were attributed to others, like "critics" or to a specific individual, rather than to the author. Thus, the author seemed to strive for a more objective stance. Only rarely did the author make his or her opinion clear, like when explaining that position three was excluded due to an "ethical difficulty."

6. Interpreting Opinions Through Question Practice

The best way to become skilled at differentiating between viewpoints in a CARS passage is to practice, especially through questions. Let's analyze some opinion-related questions drawing on the passage about brain death that we worked through in the previous section. Consider the question below:

A supporter of Position Two would most likely argue that an individual with a "consciousness-compromising condition" should be considered:

A. alive, as the patient is able to spontaneously interact with the environment.

B. alive, as a patient's whole-organism integrated functions remain intact.

C. dead, as treatment of a patient in this state causes an undue burden to the patient and family.

D. dead, as the patient is not able to spontaneously interact with the environment.

Note the patterns among the answer choices: we have to decide if a supporter of Position Two would perceive such an individual as alive or dead while also making sure our answer is paired with the proper rationale for that belief. In questions like these, it might be tempting to always evaluate the first part of the answer choices first (here, whether such an individual would be considered alive or dead) so we can eliminate two choices right off the bat. However, we shouldn't limit ourselves to that approach. In this case, we may want to move on to the second part of the answer choices because it's difficult to tell whether "alive" or "dead" should be in our answer. Let's refresh our memory on this issue and try to make a prediction. Position Two states that brain death is a decent indicator of true death. If we return to the final paragraph, we're reminded that a supporter of this position says that "work," or the drive to spontaneously interact with one's environment, is an indication of life.

This phrase, "consciousness-compromising condition," was unique enough that the author chose to put it in quotes. This refers back to Position Three, where such a condition is described as one "in which a patient can move, wake up, and groan." Does this kind of activity (moving, waking up, groaning) count as "work"? Since paragraph five defines "work" as "receptivity to stimuli and environmental signals," then someone in support of Position Two would likely believe that someone who can move and groan in response to pain is in fact reacting to the environmental stimulus of pain, and thus is capable of work. So, by this definition, this person must be alive. We can eliminate choices C and D, and now look for the explanation that best matches our prediction. Choice A explains that the patient is alive because this individual can spontaneously interact with the environment, which is exactly the definition that a supporter of Position Two would be looking for. Choice B says this patient is alive because the "whole-organism integrated functions" are intact. "Integrated functions" were presented as a component of Position One, so this is a poor and somewhat irrelevant explanation. Thus, choice A is the best answer. To summarize, we answered this question by first returning to the passage to remind ourselves what criteria Position Two looks for as signs of life. Then we returned to the definition of a "consciousness-compromising condition" to see if it met these criteria. We were also able to avoid trap answers like choice B by keeping these different viewpoints separate, as tempting as the answer choice sounds on the surface.

Let's consider another question about passage viewpoints:

The passage suggests that the author would most likely:

A. disagree with John Lizza's assertion that total brain failure involves the death of the person and the organism.

B. agree that the idea of "personhood" is not easily defined in patients with consciousness-compromising conditions.

C. assume that patients with TBF are living, based upon a lack of a "second window" to death.

D. assume that patients with TBF are deceased, based upon a lack of ability to interact with the environment.

This question could go a number of different ways, making it difficult to make a prediction. In this case, we should review each answer choice. Turning to choice A, would the author "disagree with Lizza's assertion that total brain failure involves the death of the person and the organism"? Recall that the difference between the death of the person and the death of the organism is a key distinction made by Position Three. The answer choice also mentions John Lizza, who is the supporter of Position Three. What did the author have to say about Position Three? The author simply says that there's an "ethical difficulty" associated with determining where the line falls between a "consciousness-compromising condition" and the loss of personhood, but the author makes no judgment on whether this position is right or wrong. This answer choice is incorrect not because the author actually agrees with Lizza, but simply because the author didn't really make any judgment either way.

Turning to choice B, let's consider what the author thinks about the idea of "personhood" being difficult to define in those with consciousness-compromising conditions. We just discussed the "ethical difficulty" associated with making this distinction between loss of personhood and consciousness-compromising conditions. In fact, this is one of the rare circumstances in which the author does show his or her cards and takes a position on an issue. Based on this, we can conclude the author would agree that it's hard to define personhood in those with such conditions, so choice B is looking promising.

Let's check out choices C and D to be thorough. Choice C says the author would agree that patients with total brain failure are living, whereas choice D says the author would agree that such patients are deceased. Recall that this is the exact contrast made between Positions One and Two, which hold that brain death is not, or is, indicative of true death, respectively. Where does the author stand in this debate? We have no idea. The author tries to present these positions in an objective fashion, so we can't say whether the author is inclined to agree with either position. So choice B remains our best answer choice.

Note how helpful it was for us to translate choices C and D into the ideas that they represent: choice C is really asking whether the author supports Position One, and choice D is really asking whether the author supports Position Two. In fact, we did the same with choice A, which asks what the author thinks about Position Three. While the author didn't exactly take a firm stance on any of these positions, the only time the author's perspective was revealed was when the author discussed the "ethical difficulty" of drawing a line between loss of personhood and consciousness-compromising conditions. Highlighting this portion of the passage to draw attention to this sole section where the author expressed a personal opinion could have helped you make a beeline for answer choice B, the correct answer. As always, reading critically as you go helps save you time and rack up points in the long run.

Here's one more question that draws on multiple viewpoints from the passage:

If the passage information is accurate, it can most reasonably be concluded that:

A. the Harvard Committee strongly favors Position One.

B. the debate regarding the standard of death has persisted since ancient times.

C. total loss of consciousness, cessation of spontaneous breathing, and TBF indicate death.

D. some of the patients in Shewmon's 1998 article did not follow the expected biological course following brain death.

Again, it's going to be nearly impossible to make a prediction here without first evaluating the answer choices one-by-one. For choice A, we have to determine the relationship between two parties, or two viewpoints expressed in the passage. What do we know about the Harvard Committee? Hopefully we either highlighted it, or it jumps out at us from paragraph three. This committee believes, in contradiction to Position One, that an "irreversible coma should be synonymous with death." Recall that this paragraph began with the opposing stance, to which Hans Jonas, a supporter of Position One, dissented. By simply mapping the Harvard Committee to the paragraph in which Position One was discussed, we're at risk of making the assumption that these two are in agreement when in fact they're not. Since we read carefully, though, we can eliminate choice A.

Choice B states that the debate surrounding the standard of death has been around for ages. For this choice to be correct, we would need to find confirmatory evidence. If the passage were to discuss this topic, it'd likely be found in the introductory paragraph with the other background information about this debate. Paragraph one tells us that "recent advances in science and medicine" have "raised this question," which is in direct opposition to this answer choice. Goodbye, choice B!

Choice C states that loss of consciousness, cessation of spontaneous breathing, and total brain failure indicate death. Does the passage weigh in on this? Well, a supporter of Position Two would likely agree with the idea that brain death is an indication of true death. However, supporters of Position One would clearly disagree. But what are we as readers led to conclude by the author? We're free to make our own conclusion, actually. The author doesn't lead us toward one position or the other as the more "reasonable" conclusion. Thus, the assertion in choice C cannot be reasonably concluded based on the passage. We want to be wary of such extreme answer choices when the passage doesn't clearly warrant, it especially since a supporter of Position One could argue that this is not a reasonable conclusion.

Finally, choice D refers to the patients in Shewmon's article, stating that some of them did not follow the expected biological course after brain death. Remember, we're looking for a reasonable conclusion based on the literal text of the passage. Paragraph four tells us these patients experienced brain death but continued to "survive" in terms of basic biological functions, according to Shewmon, for at least another week. However, paragraph four also says that critics argued it's actually quite rare for patients to "survive" past brain death. Thus, piecing this information together, it is reasonable to conclude, if we are to believe these critics, that these patients were a bit of a medical anomaly. Therefore, choice D is the best answer choice. It's also worth noting that choice D is quite moderate. It only says that "some" of the patients in Shewmon's article did not follow the expected biological course, but not that this was true of all patients.

As you practice, make note of the various ways in which CARS questions will test different viewpoints and the relationships between them. It's just as important to keep each viewpoint straight as it is to decipher how a supporter of one position would react to another position. It's also vital to avoid making any assumptions about the author's beliefs. Instead, critically examine the evidence: when are subjective value judgments made, and when does the author speak objectively and reserve judgment? The more easily you begin to recognize such patterns in passages, the better equipped you'll be to answer their questions.

7. Relationships Between Ideas

So far, we've been discussing the viewpoints of specific people, or schools of thought, but we can broaden our analysis to include ideas in general. In fact, if we were to completely dissect a CARS passage, we could fragment it into a collection of ideas. There's of course the singular "**big picture idea**," but there's also the **main idea** of each paragraph, and then each individual sentence and even phrase expresses its own unique idea. These ideas build upon each other in sequence, refining previous ideas with more detail and nuance. They also complement each other through similarities and contrasts. It's the relationships between these ideas that bind a passage together into a cohesive unit, and the author signals those relationships by using transition words and value words. Believe it or not, in a CARS passage, no word or sentence is wasted. Even though it might not always seem obvious, every part of a passage tells us something new. We need to track this sequence of related ideas in order to make sense of the passage as a whole.

We already do much of this in our everyday writing and speaking. We automatically know that the word "similarly" is used to indicate a comparison and the word "but" indicates a contrast without having to refer to a list of rules for English syntax. To succeed in CARS, we need to pay closer attention to aspects of word choice that we might otherwise skim over. This forces us to consciously recognize the function of important words like "similarly" and "but," and it also requires us to tap into more advanced critical reasoning skills that help us dissect assumptions, inferences, and complex relationships between ideas.

Among the most common relationships we encounter are comparisons and contrasts. "Comparison" is a very general term that can encompass a range of degrees of similarity. **Comparisons** can be simple, complex, or somewhere in between. On the simple side, a comparison can involve an author directly stating that two examples are similar. This can be done without using the word "similar," though. For example, if an author is arguing that nutritional labels should be more transparent to consumers, she might support this by citing surveys that show that most American consumers read nutrition labels before buying new products but often feel misled by nutrition labels that vastly underestimate the typical serving size. The author might then strengthen the point by saying something like "…much like how Americans report that they often look at movie ratings but don't actually understand what makes a movie R versus PG-13." Here, the phrase "much like" indicates a similarity between these two examples, which is that consumers consult a source of information without clearly understanding it. More complex comparisons arise when the author indicates, explicitly or implicitly, how two ideas compare to one another. The author might explicitly state that detailed nutrition labels are *better* or *more* informative or cause *less* confusion than do nutritional labels without as much detail. More subtly, the author might use words that indicate opinion or attitude that suggest a comparison. For example, suppose a passage states that "The decision to include a breakdown by fat type on nutritional labels gives consumers the autonomy to make informed decisions about their nutritional intake." Here, even in the absence of comparative adjectives or adverbs, the author uses language that conveys a positive attitude toward nutrition labels that include a fat breakdown. Specifically, we might point to "autonomy," which is generally considered a good thing, and "informed decisions," which is another positively-worded phrase. If a question asked about nutrition labels without such breakdowns, even if those labels weren't explicitly mentioned within the passage, we could easily draw the comparison that the author thinks nutrition labels without a fat breakdown would be worse because the consumer would have less autonomy.

Be on the lookout for other words that may introduce similarities, like "also," "too," "plus," "like," and "furthermore," although some of these words can be a little bit tricky. They can either mean that the author is just adding some extra information or that the author is pointing out a similarity. For instance, if we were to say, "Oh, you think John's a good singer? Well, don't forget, Sarah's also a good singer," then "also" points out a similarity between Sarah and John. But if we say, "John's definitely a good singer, but we should also remember that we need someone who's a good performer on stage," then "also" is indicating that there's something extra for us to think about. It's also important to be aware of comparison words that indicate specific relationships. For example, comparative adjectives that compare two ideas will use words like "more," "less," "better," "worse," or adjectives that end in "-er." Superlative adjectives that compare three or more ideas will use words like "most," "least," "best," "worst," and adjectives that end in "-est."

Whereas "comparisons" is a very broad category, **contrasts** emphasize the differences between two related ideas. You'll easily recognize contrasts from words like "in contrast," "conversely," "on the other hand," "unlike," and "however." Sometimes contrast words are not as obvious, such as "although," "while," "even though," "nonetheless," "still," "otherwise," "unless," and others. For example, the author might discuss the advantages and disadvantages of two systems for reporting sugars on nutrition labels, where *on one hand*, the first system has Pros A, B, and C, but *on the other hand*, the second system has Pros X, Y, and Z. The author might also contrast the merits of one of these systems with its own flaws. The first system might have Pros A, B, and C; *however*, it might have Cons D, E, and F.

Contrasts may also be much more subtle or discreet, like if the passage were to state: "Until the FDA issues clear guidelines on the recommended daily sugar intake, consumers are unlikely to reduce sugar consumption." In this example, a contrast can be made between sugar consumption habits *before* the FDA issues sugar intake guidelines, and the reduction in sugar consumption that might occur *after* the FDA issues such guidelines. When two things are contrasted in CARS passages, the difference between them is typically made clear and they're often crucial to understanding the larger argument being made. Note that contrasts can signal a wide range of differences, from slight disparities in the perspectives of two people to stark opposition and absolute, black-and-white contrasts. On a final note, when the words "former" and "latter" are used to refer back to two separate ideas, be sure not to confuse the ideas being referenced. "Former" is always for the one that comes *first*, and "latter" is like "last," except it's the idea that was mentioned *second*.

	Comparisons	Contrasts
Emphasis	Similarity	Difference
Signals	also, too, plus, similarly, much like, more, less, superlatives	in contrast, conversely, on the other hand, unlike, however, although, while, nonetheless, still, otherwise, nonetheless, unless
Example	Pre-med students devote much time to their studies, like their medical student counterparts.	Unlike law school, medical school is four years.
	The pre-med student also enjoyed her cell biology class, in addition to her molecular biology class.	In contrast to general chemistry, organic chemistry takes a different perspective on chemical reactions.

Figure 4. Comparisons and contrasts

Sometimes comparisons and contrasts are made between two ideas that are related temporally or sequentially. To put it simply, these comparisons are time-based; maybe one idea came first and the other is more modern. This is particularly true of passages that trace the evolution of thought on a given topic over time. For example, the author might compare how things were before and after an event or how dietary habits have changed between then and now. A word like "initially" might be used to preface a description of how things used to be. But, this word can also foreshadow that things have changed since then, so you'll want to pay close attention for words in the following sentences that indicate change. The word "historically" often has a similar effect, at times implying that things used to be different in the past, but this word might also be used to justify how a particular tradition persevered and why things are the way that they are now. An example of the former would be to say, "historically, food products did not have nutrition labels," and likely this would be followed with a contrasting statement that this is no longer true today. On the other hand, an author could say something like, "historically, the calorie has been the unit used to measure energy in food." In this latter example, the author may be explaining why we still use the calorie as our unit of energy to this day. CARS passages will always be written in a way that allows you to figure out what you need to know just from the text itself.

Sometimes what's more important than how things have changed is why they've changed. If historically, food products did not have nutrition labels, then what event or person or catalyst sparked the decision to add nutrition labels to food products? Think about this from the perspective of someone passionate enough about nutrition labels to write an entire passage on them. Such a person will likely be concerned with the reasons why food products do or don't, or should or shouldn't, have nutrition labels. Likewise, think about this from the perspective of the author's readers. Suppose the author simply stated, "well, food products used to be labeless, but not anymore!" Wouldn't you have lingering questions about who decided to change this and why?

Explanations concerning the why of a phenomenon often involve statements about causation. **Causation** has a "before" state, an "after" state, and some kind of catalyst or cause in the middle. We often like to treat the "before" state as the baseline and focus on the cause and effect parts. What this means is that some stimulus directly caused and is responsible for some outcome, which can be difficult to prove. However, our job as CARS analysts isn't to prove causation ourselves. Instead, it's to identify causal relationships proposed, endorsed, or rejected by the passage author. Be on the lookout for keywords like "because of," "since," "due to," "attributed to," "cause" or "caused by," "as a result," "consequently," "thus," and "therefore." Watch for causal verbs like "stimulated," "prompted," and "induced" as well. Make sure not to confuse the cause with the effect, which you can avoid by taking a complicated statement of causation and rephrasing it as "X caused Y." For example, a passage might state: "Since new regulations went into effect, food products were required to have nutrition labels." We could reframe this as "New regulations *caused* food products to have to have nutrition labels." In particular, keep your eyes peeled for words like "consequently," "thus," and "therefore" that typically precede an effect, and always go back to the prior sentence if the cause-and-effect relationship is unclear.

8. Cause-and-Effect Relationships

Causality is a topic worth exploring separately from comparisons and contrasts for two reasons. First of all, passages will directly describe causal events, and CARS questions will ask about them. Second, authors' arguments and assertions are often based on cause-and-effect relationships, many of which are indicated by subtle words like "consequently" or "induced," as we discussed above. Sometimes the author might not even use a specific word to indicate a cause-and-effect relationship, meaning that we have to infer it from the context alone.

This sounds highly abstract, so let's use a concrete example. Imagine that an author argues that a certain law should be passed because it will be "good for the economy." This idea reflects a putative cause-and-effect relationship because being "good for the economy" means that the law itself will *cause* certain changes that will have the *effect* of economic improvement. The evidence for an argument might contain cause-and-effect relationships too. For instance, the author might say that similar laws were passed in another country and had good effects. Therefore, we need to be on the lookout whenever an author presents evidence for a certain conclusion because testable cause-and-effect relationships may be lurking. Of course, not all arguments necessarily work this way, but it's more common than you might think.

Thus, questions can directly test cause-and-effect relationships by asking you to do things like predict the outcomes of hypothetical events. Even more frequently, questions can ask about assumptions, inferences, alternative explanations, or what evidence would strengthen or weaken a given conclusion. To do well on this variety of questions, you need to understand the cause-and-effect relationships presented in the passage. Some of these questions, especially those that ask you to assess whether new pieces of information strengthen or weaken certain relationships, can be quite tough. In order to tackle them, we'll look at several specific ways in which new information can affect a stated relationship.

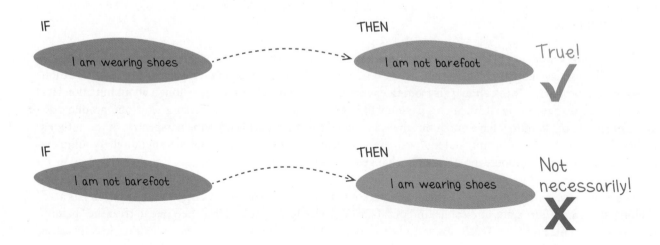

Figure 5. Testing relationships

Correctly identifying the cause and the effect is the first step in thinking about causality. If we don't get this right at the beginning of our thought process, trouble awaits. Mistakenly reversing the cause and effect can cause problems for comprehending the passage, and even worse, this misunderstanding will likely be reflected in CARS wrong answer choices. It's common for questions on this topic to include at least one option that reverses the direction of causal relationships, so we need to be careful.

The CARS section likes to test the directionality of causal relationships, particularly with respect to assumptions and premises that lead to certain conclusions. An example of a related causal error might be if you're asked for the logical conclusion of some premise X, but instead you select an assumption underlying this premise. By mapping out these relationships, either in your head or with a rough flow diagram, you'll be better able to avoid selecting a cause or premise when asked for an effect or conclusion, and vice versa.

So let's say that X causes Y. At this point, we actually need to get even more specific from a logical point of view. First, X by itself is "sufficient" for Y to occur. In short, if X occurs, it will cause Y to occur, or "if X, then Y." Let's make this discussion less abstract and more appealing to our taste buds, and use the example statement that *if* you eat an entire pizza, *then* you're going to feel full. Here, eating pizza is the cause and feeling full is the effect. So, in this case, eating an entire pizza is sufficient for you to feel full. Now, the second thing we can say is that condition Y is "necessary" for condition X to be true. A helpful way to think of this is that if condition Y is not true, it's impossible for condition X to be true. So if you're not stuffed, there's no way you've just consumed an entire pizza. We can express this as "if *not* Y, then *not* X." Technically, this is known as the contrapositive but the meaning behind the term is more important than the term itself. Basically, if you have a cause, then the effect must occur. If you have an effect, you might have the cause, or some other cause might be at play. But if you *don't* have an effect, you *can't* have the cause.

We have to be really careful here. The relationship, "if X, then Y" cannot necessarily be reversed to say "if Y, then X" (which is technically known as the converse of the original statement). For our example, the converse would be saying that if you feel stuffed, you must have just eaten an entire pizza. But that's not right, because you might have eaten something else. Similarly, we can't use the relationship "if X, then Y" as grounds for the conclusion "if not X, then not Y" (which is referred to as the inverse of the statement). This would be like saying that if you don't eat a whole pizza, you won't feel stuffed, which is wrong for the same reason we already identified: there are many other tasty ways to stuff yourself, so *not* eating pizza doesn't guarantee *not* being stuffed. As a side note, we mentioned the technical terms "contrapositive," "converse," and "inverse" just in case it rings a bell from previous studying you've done, but the MCAT will never ask you to use those terms directly. However, you will have to be very careful about the conclusions you can draw from a relationship.

The example we used with pizza is easy. Everyone knows that there's more than one way to be gluttonous. However, it can be harder to pick up on these relationships when they're embedded in a dense CARS passage. For instance, let's consider a policy change that has been made in some states to require chain restaurants to show information about how many calories are in every item. Someone in favor of that policy might say something like "if consumers see how many calories they're consuming, they won't eat as much fast food." Okay, reasonable enough. Now, let's imagine that fast food sales drop. Is that evidence that this policy succeeded? Not necessarily. Remember how we said that "if X, then Y" does not guarantee "if Y, then X"? The same reasoning applies. There might be any number of reasons why people stopped eating as much fast food.

Another thing to note about that example involving calorie labels is that we're starting to move into the domain of real-world arguments that people actually make. Let's take this a step further and embed the idea that calorie labels reduce fast food consumption into an explicit argument, which is "if calorie labels reduce fast food consumption, then chain restaurants should be required to post that information." The word "should" here is a tip-off that we're likely dealing with a strongly-worded argument. We can work through our same chain of logical reasoning, labeling the first part of that assertion as X and the second part as Y. So now we should be familiar with the idea that "if X, then Y" does not allow us to conclude "if Y, then X." In this case, that means that it would be incorrect to say that someone who agrees that chain restaurants should be required to post calorie information must agree that calorie labels reduce fast food consumption. We can think of other reasons to support requiring those labels. Someone could believe that consumers should have access to that information regardless of whether it changes their behavior, or maybe someone just thinks that all those numbers look nice on the menu. We also can't conclude "if not X, then not Y." Although we have to be careful to avoid getting confused by all the "not"'s, that would mean saying that someone who believes our original assertion would also believe that if calorie labels don't reduce fast food consumption, then we shouldn't require labeling. That doesn't follow, for much the same reason. There might be other reasons to support, or oppose, labeling.

What if we change one little word in that statement by substituting "because" for "if", and make it say "*because* calorie labels reduce fast food consumption, chain restaurants should be required to post that information"? Essentially, what the word "because" is doing here is changing how we relate to our first statement, which we labeled X. Instead of framing it as a hypothetical, we're now assuming that Y is true. So we can think of the "because" version of this statement as being logically the same as "if X, then Y," just with the extra assumption that X is true. And this, in turn, leads us to an important consideration. Premeds are trained to think empirically, so as we worked through this logic, you might have been thinking: OK, this is all well and good, but is it actually true that calorie labels reduce fast food consumption? That's a valid point, and a passage might present relevant evidence, so your task is to avoid (and identify) errors in causal reasoning based on information given in the passage. For example, a relationship is not necessarily causal just because one event precedes the other or two events occur simultaneously. For that to be the case, we need clear proof that it precipitates or causes the latter event. Statements like "consumers who read nutrition labels tend to have healthy diets" may initially appear to describe causation, but there is no indication of causality or directionality of this relationship. It could be that reading nutrition labels causes people to buy healthier food, but it could also be that eating a healthier diet makes people feel more health-conscious and have the desire to read nutrition labels. Or there very possibly could be a third variable, like a vigorous advertising campaign causing people to both eat healthier and read nutrition labels. This is simply a **correlation**. Do not assume that associations or correlations like these are causal unless stated otherwise.

To reiterate, proposed causal relationships must be evaluated in light of real-world evidence. Some of the most difficult CARS questions ask about information that would strengthen or weaken a given claim (which, we should note, is not necessarily the same as conclusively proving or disproving it since weakening a claim might just mean that an author needs more evidence). The key to answering such questions is to understand the fundamental logic that must be true for that claim to be valid. If we can weaken the underlying premises for a claim, we undermine its validity.

Let's talk about three scenarios that would weaken the claim of a causal relationship between cause X and effect Y. The first scenario is if cause X occurs, but it does not elicit effect Y. Recall that in a causal relationship, X is sufficient to elicit Y, such that if you eat an entire pizza, you will feel full. If it so happens that the effect (feeling full) does not occur after the cause (eating pizza), then the author's claim of causality here is weakened. Of course, there may be more than one effect. Cause X can result in both effect Y and effect Z. For example, if someone feels thirsty after eating an entire pizza, this doesn't necessarily weaken the causal relationship between eating pizza and feeling full, as we know one can feel thirsty and full at the same time.

A second scenario can occur when the author believes not only that cause X results in effect Y but that only cause X can result in effect Y. In other words, effect Y exists *if and only if* cause X holds true. If the author believes there is absolutely no other cause in the world that could ever be responsible for effect Y, then X must always occur when Y does, and this argument would be weakened if Y occurred but X did not. For example, suppose the author believed that the *only* cause of feeling full was eating pizza. If someone felt full but never touched a slice of pizza, the author's claim would be weakened. Of course, this situation only applies when the author explicitly states that there can only be one cause for a particular outcome.

Finally, a claim about causal relationships is weak if the evidence for the cause is flawed. If the author's entire argument is that effect Y relies on cause X and we poke holes in whether X is actually true, this casts doubt on the relationship as applied to a concrete circumstance. For example, one could argue that an individual feels full because that person just ate an entire pizza. If, however, it turns out that that person actually didn't eat the entire pizza but instead shared it with friends, then this relationship wouldn't be supported. For a more CARS-like example, let's work with our earlier argument that calorie labels on fast food menus improve health outcomes by causing consumers to eat less fast food. This argument relies on two premises: first, that calorie labels on menus result in consumers eating less fast food; and second, that eating less fast food results in better health outcomes. Now, if a study showed that calorie labels made no difference in fast food consumption, or if an experiment proved that fast food was in fact as healthy as it is delicious, then the author's argument would be significantly weakened. Diagramming these relationships and identifying how each component is affected individually by new information can be quite helpful for connecting each sub-point to the larger argument at hand.

9. Relationships in a Practice Passage

There's no better way to learn how to analyze relationships between ideas in CARS passages than to go straight to the source itself. Let's take a look at a CARS passage that contains a range of comparisons, contrasts, and cause-and-effect relationships throughout its text:

Community health workers (CHWs) have been widely deployed to expand access to treatment for malaria and other common infectious diseases, to encourage participation in health screening programs, and to promote a variety of pro-health behaviors. These programs are best known in resource-poor countries, but they have also been officially recognized in several states in the US as ways to extend access to care to underserved communities.

CHW programs have shown considerable success in promoting child immunization, improving the diagnosis and treatment of malaria, ensuring adequate treatment for diarrhea in children, and improving adherence with treatment for active pulmonary tuberculosis. These diseases have an impact on mortality that is disproportionate to the relatively low level of interest that they attract, both among the general public as a whole and, to a significant extent, among researchers and funding bodies. This may be because their treatment is relatively well understood, and success at the population level is largely a matter of execution. The positive impacts of CHWs have also been linked to their ability to interact with other community members on an equal footing, in a culturally competent and down-to-earth manner.

However, the effectiveness of CHWs for other conditions is less clear. A recurring theme is that CHW programs encounter difficulties with conditions that require hands-on diagnoses, even in seemingly simple settings such as diagnosing pneumonia based on an elevated respiratory rate. Studies have repeatedly shown that CHW programs require careful training and supervision. This leads to two important points. First, CHWs are not substitutes for investments in strengthening and expanding the scope of nationwide health systems. Treating them as such would both be ineffective, due to the limitations of CHWs' scope of practice, and an abnegation of the responsibility of civil society to extend care to community members living in far-flung, poorer regions. Second, the effectiveness of CHW programs must be considered in terms of trade-offs because the cost of adequately running and supporting CHW programs is non-negligible.

In fact, the cost-effectiveness of CHW programs is very much an open question, although the issue has been investigated by several studies. However, the results are inconclusive, largely because of methodological difficulties. Cost-effectiveness analyses require extensive assumptions about the value of interventions over time. For example, how many deaths are averted by ensuring suitable treatment for childhood diarrhea, and how can the value of those saved lives be quantified? Methodologies do exist for these dilemmas, but the underlying assumptions are certainly subject to question. Some studies have attempted to address these uncertainties by conducting robustness analyses in which the assumed or extrapolated values of key parameters are varied to determine the effect of uncertainty in those parameters on the studies' conclusions, but this practice is unfortunately far from universal.

Furthermore, some ethical concerns have been raised about CHW programs. CHWs are generally either volunteers or minimally compensated, which can be a source of dissatisfaction for them personally, but also suggests the possibility that CHW programs may, paradoxically, reinforce the structural patterns of health inequalities that they are ostensibly designed to address. Another concern relates to CHWs' role in mediating between community members and formal systems of healthcare; as has been noted for medical interpreters, information transfer between medical professionals and patients is not necessarily neutral or entirely objective. These concerns should not be taken as invalidating the contributions of CHW programs, but they certainly deserve more attention from the global public health community.

From this first paragraph, we can already appreciate that this is a social sciences passage with a public health focus. Let's focus on identifying comparisons, contrasts, and cause-and-effect relationships for this passage. This first paragraph introduces the notion of community health workers as agents who advance causes of public health in certain countries and parts of the US. Notice how the contrast word "but" in the last sentence of this paragraph draws a contrast between "resource-poor countries" and the US, suggesting that the US is not a resource-poor country as a whole, even if underserved segments of it may be considered as such. Now, this particular point may or may not be a major focus of the passage, but what this example demonstrates is an underlying assumption implied by this contrast. Without explicitly stating that the US is not a resource-poor country, the author requires us to assume this is true for the rest of this statement to make sense.

In paragraph two, we're told that programs for community health workers have been successful in several areas related to the prevention and treatment of infectious diseases. You might not automatically think of words like "promote" or "improve" as causal verbs, but let's think about why we should treat them this way. First of all, a causal relationship requires directionality from the stimulus to the effect. Words like "promote" and "improve" indicate that some stimulus (in this case, community health workers) has an effect on some outcome (say, child immunization or malaria treatment). Causation requires the stimulus to directly result in that changed outcome, which is exactly what is indicated here: community health workers are themselves responsible for higher immunization rates, or better malaria outcomes. These causal verbs were chosen deliberately by the author to credit community health worker programs with these results. If the author had instead chosen to state that these programs were *linked with* or *associated with* improved measures of public health, this would become a very different statement. We'd no longer have a causal relationship but, instead, a correlation between the two, leaving open the possibility that something else could be causing these improvements.

A causal statement, however, is more assertive, which can be a bit of a double-edged sword. On one hand, it makes clear the causal nature and direction of this relationship. On the other hand, proving causality requires evidence. This means it can be strengthened by supportive findings, but it's also vulnerable to new information that challenges or weakens the relationship. For example, if it were discovered that study findings showing higher immunization rates among children treated by community health workers were based on flawed data collection, or that child immunization rates had been increasing long before such programs were in place, we might predict that such information would damage this stated claim. So when we identify causal statements in CARS passages, we should be primed for questions that ask about information that might strengthen or weaken such claims.

Moving further into this same paragraph, the author introduces a new contrast between the mortality burden of the diseases treated by community health workers and the "relatively low level of interest" in these diseases among the public and among scientists. Based on this contrast, we can assume that diseases like malaria, childhood diarrhea, and tuberculosis have carried a significant death toll, at least more so than you'd expect based on how much attention they receive from the public and from the coffers of funding bodies. This contrast is a very important turning point in this passage for several reasons. For one, this is an opinion. Not all contrasts are opinions, but many of the interesting ones are. What the author is suggesting is either that, in the author's opinion, these diseases really deserve more funding or that there is some underlying explanation for this surprising disparity. Contrasts often create this kind of tension that needs to be resolved. Sometimes they'll pose a problem to be solved or, in this case, some disparity that has yet to be explained. This raises the question: why do diseases that carry such a significant public health burden attract such little interest? The author answers this question in the following sentence: it's possibly because their treatments are well understood, and because succeeding in treating them is more a matter of going out there and doing it, rather than developing effective treatments. Now, since these are the author's beliefs, we might be asked to extrapolate to new contexts and predict what kinds of diseases the author believes would or wouldn't attract research attention. The implication of this pair of statements, of course, is that diseases whose treatments are well understood and whose outcomes depend on execution will attract less attention relative to those whose treatments remain elusive and still need working out in the lab.

The next paragraph starts out by contrasting the effectiveness of community health workers in the treatment of malaria and tuberculosis with their effectiveness in the treatment of "other conditions." First, notice the use of the contrast word "however," especially at the beginning of a new paragraph, and how it signals a transition from one idea to another. Also, notice how this contrast continues to provide a passage roadmap. Now we know that the previous paragraph was setting us up to perhaps be perplexed or at least intrigued by their mixed success in treating other diseases. Knowledge of community health workers' success in certain settings allows us to interpret their lack of success elsewhere in that context. This establishes a problem and a question: why aren't community health workers effective in the treatment of other diseases?

One clue to this is that community health worker programs seem to have trouble with hands-on diagnoses, and the author adds that such programs require "careful training and supervision." Notice here that the causal phrase "leads to" doesn't point so much from a cause to an effect as from evidence leading to a given conclusion. The directionality from evidence to conclusion models the directional relationship between a cause and its effect, which is also significant. Just as we might face questions about information that reinforces or challenges a causal claim, we might also be asked to evaluate the logical steps leading to a particular conclusion and the evidence upon which that argument is built. Therefore, as a result of this evidence, the author concludes two things: (1) that community health workers are not substitutes for a robust healthcare system, and (2) there are tradeoffs in employing such programs in terms of cost-effectiveness. The CARS section is not going to ask you whether you think the evidence the author used for this argument was good. However, you're much more likely to be asked about what kind of information would make the author's argument less sound. For example, we might be able to poke holes in the author's evidence if it were shown that community health worker programs were self-sufficient and required minimal supervision or that for every dollar it cost to train a community health worker, three dollars were saved in the national healthcare budget. Therefore, be on the lookout for causal relationships and evidence used in support of the author's conclusions, as these are ripe pickings for CARS questions.

The next paragraph zeroes in on the issue of cost-effectiveness, which itself poses an inherent contrast between the cost and the perceived value of community health worker programs. The previous paragraph deliberated the trade-offs between the costs of running such programs versus their effectiveness, and this becomes a major unanswered question central to the passage, which the author explores using rhetorical questions. How many deaths are prevented as a direct result of community health worker programs? How do we measure the value of these lives? We don't have to answer these questions, but we do want to know what the author thinks. This paragraph begins by framing this as an open question, and it closes by highlighting the few studies that have started to investigate these questions. However, these questions are largely left unanswered.

And finally, let's see if we can identify any contrasts in the last paragraph. The passage makes this relatively easy by calling this contrast a paradox, specifically referring to the inconsistency between community health worker programs' supposed role in addressing health inequities and their part in perpetuating them. After all this time talking about community health workers' role in improving health outcomes in underserved and resource-poor communities, it turns out that community health workers themselves are paid poorly or not at all! This is again an example of a contrast indicating a strong opinion held by the author. Mortality statistics and community health workers' compensation rates are verifiable, factual pieces of information that we could theoretically look up. However, it's an opinion that the pay of community health workers doesn't match their level of impact and serves to further exacerbate the health disparities they were designed to address. Given that the conclusion is where the author will tend to present closing arguments, we should assign quite a bit of importance to this concern, as well as to the following concern about community health workers' non-neutral role as mediators between communities and systems of healthcare.

Looking back on this passage, the author first presented the concept of community health worker programs and showcased their success in the treatment of a limited number of diseases. But then the author pivoted to question the effectiveness of community health worker programs for other conditions, particularly in light of the training, supervision, and costs required of such programs. All this is followed by a pursuit of certain ethical issues they pose. It's not at all uncommon for a CARS passage to present two opposing or contrasting sides on an issue, but fortunately, we know a lot about the author's stance from the opinions we identified throughout the passage. Furthermore, the passage ends by assuring us that the concerns raised don't invalidate the contributions of community health worker programs, but they're serious enough to be worth looking at.

Let's take a moment to review the takeaways from what we've discussed. First, note how words like "improve" and "promote," among others, often indicate causality, and words like "but" and "however" are commonly used to introduce contrasts. We've also seen how investigating contrasts can reveal underlying assumptions, differing viewpoints, conflicts or problems to be solved, and questions that have yet to be answered, often leaving us a roadmap for where the passage is headed. And finally, actively looking for contrasts and causal statements and studying the relationships between ideas helps us understand main ideas and the fundamental structures of passage arguments more thoroughly. Plus, you're bound to be asked about comparisons, contrasts, and cause-and-effect relationships in the CARS section, so being able to identify them as you read will mean you are even more prepared to answer those questions.

10. Must-Knows

> Facts vs. opinions: facts = verifiable statements rooted in objective reality; opinions = non-verifiable, subjective statements.
> Indicators of opinions:
> - Qualifiers ("may," "might," "probably," etc.).
> - Adjectives ("good," "bad," "beautiful," etc.).
> - Comparisons ("worse/worst," "better," "similar," etc.).
> Questions to ask when you encounter an opinion:
> - Whose opinion is it? The author's? Someone else's?
> - What does this tell me about what the author believes?
> - Why might the author believe this?
> - Is this consistent with the passage as a whole?
> - How does this contribute to the author's agenda and the main arguments of the passage?
> - Based on this, what other ideas might the author support, and what other positions is the author likely to disagree with?
> Personal opinions: beware!
> - Outside knowledge/opinions can seep in around the edges, causing bias.
> - Boredom or negative opinions towards passage/author can impede efficiency.
> Passages often contain multiple viewpoints:
> - Keep careful track of whose opinion is whose.
> - Watch out for shifts in ideas in passages.
> - Be on the lookout for transition words ("however," "but," "in contrast," "nevertheless," etc.).
> Comparisons and contrasts:
> - Similarity-indicating language: "similar," "also," "too," "plus," "like," "furthermore," etc.
> - Comparative adjectives: words like "better," "worse," or ending in "-er"; superlative adjustives (the "most"/"worst"): end in "-est."
> - Contrast-indicating language: "in contrast," "conversely," "on the other hand," "unlike," and "however," "although," "while," "even though," "nonetheless," "still," "otherwise," "unless."
> Causation versus correlation:
> - Causation: two phenomena linked by cause and effect, with a before state, an after state, and a catalyst or cause in the middle.
> - Causation-indicating language: "because of," "since," "due to," "attributed to," "cause" or "caused by," "as a result," "consequently," "thus," and "therefore," also causal verbs like "stimulated," "prompted," and "induced."
> - Logical structure of causality: "if X, then Y" implies "if not Y, then not X." "If X, then not Y" and "if not X, then not Y" are not valid inferences.
> - Correlations: two events just happen to co-occur, without causal relationship.

Applied Practice

The best MCAT practice is realistic, with detailed analytics to help you assess where things went wrong. For those reasons, we recommend completing practice questions in an online setting that simulates the real MCAT interface, and using the analytics provided to help you decide how to best move your studies forward.

CARS does not require knowledge of specific subject areas, but it does require development of strong test-taking skills. To ensure you are honing those skills as you work through this book, we suggest you go online after wrapping up each chapter and generate a Qbank Practice Set of 2-3 CARS passages to practice and review. While not every chapter of this book is directly applicable to CARS, regular CARS practice is key to test day success.

As a further supplement, given the importance of active learning for effective studying, we also suggest that you consult the Must-Knows at the end of each chapter of this Reasoning text as a basis for creating a study sheet. This is not a sheet to memorize in the more traditional sense of content memorization, but rather a quick reference of the most important strategies for you to refer to during and after practice in your early prep. Frequently revisiting the most important strategies for the MCAT - in both CARS and the Sciences - will help you continue to improve your performance.

This page left intentionally blank.

This page left intentionally blank.

Arguments in CARS Passages

1. Arguments in CARS

Every CARS passage was written by a real human being with an agenda. Even in a dry, neutral passage that mostly conveys factual information, there's some message the author is trying share. It's your job to *critically analyze and reason* through the major arguments of the passage. To evaluate an argument, you have to do two things: identify it, and then critically analyze the evidence that supports it.

In contrast to the looser usage that can occur in real-world contexts, the word "**argument**" in context of the MCAT specifically refers to a claim that can be asserted and backed with evidence to persuade others. Arguments that are assertable must be evidence-based judgments, so, there are several types of statements that don't count as arguments in this sense. For one, an established fact is not an assertable argument: you don't need to persuade anyone that the sky is blue or that ocean water is salty. Likewise, even theoretically arguable statements with which pretty much everyone would agree also don't make for good arguments, like that brussel sprouts are good for you. There might have been a debate about this once, but it's been settled. Personal feelings are also not assertable arguments: you don't need to convince anyone that *your* favorite color is blue. No one's going to argue that you feel differently.

Now, wait a minute, you might think: people argue about stuff like their favorite colors all the time. There's a couple different issues at stake here, and this example is helpful for untangling some of them. First off, we need to distinguish between *your feeling* that a particular color looks nice *to you*, which is a purely factual statement about what you feel, versus a hypothetical argument that everyone else must feel that way, too, or that blue is objectively better than other colors. Therefore, feelings and facts aren't arguments in and of themselves, but they can sometimes serve as a starting point to build one or as support for an argument. An "argument" in everyday life about something like this is probably just going to involve people loudly stating their preferences at each other, not anything resembling actual evidence. Thus, the point here is that the kind of arguments we might have in our daily lives don't really carry over to the arguments that we evaluate in CARS. For the MCAT, we have to get serious, and only focus on the kind of arguments where **reasonable disagreement** is possible and one or both sides can be supported by **evidence**. If either of those criteria fails (that is, if reasonable disagreement is impossible, or if there's no real evidence one way or the other), we don't have a viable argument.

CARS passages can be complicated because they generally contain more than a single argument. Of course, the main thesis of a passage is the argument you should be most concerned with, although you'll also want to consider each of its supporting sub-arguments found throughout the text. Just like opinions, arguments may not be as explicit as you might hope, but they're definitely there. This means we must be vigilant for any words that indicate evidence or conclusions throughout the text.

It's important to be able to deconstruct CARS arguments, if for no other reason than you're going to be asked about them on the MCAT. You'll be asked to identify arguments, including the main argument of the passage. You'll also be asked to identify support for arguments within the passage and whether new information weakens or strengthens those arguments. Thus, part of skillfully reading CARS passages is always trying to ascertain what the author's end goal is, what the author wants to prove to you, what assumptions the author wants you to agree with, and how convincing each level of support is.

Let's consider the anatomy of an argument. Typically, the author will state a position and then back it up with evidence. When a position (or conclusion) is asserted and then followed by more specific pieces of evidence leading to that conclusion, it follows a **top-down argument structure**. This is a common structure in CARS passages (and probably your fair share of school essays and term papers), as it's an organized way of presenting a clear thesis before establishing support for it. This support should seem to logically support that the original thesis is true, so in presenting it after the thesis, the author lends credibility to his or her original statement. Alternatively, a **bottom-up argument structure** begins with the evidence, from which patterns emerge and lead to a certain conclusion that becomes the thesis statement. This approach is more common in the humanities, especially literature and art criticism, where the author might want to take you on a journey through various observations about a piece of writing or work of art before arriving at a conclusion. For example, the author might outline two or more viewpoints, observations, or pieces of evidence in the body paragraphs of an essay and only reveal his or her ultimate conclusion in the final paragraph.

A persuasive essay considers its audience and tailors its arguments to its readers, providing the right amount of **support** to be convincing yet also concise. What is considered sufficient evidence for an argument depends on the field. In science, for example, we're often concerned with empirical data and statistics. To demonstrate the harms of driving under the influence, we could conduct a study on the effects of alcohol on motor function, or we could cite statistics about fatalities due to drunk driving. In contrast, a passage with a literature focus may rely on textual evidence, specifically quotes and summaries from the literature in question. A passage about history might point out relevant events, or a passage about philosophy might even use some other author's argumentation as an example of how people have thought about a question of interest. CARS passages can also be about social sciences, including economics and linguistics, and the "science" part of "social sciences" might be reflected by passages that cite relevant studies, much like we'd see in a biomedical research article.

Another form support might take is the expert opinion. A passage on the possibility of head transplants has little credibility without the authoritative voice of an expert neurosurgeon, someone with relevant credentials who can interpret factual information. For example, if an author argues that head transplants are the way of the future and then backs this up with scientific information about the intricate network of nerves and blood vessels that must be severed and rejoined during such a procedure, most of us aren't going to be able to do much with that information without input from an expert in the field. Such a position might be incorporated as a direct quote, a paraphrase, or a summary of the expert's position. We (and the author, for that matter) don't necessarily have to accept the expert's conclusion as our own, but expert opinions help us make sense of information in a place where the factual material is so technical or dense that a non-specialist reader might have trouble assessing the situation. It's worth noting that this can occur in a very wide range of fields. For instance, although history might not be technical in the same way that neurosurgery is, it still might be the case that relatively few people have immersed themselves in a given subject, like the Napoleonic Wars, to the point of really mastering all the information.

An expert opinion is an example of a secondary source. Sources of support can be either primary or secondary. **Primary sources** include research data, original documents, and other first-hand accounts. In contrast, **secondary sources** analyze or interpret primary sources. On one hand, secondary sources can be tremendously valuable, like when an expert opinion helps us make sense of a very particular, detailed subject. In these areas, secondary sources facilitate a deeper understanding of such enormous factual information and let us reach an informed opinion without having to become a master in the field. On the other hand, we do have to keep in mind that secondary sources involve a degree of interpretation. Remember what we went over last chapter: there's no such thing as an author without an opinion, so we have to think about the source's (and the passage author's) perspective and potential bias.

Practically speaking, for CARS, every passage is a secondary source. The CARS section isn't going to give you a historical treaty or a piece of literature and ask you to interpret it directly. But part of being an attentive reader is being aware of when an author is using another secondary source to support an argument versus using primary sources of data. You won't be asked a direct question about identifying primary versus secondary sources on the MCAT (we promise nothing like "which of the following is NOT a primary source?" will pop up in the CARS section). However, being aware of the basic difference between primary and secondary sources is helpful for tracking which assertions an author does back up with evidence, which *is* something you can be asked about.

A skilled debater will not only present a strong argument but will also anticipate and refute potential counterarguments. You can often spot a counterargument's introduction by transition words like "while" or "however." This is a common strategy you'll encounter in CARS passages. A passage may present a thesis supported by the author right off the bat and later present and swiftly defuse counterpoints. Alternatively, a passage may begin with a common belief or position, and then counter with how this position is flawed, before leading into what the author believes. Be aware that we need to interpret the text to understand which position the author supports. For example, if a passage argues that daylight savings should be held year-round, the author might predict the counterargument that one less hour of daylight in the morning makes it unsafe for kids to commute to school in the dark during the winter months. *However*, the author might retort that the transition between daylight savings and standard time actually poses a greater risk to kids' safety. Or perhaps kids could begin school one hour later to better align with the times at which they are most alert, which would provide more support for the author's pro-daylight savings argument. See how much stronger this argument is now? Note how similar this is to what we've discussed elsewhere about watching out for different viewpoints, and carefully distinguishing between them, especially the author's opinions from those the author mentions. Being able to identify arguments well will help you identify different opinions or perspectives more easily, and vice versa.

2. Arguments in Practice

Let's see if we can identify arguments, find their supporting evidence, and determine their functions within a CARS passage. Let's consider a passage about the relationship between health and religion.

A positive relationship exists between functional health and religion, and there has been a proliferation of studies investigating this relationship over the last decades. As an example, a review of faith-based physical activity interventions indicated that significant improvements were observed in indices related to cardiovascular disease. In regard to compliance or participation, faith-based studies have found that pastoral support, which is modeled on the paternal role, was associated with higher rates of follow-up participation for physical activity.

While the results of these studies are intriguing, a number of criticisms have been leveled at them, related to the fact that religion is considered to be a multidimensional or multifaceted phenomenon. Controlling all the independent variables is problematic. It is not clear what mechanisms might underlie the connection between the independent variable, religion, and the dependent variables such as increases in social support, discouragement of certain risk behaviors, and psychological effects related to the performance of rituals. A related problem, however, is that we have not defined religion, other than to provide a laundry list of common components, such as beliefs, feelings, attendance, rituals, feelings, and supernatural beings.

One universal characteristic of religion is the use of kin terms. For example, a priest may be called father while a nun may be addressed as mother or sister. Members of congregations may refer to one another as children of God, and as brothers and sisters to one another. The widespread use of these kin terms in situations that do not involve biological kin seems to have a common effect: it helps create a metaphorical family, the members of which tend to act as kin, preferentially cooperating with and sacrificing for their metaphorical relatives. This particular characteristic of religion is ancient and found around the world in all societies.

In this discussion, we may borrow from Steadman and Palmer, who see religion as a form of communication involving the making and acceptance of supernatural claims, one of which is that all members of the religious group share a supernatural father. While religion may be much more than this, what this definition allows us to do is begin to examine the effects of the claim that all members are metaphorical kin. What Steadman and Palmer argue is that one effect is a growing development of kinship-like cooperation. Religion, they argue, appeared very early in human evolution, a time when humans lived in small groups of kin, practiced traditions that were honed through time, and honored their ancestors, who were said to be the ancestors shared by everyone in the religion. In religions, as in families, brothers and sisters are encouraged to behave altruistically toward one another. Furthermore, the shared metaphorical ancestors (e.g., a supernatural being who is a father or perhaps a mother) are used to provide authority to rules of social behavior and their enforcement. When two individuals identify one another as kin, their social relationship is strengthened.

This discussion suggests that part of the importance of religious involvement may lie not in "unspecified psychosocial influence" but rather in the close, trusting, and enduring social ties—kinship-like relationships—regularly encouraged by religions. Research indicates that not only do religions regularly encourage social ties, but that social ties and the lack of such ties are related to health and its absence.

Adapted from Coe, K., Keller, C., & Walker, J. R. (2015). Religion, Kinship and Health Behaviors of African American Women. Journal of Religion and Health, 54, 46–60 under CC BY.

The author's very first statement posits that there is a "positive relationship" between functional health and religion. This is somewhat of a provocative, or at least unexpected, position since the author's making an arguable claim here, not just reporting an objective fact. It's safe to say that the successive sentences will likely seek to support this thesis.

In fact, within the same breath, the author claims that there have been numerous studies looking into this relationship, which is exactly the kind of evidence we're looking for. For example, one paper showed that faith-based exercise interventions were associated with improved cardiovascular health. Note that a "review" tells us that this paper analyzed a series of related studies rather than presenting the results of a single study, so it reveals broader patterns across the research literature. The next sentence introduces a separate example: that pastoral guidance is associated with more follow-up, suggesting that faith or religion may play a role in improving compliance or participation. Is any of this relevant? Absolutely, since both the review of interventions and pastoral guidance support the opening claim that religion or faith may be related to better functional health outcomes. These are good examples of support because they provide mechanisms by which religion or faith can improve health outcomes: either by directly improving health measures or by resulting in greater compliance with treatment.

Recall that the author seeks to support the idea that there is a "positive relationship" between functional health and religion, which simply means that as one goes up, the other does, too. We have to be careful not to extrapolate too far beyond the text. The author isn't arguing that religion is good or bad or that everyone should join a church to see soaring cardiovascular health. The claim is merely that there appears to be a relationship between religion and health, and the two examples cited in the opening paragraph appear to support this. So we have a good argument, but what do we know about how the author feels about all this? Note the verbs used in this paragraph: "a positive relationship *exists*," "a review...*indicated*," and "faith-based studies have *found*." These are assertions made by the author, without using qualifiers like "might" or "possibly" and without framing them as others' beliefs. So we don't have any reason to believe the author doubts this evidence.

The next paragraph, however, pivots with the transitional phrase, "while the results of these studies are intriguing." This doesn't outright dismiss the previous studies mentioned, but it does suggest that we're about to encounter some counterarguments or conflicting results. In this instance, we're faced with "a number of criticisms" leveled against the purported positive relationship between health and religion. These criticisms have to do with the fact that religion is multidimensional, meaning that if religion is shown to improve health, it's very difficult to determine, and control for, the various specific factors, or independent variables, that may have resulted in better health outcomes. The author lists a few examples of some of the outcomes of religion, including greater social support, reduced risk behaviors, and psychological benefits, highlighting the complex nature of this relationship. Another problem is that religion needs to be better defined so we can more clearly assess the relationship.

Paragraph two opens by stating that others have critiqued the studies showing a relationship between health and religion. However, the examples provided are stated matter-of-factly. "Controlling all independent variables is problematic." "It is not clear what mechanisms might underlie this connection." "A related problem is that we have not defined religion." Thus, it appears that the author does not dismiss these critiques but instead finds them legitimate. Does this mean that the author has gone to the other extreme, and thus we can conclude there's absolutely no relationship between health and religion? Not necessarily. All we know is that the author has conceded some points from the opposing side, so perhaps we need to define religion more precisely or consider one independent variable at a time. So the author began with an argument in paragraph one and now is further refining it and developing nuance in paragraph two. Specifically, the current claim is something akin to, "There may be a relationship between health and religion, but in order to investigate this, we have to dive deeper, sort out the independent variables and agree upon a clear definition for religion."

With this in mind, let's take a look at the next paragraph, which tells us about a "universal characteristic of religion... the use of kin terms." The previous paragraph left us with a problem (the need to define religion) and this paragraph gives us a potential solution (a common element that might be used to define religion). We might ask ourselves, what does the author mean by this? And is this universally true of religion? The author provides a few examples: the use of the term "father" or "mother or sister" for holy persons or "brothers and sisters" for peers of the same faith. The author then argues that this results in a "metaphorical family," creating kinship ties that promote cooperation. Finally, the author states that this kinship has been a component of religions across societies and across time. CARS questions often ask which arguments are or are NOT supported by evidence, so it's good to get into the habit of spotting ones that have an abundance or lack of support.

This last claim of the enduring nature of kinship as a religious component is a good example of the latter. While the use of kinship terms in religious faiths is mentioned, technically the author doesn't show us evidence that proves this has been true across all societies and in ancient times. This isn't a hard-and-fast rule, but on the MCAT, arguments supported by evidence will often be immediately followed by that evidence in the same paragraph, so sentences at the end of a paragraph, like in this case, tend not to be well-supported by evidence. In fact, the paragraph that follows this one focuses on a subtly different point rather than providing direct evidence for the ancient and universal nature of kin terms. Again, it's essential to keep in mind how each argument within the passage relates to the overall thesis. In other words, somehow the idea of this "metaphorical family" we were just talking about must return to the relationship between religion and health and perhaps provide a mechanism by which religion results in improved health outcomes.

Next, the author mentions Steadman and Palmer and their definition of religion as a type of communication that has to do with the supernatural, including a supernatural father as an example of the previous point about kinship terms. Here, the author cites specific persons, possibly scholars or theologians, and we must distinguish between their claims and the author's. The transitional phrase "while religion may be much more than this" tells us that the author views this definition as a bit oversimplified, which ties back to the previous caveat that religion as a whole is too complicated to neatly study its effects on functional health. However, this simplistic definition helps us examine the claim about the use of kinship terms, the effects of such a claim, and the mechanisms by which this may relate to health improvements. For one, Steadman and Palmer suggest that religion encouraged kinship-like cooperation and altruistic behavior early on in human evolution, as supported by evidence from anthropology. Second, a supernatural father provides an authority figure to codify and enforce social behavior. It's one thing to disobey your tribe's leader. It's quite another to disobey your own parent or literal kin. Thus, a belief of kinship to one another through religion promoted cooperation, altruism, and stronger social bonds.

Again, we should ask ourselves, how does this relate to the bigger picture? To make the leap from religion to health improvements, we need some sort of mechanism. The author stated that religion creates a metaphorical family, and then argued that this kinship results in cooperation and stronger social relationships, which may result in more desirable health outcomes. Although the author's position might not seem completely clear when we're hacking our way through the middle of a passage, it usually becomes clear by the conclusion. Here, the author explicitly states that the importance of religion (in relation to religion and health) probably has to do with the kinship-like social relationships fostered within religious communities and, furthermore, that these relationships are closely tied to health.

The structure of this passage is not uncommon among CARS passages: a position is stated, then refined in response to critique. Specifically in this passage, in response to the criticisms leveled against the evidence for the positive relationship between religion and health, the author identifies a problem (that religion needs to be more clearly defined) and then provides a solution by defining religion through its use of kin terms and creation of a metaphorical family. This lays the groundwork for successive paragraphs to discuss how feelings of kinship may account for the health benefits associated with religion. At each step, the author provides some type of support in the form of research results, the opinions of experts like Steadman and Palmer, or examples from anthropology and religion. At the same time, some assertions were not directly supported, so it's up to the reader to evaluate the merit and strength of those statements. More critically, it's important to be able to identify the function of each argument and each example of supporting details within the context of the passage as a whole. Consider how each relates to and supports, or contradicts, the passage thesis. Be sure to identify transitional phrases, which signal when a new argument is introduced, and try to distinguish the author's beliefs from those of others or your own. By doing so, you'll be able to predict where a passage is headed, enabling you to answer any questions about the major arguments of a CARS passage.

3. Argument-Related Questions

There are a number of ways in which questions about arguments might be asked in the CARS section. The first category of questions will ask you to identify **arguments within the passage**. For example, a CARS question might ask you to identify the **main idea** or **main assertion** of a passage. When reading a passage like the one above, you may need to have an understanding of the entire passage to identify the main assertion, which is that religion may be associated with improved health as a result of stronger kinship-like social relationships. You may also be asked to identify individual arguments embedded within the passage. In this case, a question might ask what the author thinks about the criticism that the multidimensional nature of religion makes it difficult to interpret studies that show an association between religion and health outcomes. If you were reading carefully, you'd likely remember that in paragraph two, the author asserts that, as a result of the multidimensionality of religions, controlling all independent variables is "problematic." So it appears that the author agrees at least to some extent with this critique.

Another category of CARS questions is concerned with the **function or purpose of an argument** or the **support for an argument** within a passage. For example, we might be asked about the author's purpose for stating that "members of congregations refer to each other as children of God" or the function of the argument that religion involves a metaphorical family, as shown by the use of kinship terms. By zooming out to the passage as a whole, we can point to the overall goal of the passage, which is to argue for a mechanism by which religion has a positive relationship with functional health. Thus, the purpose of this particular claim about a metaphorical family, and the support for this claim, is intended to establish a mechanism of kinship and social support that could explain this relationship. We might also be asked why the author holds a particular belief or puts forward a particular claim. In these cases, it is usually helpful to go back and look at the text directly for where this belief or claim is mentioned. For example, suppose we were asked what best explains why the author believes the "involvement of religion [for health lies in]... close, trusting, and enduring social ties." We'd want to return to previous paragraphs where the author laid out this case for religion creating feelings of kinship among its members.

MCAT test-writers aren't just interested in your ability to identify arguments and determine why they're there; they want you to be able to dissect them and to examine the support for each argument. For example, a CARS question might ask, which of the following statements from the passage is directly supported by specific evidence in the passage? Or alternatively, it may ask the opposite (which passage statement is NOT directly supported by specific evidence?) In paragraph three, for example, let's examine the first statement, "One universal characteristic of religion is the use of kin terms." This statement is followed by evidence in the form of examples (priests are called 'fathers,' nuns 'mothers' or 'sisters,' and fellow congregates 'brothers and sisters'). On the other hand, the last sentence of paragraph three states, "This particular characteristic of religion is ancient and found around the world in all societies." Here, it's not immediately clear what the pronoun "this" refers to, so we need to glance back in the passage to see what the author mentioned recently as a specific "characteristic" of religion. We find this in the first sentence of the paragraph, which again states that the use of kin terms is a universal characteristic of religion. True or not, this statement is not directly supported by specific evidence of metaphorical families created by religion in all societies and in ancient times.

You could also see an argument question cite an example from the passage and ask what idea it supports. For example, we might be asked why the author describes "traditions honed through time" in paragraph four. This description is part of a larger example in paragraph four of the early development of religion in human groups, describing how those traditions were intrinsically linked to the honoring of ancestors and eventually evolved into what we would consider religious traditions. On a larger scale, this example is used to support the idea of metaphorical ancestors and kinship felt within a religion.

Finally, a common strategy employed by CARS questions is to ask you to evaluate **new information**, going beyond the text to do one of two things: either apply the information in the passage to a new context or take new information and integrate and evaluate it in the context of the passage. The first skill may be tested by asking whether a new argument or piece of information is consistent with passage assertions, whether it is or is NOT supported by evidence in the passage, what the author would think about this new information, or how the author would best clarify or support this statement. For example, we might be asked how the author would react to the claim that meeting close friends and family for a biweekly dinner would yield more beneficial health outcomes than would participating in a religious retreat that focuses on silent meditation. The author argues in the last paragraph that social ties, or their absence, is what leads to the presence or lack of good health. The author also states that religion encourages these ties by building familial relationships between members. Therefore, a biweekly dinner with friends and family, which clearly features social ties and familial relationships, would be more likely to promote good health than would a meditation retreat, at least according to this author.

The second CARS question type that requires you to reason beyond the text asks you to accept new information and interpret the passage text in light of that information. You'll essentially be asked what impact a statement, or a series of statements, might have on the assertions within the passage. For example, you might be provided a series of examples and asked which would most strengthen or weaken, or challenge or support an assertion within the passage. A specific example of this would be the question: If a new study shows that negative relationships between children and their parents can cause a decline in physical health, what impact would this have on the author's main argument? First, let's recall the author's main argument: the metaphorical kin encountered in religious contexts, as manifested by the widespread use of terms such as father and brother, can lead to increased social bonds and improved physical health. The author never claims that family is always a positive influence or always has health benefits, only that the familial ties formed in religious contexts are generally positive and beneficial. Therefore, we'd expect this new information about the negative impacts of toxic familial relationships not to have much impact on the author's main idea.

If you focus on thoroughly understanding the arguments presented in CARS passages and their main ideas, such as by asking yourself whether these claims are backed up by evidence, then answering the questions will come much more easily to you.

4. Logic in the CARS Section

The logic inherent to arguments in CARS passages is often tested in the form of Inference questions. These questions will ask about assumptions and implications that can be drawn from the passage text. An **assumption** is unstated evidence that must be true for the author's argument to be valid. In other words, an assumption is necessarily implied by the author, even if not explicitly stated. For instance, imagine that a CARS author states that ancient Chinese architectural design influenced much of Southeast Asian architecture. For this argument to be valid, we must assume that ancient Chinese architecture pre-dated much of Southeast Asian architecture. If this were not true (i.e., if instead Southeast Asian architecture pre-dated ancient Chinese architecture), then this argument would very quickly fall apart. After all, how could Chinese architecture have had this influence if it didn't even exist yet?

An **implication** is an unstated conclusion that must also be true if the author's argument is valid. So again, if the passage claimed that ancient Chinese architectural design influenced much of Southeast Asian architecture, then we could logically infer that there must be some architectural works in Southeast Asia that resemble or in some way draw upon ancient Chinese architectural styles. This is a very direct, logical conclusion based on the stated premise that doesn't require any leaps in logic. On the other hand, if the passage simply stated that ancient Chinese architecture pre-dated much of Southeast Asian architecture, we could not infer from that alone that there must be Southeast Asian architecture that resembles ancient Chinese architectural styles. While that certainly could be true, it's not necessarily true, so this is not a valid implication based on this premise alone. Be careful to distinguish explicit assertions from valid assumptions and implications. Further, you should also be very careful not to make assumptions or implications that are not supported by the passage at all! Trap answer choices on inference questions will often include implications that go too far beyond the passage text, so avoid extrapolating too far. Instead, focus on using what the author explicitly states to identify what must be true in order for the author's argument to be true (an assumption) or what must also be true if the author's argument is valid (an implication).

While both assumptions and implications are unstated parts of an argument, this doesn't necessarily mean the author is trying to trick you by making disconnected logical jumps or that the author's simply lazy for not spelling out what exactly is being assumed. Rather, we do this kind of thing all the time in writing and in everyday life. Even a simple everyday question like "How was your commute today?" has some assumptions - first, that the person you're talking to regularly travels to and from work or school, and second, that transit conditions can either be relatively good or relatively bad. If either of those assumptions doesn't hold, the question just doesn't make sense. To visualize this, imagine asking that question to a four-year-old or to your retired grandparents. You'd get a pretty weird look, right?

Similarly in CARS, if you're not reading critically, it's all too easy to accept an argument without dissecting its assumptions, which, if flawed, could dismantle the entire premise of the argument. The best approach to questions that ask you to identify the assumptions made by an author's argument is first to return to the passage. Locate the argument or premise in question within the text. Next, examine each answer choice one by one and ask what would happen to the argument if each choice, or assumption, were not true? If invalidating the assumption causes the argument to fall apart, then the assumption must be true for the argument to be valid. In our previous example, suppose the assumption that ancient Chinese architecture predated much of Southeast Asian architecture were untrue; in fact, suppose most Southeast Asian architecture had been around long before ancient Chinese architecture. There would then be no way that ancient Chinese architecture could have influenced much of Southeast Asian architecture! Be careful with irrelevant, extreme, or overgeneralized answer choices here. For example, we can't assume that ancient Chinese architecture influenced all of Southeast Asian architecture or that specific elements in particular were highly influential. Stick to the passage text. The best way to avoid choosing the wrong answer is to go through the answer choices one by one and identify the answer choice that, if false, must invalidate the argument in question.

Inference questions might ask you to reason within the text about what can be inferred directly from the passage, but they might also ask you to reason beyond the text about conclusions that can be drawn from passage information and/or new information. For example, you might be asked, if X piece of information were true, how would that affect Y in the passage? Or if the author believes X, what would the author believe about Y? You might also be asked how a new piece of evidence would strengthen or weaken an argument in the passage. The key to answering these questions isn't to make logical leaps or to choose an answer that just sounds good. Rather, you need to rely on what the text literally says and what assumptions and implications must follow logically. For such questions, focus on each answer choice one at a time, asking yourself what would be the logical result if each were true or false.

Inferences come in two flavors: deductive and inductive. Although you won't be asked to identify examples of deductive and inductive reasoning on the MCAT, these concepts are useful in framing our conversation about making logical inferences, which begin with at least one premise and use logic to then arrive at a conclusion.

Deductive reasoning involves starting with a broad, generalized hypothesis and then making specific observations that follow from that hypothesis until a conclusion is reached. **Inductive reasoning** is, in a way, the opposite, beginning with specific observations that lead to a broad generalization. The scientific method is an example of using deduction, since you start with a hypothesis and then examine the evidence, leading to a conclusion that supports or refutes the hypothesis. In formal logic, we call both the hypothesis and the pieces of evidence "premises" because they're pieces of information that lead to the conclusion. With deductive reasoning, if the premises are true, we can infer conclusions we know to be certain. For example, suppose we begin with the premises that bats are mammals and all mammals have mammary glands. These premises, of course, would be invalidated if we found a bat that wasn't a mammal or a mammal without mammary glands. However, provided these are true, we could properly infer that bats must have mammary glands.

In CARS, deductive reasoning might look something like this: if we begin with the generalization that ancient Chinese architectural design influenced much of Southeast Asian architecture, what must we be able to conclude from this? If ancient Chinese architecture influenced Southeast Asian architecture, there must be Southeast Asian architecture that looks a lot like ancient Chinese architecture. As long as the premise is true, the conclusion must be true as well. Of course, we can't know that the premise is true: after all, we don't need to know anything about ancient architecture! We just need to understand that as long as it is true, the conclusion logically follows.

Inductive reasoning works in the opposite direction, beginning with specific observations that lead up to a generalizable hypothesis based on this evidence. This is often how scientific hypotheses are formed: Gregor Mendel must have observed the inheritance patterns of scores of pea plants before coming up with his principles of genetic inheritance. We draw conclusions all the time about life based on a relatively limited set of personal experiences. In contrast to deduction, the conclusions drawn from inductive inferences are not certain. For example, you might observe 10 bats and note that all have mammary glands, and then you might realize that all mammals you've ever seen have mammary glands. Therefore, you might infer that bats must be mammals. This conclusion just so happens to be true, but that's not always the case. For example, if you observe that all 10 bats have brown fur, you might be tempted to conclude that all bats have brown fur. But in reality, there are bat species that have black, orange, white, gray, or red fur, so we have to be careful about making inductive inferences. Returning to our example of architecture, a relevant example would be if you traveled to Vietnam and noticed that a lot of the architecture resembles the style of ancient Chinese temples. Then you might infer, based on these observations, that ancient

Chinese architecture influenced Southeast Asian architectural styles, although your observations do not definitively prove that this is true.

The figure below summarizes the distinctions between deductive and inductive reasoning, as applied to our examples of the mammalian nature of bats and the potential influence of Chinese architecture throughout Southeast Asia.

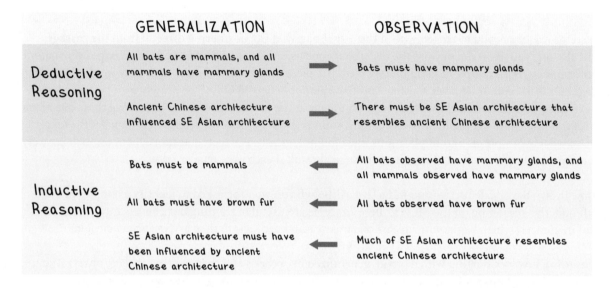

Figure 1. Deductive vs. inductive reasoning

Here's another example that may help clarify the difference between inductive and deductive reasoning: "If I drive fast, I will get a speeding ticket". With deductive reasoning, this general principle would then lead to specific observations or predictions, like if I drive too fast today, I will get a ticket. Same thing tomorrow. And the next day. Inductive reasoning starts with specific examples and moves to a general conclusion. For example, let's say I drive too fast today and get a speeding ticket. Same thing tomorrow. And the next day. This might lead me to conclude that if I drive too fast, I will get a speeding ticket. Now, of course, as we might know from our own personal experiences, it is not the case that driving too fast automatically results in a speeding ticket. From the point of view of deductive reasoning, this means that our initial premise must be flawed, or at least in need of some revision. From the perspective of inductive reasoning, though, it's our conclusion that was falsified. The point we're working towards is that both types of reasoning are falsifiable, but that the possible discrepancy between our reasoning and reality affects different parts of the argument: the premise for deduction and the conclusion for induction. The most important takeaway point here is that the conclusions we reach using inductive reasoning are always somewhat tentative. That is, there could always be some empirical fact that proves us wrong.

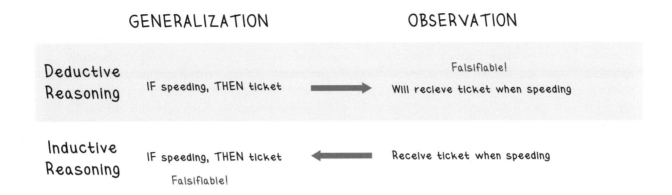

Figure 2. Falsifiability of deductive and inductive reasoning

As discussed earlier, you're not required to identify examples of deductive or inductive reasoning for the CARS section, but you'll be using such reasoning skills to analyze CARS passages. Passage arguments will involve some kind of conclusion, which is usually a main idea of the passage. The passage will also outline the evidence leading up to that conclusion. Our job is to identify the assumptions necessary for the author's premises to be true and to draw valid implications based on the passage text.

It's also crucial to be aware of **flaws in logic**. For example, be careful not to confuse the conclusion "all A are B" with "all B are A" or "only A are B." For a real world example, we know the conclusion "all dogs are animals" to be true. However, this does not mean that all animals are dogs or that only dogs can be animals. A more obvious, but still highly important, point is that moderate words like "some" are very different from extreme words like "all." So if a CARS author argues that some Southeast Asian architecture resembles ancient Chinese architecture, don't conflate this with all Southeast Asian architecture resembling ancient Chinese architecture. Even if we were told that all Southeast Asian architecture resembled Chinese architecture, this still wouldn't mean that only Southeast Asian architecture can resemble ancient Chinese architecture nor that all ancient Chinese architecture resembles Southeast Asian architecture.

To recap, while assumptions and implications are not explicitly stated in the passage, they are explicitly implied. In other words, you should be able to literally point to or highlight specific text within the passage and directly come up with an assumption or inference that would also be made by anyone else reading the exact same passage. There must be textual clues you can point to that help "prove" the correct answer choice. Thus for these questions, it can be extremely beneficial to re-examine the text so you can feel confident.

5. Arguments in a Practice Passage

Let's consider what we've learned while we read this passage on Daoist rituals:

> On the basis of the protagonist Yuanshuai and the lyric "luo li lian," it may be tentatively inferred that the origins of Tapeng are deeply rooted in Daoism. Of course, this is just a partial comparison and investigation. Because Tapeng is a part of the ritual for purifying the stage prior to a Puxian opera performance, we will use the motives and sequence of this ceremony as a basis for comparison with the Daoist rite for purifying the altar.

> British anthropologist Victor Turner advanced the theory of liminality in a ritual context. In his view, the period of liminality within the ritual process eliminates the inequalities of social status, causing a unique bond to form among the ritual's participants. This is a kind of "communitas." In Daoist rituals, this kind of communitas can be viewed as an equality of communication and exchange

between humans and spirits. Furthermore, the Daoist ritual area seeks to develop the distinctive space of these exchanges. Due to the sacred nature of this space, one must ensure its purity. The rite for purifying or cleaning the altar is one of the important rituals found within the repertoire of Daoist zhai and jiao ceremonies. Daoism holds the ritual space of the altar to be the site where the three effulgences open and enliven an icon's eyes, where the five phases pervade, where myriad patterns are restored and proliferate, and where yin and yang arise and descend. Prior to performing a zhai rite for communicating with spirits or petitioning the gods to offer protection from calamity, the Daoist master will want to observe divine law by dispelling any impure vapors from the space of the altar.

The stage of the theater is also a mystical space where the joys and sorrows of life play out year round: love and hate, passion and enmity, fantastic encounters with gods and ghosts and the myriad conditions of living things. Sometimes, these events unfold in the mundane world; at other times, they transpire in the abodes of transcendence or even the netherworld. The actors on stage and the audience together have lived through the variations of life. Theater uses ritualistic performances to transport actors and the audience into an imagined domain. Within a set time and space, both groups are pulled into this fantastic realm where they realize the significance of life itself. This kind of theatrical stage, which can be likened to a threshold, similarly requires the implementation of effectual measures to maintain its purity. Through investigation of the ritual for purifying the stage in Puxian opera, we have discovered that this ritual bears many similarities with the Daoist rite for purifying the altar, including congruent sequences and procedures, such as: setting up the altar or stage, talismans and incantations recited by ritual masters and actors alike, and the petitioning of the spirits.

The first paragraph is an introduction to the premise of this passage, followed by a paragraph about Daoist rituals for purifying the altar, which are then compared in the final paragraph to rituals for purifying the theater stage. There are plenty of unfamiliar terms in that first paragraph (Yuanshuai, luo li lian, Tapeng, Daoism, and Puxian opera) but we aren't expected to know what each means. Instead, we can use contextual clues to interpret how they fit into the meaning of this paragraph. The first sentence basically says that based on certain information, it may be "tentatively inferred" that Tapeng's roots are in Daoism. That language "tentatively inferred" is important because it tells us something about what the author thinks about this. The author is being cautious, for one reason or another, in making this connection between Tapeng and Daoism but still asserts that Tapeng arose out of or was heavily influenced by Daoism. Of course, we aren't told what Tapeng is until the third sentence, where we learn that Tapeng is apparently a "part of the ritual for purifying the stage prior to a Puxian opera performance." We don't need to know what a Puxian opera performance is, specifically, but the bigger takeaway is that Tapeng is a ritualistic element that has to do with purifying a stage, specifically an opera stage.

So maybe you've heard of Daoism before; if not, it's mentioned again at the end of this paragraph as involving rites for "purifying the altar," which gives us a big hint that Daoism is a spiritual or religious tradition. Next, the author more explicitly outlines the comparison being made between Tapeng (rituals for purifying theater stages) and Daoist rituals for purifying the altar. More specifically, the author states that we'll be examining the "motives and sequence" of Tapeng to compare it to Daoist rituals. In other words, we now have a passage goal: this passage will argue that Tapeng's origins are rooted in Daoism by comparing the motives and sequence of these two rituals.

Next, we're given the name of an anthropologist, which tells us that this passage at least considers an anthropological perspective. Thus we can assume that Turner must be especially interested in human societies and cultures, and so must the author, who expands upon Turner's ideas. Turner advanced what's referred to as the "theory of liminality." Since "liminality" is another uncommon term, it may be tempting to glance ahead to see if liminality is defined later in this paragraph. Unfortunately, it's not, so we must rely on contextual clues. For now, we can replace "liminality" with "something that has to do with a ritual context" and at least try to understand why liminality is important, even if we're not yet completely sure what it means. The author states that, according to Turner, liminality abolishes social inequities and forges bonds, or a "communitas," between people sharing in the same ritual. In other words, in a ritual, everyone is on the same social playing field, which results in the formation of stronger connections.

There is some elaboration on this point in the next sentence, but notably, this is also the first mention of Daoism in this paragraph. So while Turner may have applied the theory of liminality to any number of ritual contexts, here the author is explicitly applying this to Daoist rituals, stating that in Daoism this bond forms between humans and spirits, and once again reminding us to stay centered on the big-picture comparison between Tapeng and Daoist rituals. Notice how the transition word "furthermore" introduces the next point: that the "space" in which these rituals are practiced must be pure. In the successive sentences, the author explains the importance of such altar-purifying rituals, which gets at the motives the author was talking about earlier. But we don't want to get too stuck in the weeds here either; we can return for the details later, if needed.

In the next paragraph, we switch gears to the theater stage, a reference to Tapeng. The word "also" helps us make an explicit comparison between the theater stage and the Daoist altar as mystical spaces where life events and fantastical encounters occur, either in our world or in another world, that pull the audience into a mystical setting. Then, if we're asked about similarities between the two, we've got a lot of material to work with here. Recall, however, that we're looking for ties between the stage- or altar-purifying rituals of Tapeng and Daoism, which is touched on about halfway through this paragraph. Specifically, like the Daoist altar, the theater stage must be purified; the author even says, "we have discovered that this ritual bears many similarities with the Daoist rite for purifying the altar." That word "we" is slipped in discreetly here, but notice how the author and colleagues take credit for this comparative analysis. This is important because it means these are the author's own convictions, not a recounting of what someone else believes. A series of similarities between these two types of rituals is then listed, which normally might be considered a detail you can skim to some degree and return to later. However, I want to point out the word "sequences" here, which alludes to the similarities in sequence between Tapeng and Daoist rituals mentioned in the introduction. Once again, these specific examples are details that, while important, should principally be thought of as support for the larger claim that the procedures are similar between Tapeng and Daoist rituals.

Let's go back and examine the arguments made in this passage. In the first paragraph, the author outlines that "it may be inferred that the origins of Tapeng are deeply rooted in Daoism." Let's imagine that our only goal in life is to find out, once and for all, what the roots of Tapeng are. To do so, we need to be able to partition opinion from fact. This passage contains a lot of details that explain the how, and why, of rituals, but it's the opinions that will lead us to the author's perspective and biases. In that thesis statement, the qualifier "deeply" tells us that the author thinks that this is a serious, important connection that goes beyond surface-level similarities.

We also need to identify the assumptions upon which the author's arguments rest and the implications that can be made based on the stated premises in the passage. For example, the claim that Tapeng's roots are in Daoism assumes that Daoism originated before Tapeng. That's an example of an assumption that anyone should be able to make based on this statement, so it's excellent fodder for CARS questions.

In this first paragraph, the author claims that Tapeng and Daoist rituals can be compared on the basis of "motives" and "sequence." Let's stop for a moment. How compelling is the author's argument so far? There was that one reference to Yuanshuai and the lyric "luo li lian" (in fact, this is the premise upon which the author inferred Tapeng's roots in Daoism), but, without more context, we don't have much else to work with, so let's take a look at the following paragraphs.

What motives exactly was the author referring to? This is to say, for what reasons are these two types of rituals performed? In paragraph two, the passage states that Daoist rituals supposedly eliminate social inequities and forge bonds between ritual participants. This paragraph also claims that this requires a "distinctive space" where three effulgences open and where "impure vapors" must be dispelled. This gives us a reason why a ritual to purify the altar is necessary to create this distinctive space. From that last sentence, we can infer that dispelling such impure vapors allows ritual participants to communicate with spirits and gods, who may offer them protection.

Of course, there are claims made in this paragraph that we can examine individually. For example, consider the idea that "liminality eliminates the inequalities of social status." This assumes that inequalities in social status must have existed prior to this process of liminality. This opens the door to seeing assumptions everywhere. For this reason, it's less important that you identify every possible assumption as you read through a passage than it is to identify assumptions for specific statements when asked about them in the context of a CARS question. Furthermore, you don't have to know what the word "liminality" means in order to identify this assumption. Even if we had replaced it with an algebraic variable, we still could recognize that for thing A to eliminate thing B, thing B must have existed before thing A.

Now that we've identified the motives for purifying the Daoist altar, let's take a look at the comparison in motive the author draws to Tapeng. Paragraph three states that the theater stage is a "mystical space where the joys and sorrows of life play out year round" and that ritual practices "transport actors and the audience into an imagined domain." This provides a motive for the purification of the theater stage.

Then, in paragraph three, the author also lists similarities in the actual sequence or procedures of Tapeng and Daoist rituals, including "setting up the altar or stage, talismans and incantations recited by ritual masters and actors alike, and the petitioning of the spirits."

So, moving back to the big picture, are we convinced that the origins of Tapeng are deeply rooted in Daoism? There are some fairly compelling similarities between the reasons for purifying the stage or altar, respectively. More specifically, the author promised to detail the similarities in motive and sequence between Tapeng and Daoist rituals, and the author did deliver on this. It's up to us, of course, to identify if we think these motives are similar enough or if there are any flaws in the author's argument. For example, the author claims that the talismans and incantations involved in Daoist rituals and Tapeng are an example of a procedural similarity. However, a critic might want more specific evidence of this to be persuaded, believing this textual support to be insufficient.

Furthermore, a CARS question might ask us, if it turns out the Tapeng arose long before Daoism, how would this strengthen or weaken the author's argument? If this were true, then no matter how similar the motives or sequences are, this would be a pretty major flaw that could bring down the entire argument. It's totally fine if you can't predict such assumptions or flaws on the fly, so long as you're prepared to evaluate them critically in the context of a CARS question.

When a passage becomes a logic puzzle, it's a lot more fun to navigate and dissect, regardless of the topic. Depending on your interests, this might or might not be the most riveting subject in the world, but it doesn't have to be for you to remain engaged. You also don't have to be an expert on Daoism or Puxian opera to be able to do well on a passage like this, so the more practice you get with passage topics you're not terribly familiar with, the more equipped you'll be to handle anything that comes your way in the CARS section.

6. Must-Knows

> Arguments in CARS must be evidence-backed, with which others might reasonably agree or disagree.
  - Top-down argument structure: position is stated, followed by supporting evidence.
  - Bottom-up argument structure: pieces of evidence are drawn together to lead to a conclusion.
> Forms of support:
  - Empirical evidence.
  - Expert opinion.
  - Primary/secondary sources (primary: direct; secondary: indirect).
> Authors will frequently anticipate and refute potential counterarguments.
> Argument-related questions may include the following tasks:
  - Identifying arguments within the passage (e.g., main idea).
  - Reasoning about the function or purpose of an argument.
  - Identifying support for an argument within a passage.
  - Evaluating the implications of new information for passage arguments.
> Assumption: unstated evidence that must be true for the author's argument to be valid.
> Implication: unstated conclusion that must be true if the author's argument is valid.
> Deductive reasoning: start with a broad, general hypothesis and then make specific observations that follow from that hypothesis until reaching a conclusion.
> Inductive reasoning: starts with specific observations that lead to a broad generalization.
> Common logical flaws:
  - Confusing "all A are B" with "all B are A" or "only A are B"—not true!
  - Violation of unstated assumptions.

Applied Practice

The best MCAT practice is realistic, with detailed analytics to help you assess where things went wrong. For those reasons, we recommend completing practice questions in an online setting that simulates the real MCAT interface, and using the analytics provided to help you decide how to best move your studies forward.

CARS does not require knowledge of specific subject areas, but it does require development of strong test-taking skills. To ensure you are honing those skills as you work through this book, we suggest you go online after wrapping up each chapter and generate a Qbank Practice Set of 2-3 CARS passages to practice and review. While not every chapter of this book is directly applicable to CARS, regular CARS practice is key to test day success.

As a further supplement, given the importance of active learning for effective studying, we also suggest that you consult the Must-Knows at the end of each chapter of this Reasoning text as a basis for creating a study sheet. This is not a sheet to memorize in the more traditional sense of content memorization, but rather a quick reference of the most important strategies for you to refer to during and after practice in your early prep. Frequently revisiting the most important strategies for the MCAT - in both CARS and the Sciences - will help you continue to improve your performance.

This page left intentionally blank.

This page left intentionally blank.

CARS Question Types

CHAPTER

6

0. Introduction

The CARS section tests your ability to critically analyze and reason through a humanities or social sciences passage, but what does that mean specifically? On one level, it's about assessing whether you understand what the passage was about and its main purpose. Moving beyond basic reading comprehension, do you understand why the author used specific examples, various forms of support, and rhetorical devices to make certain points? What opinions and arguments does the author put forward, and how are those arguments supported? Moving even further afield, how can we extrapolate the precise text of the passage to external, real-world situations?

All of the above skills are very important, but they're open-ended, and on a very practical level, the CARS section boils down to answering questions. Therefore, in this chapter, we'll review the common question types that you will encounter in the CARS section

1. CARS Skill Categories

The AAMC has specifically designated three broad categories of reasoning skills that CARS questions test: **Foundations of Comprehension**, **Reasoning Within the Text**, and **Reasoning Beyond the Text**. About 30% of questions fall under Foundations of Comprehension, 30% fall under Reasoning Within the Text, and the final 40% fall under the Reasoning Beyond the Text skill category. First we'll talk about each of these skills broadly, and then we'll zoom in more closely to explore specific question types.

It is important to reflect on why we're embarking on this exercise. The point of defining reasoning skills and question types in the CARS section isn't to try to confuse you, or to force you to memorize a list of question types. Instead, there are a limited number of skills that will be tested on the CARS section, and, consequently, there are a limited number of ways in which questions can be asked. By appreciating this point and understanding the logic and rationale behind CARS questions, you'll start to recognize patterns and become better at predicting the questions associated with CARS passages.

To reiterate, we're *not* saying that the end goal is for you to explicitly classify the type and subtype of every question you encounter in your practice or on test day. Instead, it's valuable for you to be able to appreciate how questions fit patterns you've seen and practiced with before. If you can understand whether a question is asking about opinions, relationships, main ideas, or arguments within the passage, then you're bound to experience less uncertainty, even when dealing with unfamiliar passage topics.

Furthermore, building practical expertise with CARS questions goes hand in hand with refining your ability to read CARS passages skillfully. For instance, as you analyze which parts of the passage various types of CARS questions tend to draw on, it'll become more evident how key themes tend to appear frequently in introduction and conclusion paragraphs. You will also become more aware of when the author uses examples to support claims, and when supporting evidence is conspicuously absent.

Returning to the AAMC's established reasoning skills, **Foundations of Comprehension** questions test whether you understood the passage as a whole, as well as specific components within the passage. The basic theme with these questions is that they ask about what's explicitly stated or directly implied by the passage. Within Foundations of Comprehension there are two skill subtypes, depending on how direct the question is.

The first subtype asks about the **basic components of the text**. For example, do you understand the overall point and thesis of the passage? What did the author mean when using a specific phrase or example? Which statements make major passage arguments? Do you recognize when multiple different perspectives are given, and can you distinguish them from the author's? Do you understand the purpose of certain elements of the passage, and how they relate to the big picture? Which statements reflect the main argument, and which are subpoints? To summarize, if you can identify what's what in the passage text, you've got this skill subtype covered.

The second Foundations of Comprehension skill subtype is the ability to **infer meaning from the text**. This subtype requires you to understand what is implied, but not necessarily explicitly stated by the author. It also requires you to understand *why* the author used certain rhetorical techniques, like transitional phrases, causal or chronological language, or a specific tone, to make a point. Because of this, you may need to first identify what assumptions the author makes, what the intended purposes or effects of those assumptions are, and how this relates to the passage thesis as a whole. This skill also requires you to not just point out differing points of view, but also to identify when the author paraphrases or implies positions. This skill focuses on why the author made certain decisions when crafting the passage, based on the relatively predictable ways that authors set up their discussions. Overall, the common thread of Foundations of Comprehension skills is knowing where to look and using specific wording to answer questions.

The next skills category, **Reasoning Within the Text**, requires you to analyze the text in greater depth. After all, CARS passages are all about persuasive arguments, and this CARS skill tests how well you evaluate passage claims based on their inherent logic, the quality and quantity of supporting evidence, errors in determining causality or drawing conclusions, and the relevance of specific information presented. You may need to integrate information from multiple places, including understanding relationships between separate ideas presented in the passage, such as how someone mentioned in one paragraph might feel about a new theory discussed in a subsequent paragraph. Reasoning Within the Text questions are also concerned with whether an author uses credible sources and evidence. Based on the language that the author employs, do they present ideas objectively, or do they use exaggerated language that suggests personal bias? In other words, these questions are asking you to be skeptical and analyze the author's arguments with a critical eye.

Even as you act the part of a skeptic, it is important to remember that evaluating the credibility and reasonableness of an argument is distinct from whether you agree with it. Even if you're reading an opinion piece that you sharply disagree with, it's important to recognize that a reasonably-worded argument drawing on expert opinions and scientific studies is more credible than an argument that insults opponents and cites random angry people from the internet. On the flip side, an author might use slipshod rhetorical techniques and dubious logic to support a topic you do believe in, and, in such a case, you shouldn't let your support prevent you from recognizing deficiencies in the author's reasoning.

Finally, as you might predict, **Reasoning Beyond the Text** questions go *beyond* the passage, requiring you to re-contextualize the passage text in light of new information. This means that you will be doing one of two things: either applying passage information to new contexts, or incorporating new information into your interpretation of the passage. The former asks you to make predictions and generalizations based on the author's positions as stated in the passage. To do this well, you need to understand the author's position AND be able to apply it to new contexts. The latter question subtype works in reverse, by asking you how new information might affect the passage itself, and invites you at times to be critical of the passage and recognize potential flaws or vulnerabilities in the author's claims when confronted with conflicting information. This includes questions that ask you what information might *strengthen* or *weaken* a claim made in the passage. As you can probably tell, the better your foundational understanding of the passage, the better equipped you'll be to handle Reasoning Beyond the Text questions, which admittedly are some of the toughest in the CARS section.

So now that you have an idea of the analytical skills you'll need to bring to the CARS section, our next step is to discuss the exact types of questions you'll encounter in the CARS section. As a brief introduction, there are eight basic categories of CARS questions:

> **Main Idea** questions ask about major themes and the purpose of the passage.
> **Opinion** questions ask about the author's opinion, as well as the opinions, attitudes, perspectives, and motivations of other people mentioned in the passage and how these are related.
> **Detail** questions ask you about specific terms, facts, assertions, and relationships that are *explicitly* stated in the passage.
> **Inference** questions ask about passage assertions, relationships, assumptions, and implications that are *inferred*, requiring an extra layer of interpretation.
> **Function** questions get at *why* certain examples and rhetorical devices are used in the passage, largely focusing on how they ultimately further the main argument.
> **Support** questions ask about support provided for arguments in the passage. That is, what evidence is used, if any, and how well does it bolster passage claims.
> **Application** questions require extrapolating passage information and opinions to new information.
> **Incorporation** questions ask you to assess how new information affects your interpretation of the passage.

The latter two question types exclusively require the Reasoning Beyond the Text CARS skill, but the other question types may involve one or more CARS skills. There may also be some overlap between question types, such as questions that require you to *apply* passage *opinions* to new contexts, or Function questions that rely on your understanding of main ideas. Therefore, at the end of the day, success on CARS largely comes down to understanding what each question asks and what information and reasoning skills you need to get to the answer.

Throughout this chapter, we'll cover each of the eight CARS question types, and the discussion will be as follows: First, we'll define each question type. Then we'll provide examples modeled after real CARS questions. Next, we'll get into the details of the reasoning skills each question type assesses. By working through relevant examples associated with a CARS passage, we'll demonstrate the analytical processes that lead to success, and give you hands-on, practical advice about common pitfalls. Our goal is *not* to present shortcuts and gimmicks that don't work. Instead, we'll focus on developing your reasoning skills, because investing in core reasoning skills, rather than relying on shortcuts, is what ensures success in your CARS performance.

2. Sample Passage

There's no such thing as a CARS question without a passage, so throughout this chapter, we'll make reference to the sample passage below. As we read the passage, we'll want to reflect on main ideas after reading each paragraph, and highlight key words and phrases that capture the big picture. We can do this by asking probing questions about how the topics discussed in each paragraph relate to the thesis. But that's not all we care about - we want to consider what point the author tries to argue and the *opinions* and *arguments* the author intends to convince us of.

There is renewed interest in understanding how people use buildings. This interest is, in part, driven by the low-carbon agenda, which posits that there is a known knowledge gap between what is built and our understanding of how buildings perform. There is a gulf between the energy performance of buildings as simulated at the design stage and the actual energy consumed in use. The occupants of buildings are seemingly doing something different within the built form than what the designers of the simulation programs assumed and different from the in-use conditions that the software algorithms model. This performance difference continues to attract research attention. There are a number of studies of living in low and zero carbon (LZC) homes that report difficulties some occupants have with building controls and understanding the operation of heating and micro-generation technologies, including instances when the process of learning how to use eco-features in new homes was specifically mentioned.

In a persuasive argument, Vales take the sustainable futures debate further, building on the seminal views of Whole Earth and the agitprop Street Farm movement, emphasizing that it takes more than efficient space heating and housing design to reduce our impact on the planet. When housing is constructed with ample insulation, is orientated in the right direction, and is free-running, then its energy demand stems from the use of stuff, the technical artifacts people use within houses, and not primarily from the material fabric and building of the home. Indeed, knowing how to build passive houses is no longer a technical problem. To reduce our impact on the environment by moderating some small habits, everyday practices and lifestyle are important. Technological change in the built form matters, but one cannot ignore these lifestyle issues. Local habits and practices are now written into larger-scale assessments of environmental impact: habits relating to how clothes are washed and dried, access to public transportation, and sourcing electricity locally. These practices take place within the home, in the community, and at a city scale, all of which are now entangled in the way housing efficiency ratings are calculated and in the assessment of a green city. This increase in scale needs more explanation.

There is debate as to whether individual change, or numerous individuals' actions, will make a difference. Bookchin's philosophy seems to anticipate this critique. Bookchin was committed to local democratic participation and community scale production. His philosophy of technology placed emphasis on the social matrix within which technology operates, re-embedding technology in a web of communal social relations and ethics. He stressed the need for technologies to be compatible with face-to-face decisions made in assemblies, where "an authentic community is not merely a structural constellation of human beings but rather a practice of communizing through shared experiences." This is a shift in the unit of analysis from the individual to the actions of a community; this way of thinking has a history.

Forty years ago, it took high levels of personal commitment for the pioneers of progressive initiatives at Cat and Vauban in Freiburg to live in settlements with less impact on the environment. In today's mainstreaming of many of these co-evolution ideas, there is an upscaling of what were once viewed as alternative lifestyles, through citizen-led initiatives in the community and intervention at a city scale. Bookchin's ideas preceded the local heat and power generation solutions and the potential for local production that are currently promoted.

Adapted from Luck, Rachael. 2014. "Learning How to Use Buildings: An Exploration of the Potential of Design Interactions to Support Transition to Low-Impact Community Living." Buildings 4, no. 4: 963-977 under CC BY 4.0

As a brief summary, the author discusses an energy performance gap, which is explained by how the people who live in these buildings affect their energy performance. After weaving through the views of Vales, Bookchin, and others, the author ultimately builds to the thesis that, in order for green technologies to reduce our environmental impact, we ought to consider the ways in which they are used by individuals.

3. Main Idea Questions

All **Main Idea** questions rely on the Foundations of Comprehension CARS skill, which reinforces how important it is to have a clear idea of the key themes of each passage. Such questions ask about the thesis and purpose of a passage. These are two closely related but technically distinct concepts: the **thesis** is the main idea of the passage as a whole, and the **purpose** has to do with the author's intent and motivation for writing the passage. Some Main Idea questions include:

> > What is the main idea of the passage?
> > What is the author's central thesis?
> > What is the primary purpose of the passage?
> > What title would best fits the passage?
> > What is the most likely background or profession of the author?
> > Who is the intended audience?

While some of these questions are more straightforward than others, even those that ask about the audience, the title of the passage, or the background of the author are still asking about the passage's main ideas. Some questions focus on the passage thesis; if you understand the big picture and can paraphrase it in a sentence, you've got these questions in the bag. Others target the related idea of purpose; if you understand why the author cared to write a passage on this topic, you can probably predict the primary purpose, and make assumptions about the author, or take a stab at the intended audience.

If you find yourself having trouble with Main Idea questions, here are a few things you can try during your practice. First of all, pay attention to what the author spends the majority of the passage discussing. In other words, what ideas, themes, or arguments are repeated. In particular, pay special attention to opinionated, arguable assertions in the introduction and conclusion, when present. Some passages present a counterargument in the introduction, and others might end with caveats or outstanding questions in the conclusion. Once we think we've identified the thesis, we can check our work by seeing whether we can complete the sentence: "The author argues that _____." This both verifies that we spotted an arguable assertion and gets us in the habit of paraphrasing any theses we find—a trick that will come in handy when we start attacking those Main Idea questions.

Although we don't generally recommend note-taking while taking CARS passage, if Main Idea questions regularly cause you trouble, you can try jotting down main ideas while you practice. Then, while reviewing the passage as a whole, summarize the passage using a very brief phrase, and see how many questions you can answer using that summary alone. Afterwards, ask yourself what other information you should have included that would have helped you answer more questions correctly. In other words, what ideas or opinions in the passage were more important than you originally thought? This exercise will give you an appreciation for how many CARS questions relate to the passage thesis, even questions that don't directly ask about the main idea.

A third technique to test in your practice is scrolling to the very bottom of the passage to read the title of the work it's derived from (if that information is presented) before reading the passage. Sometimes this doesn't give you much useful insight, but at other times, it at least gives you an anchor for what's to come, allowing you to frame your reading of each paragraph around the likely central idea of the passage. The passage title we're analyzing in this chapter is "Learning How to Use Buildings: An Exploration of the Potential of Design Interactions to Support Transition to Low-Impact Community Living." This gives us a sense of the passage topic, hinting that it will explore the actions of individuals beyond building design with the word "interactions," and it also tells us something about the author's position on such design interactions "supporting" or enabling the transition to "low-impact community."

For CARS questions, falling for **trap answers** is a common pitfall, and each question type tends to have its own typical examples of trap answers. For Main Idea questions, trap answer choices might be too narrow, focusing on a sub-point of the passage rather than on the main idea. Such an answer choice can be especially tempting if it focuses on a topic in the introduction or conclusion, like the history of green technologies, or how alternative lifestyles are defined. These are certainly important components of the passage, but they do not reflect the thesis.

On the other end of the spectrum, some wrong answer choices will be too broad or take the author's position too far. For example, note how, in the introduction, the author discusses how occupants' use of building controls affects the energy performance of these buildings. A wrong answer choice might suggest that the thesis of this passage is that low and zero carbon homes are constructed in such a way to be non-intuitive to use. Even though more intuitive controls might improve the energy performance in some cases, this ultimately takes the author's claim past its logical limits.

Finally, wrong answer choices might be on the right topic and even be on the right track, but one detail might misinterpret or exaggerate the author's position. An example of this would be an answer choice that states that the individual actions are the *only* or *primary* factor affecting the environmental impact of green technologies. While the author certainly believes that individual actions have an effect, nowhere in the passage does the author express the belief that this is the only or primary factor impacting the environment. We have to take the author at his or her word. The language in this answer choice too extreme in the context of the passage. So, be wary of answer choices that sound good, but don't get the author's position exactly right. In such cases, take a careful look to see if another answer choice might be a better fit. If you're only left with an option that you cannot defend as the main idea, don't jump to pick it! Instead, check for other answer choices you might have eliminated for wrong reasons, like a small detail that seemed out of place but in reality wasn't.

4. Opinion Questions

As we've discussed, opinions and arguments are at the heart of CARS passages. Therefore, as you work through the CARS section, you'll be met with a deluge of **Opinion** questions. To give you a preliminary sense of what we're dealing with, here are a few examples of Opinion questions:

> What is the author's response to X within the passage?
> Which most accurately describes the author's attitude towards X in the passage?
> X assertion in the passage is *least* or *most* consistent with which point of view?

Opinion questions in the CARS section vary in difficulty. Some require only the most basic level of passage comprehension, the Foundations of Comprehension CARS skill. Others involve an added layer of inference when an attitude or opinion is implicit, requiring the Reasoning Within the Text CARS skill. What this means is that, for some questions, going back and gleaning the author's attitude through value words will suffice. However, more often than not, you'll be rewarded by digging deeper as you read, peeling back the layers to reveal the author's true feelings or potential motivations.

One way to set yourself up for success on Opinion questions is to thoroughly read the passage. In particular, focus on the main idea of the passage and try to have an idea of where it's going by the end of the first paragraph or the start of the second paragraph. As you read, take a moment to identify the crucial arguments made in each paragraph, the purpose of that paragraph in the passage as a whole, and any language that indicates attitudes and opinions. It's common for trap answer choices to misattribute opinions, so be sure to keep an eye out for which opinions are the *author's* and which opinions are held by other people.

One of the most common pitfalls on Opinion questions is misinterpreting the author's opinion. More concretely, this can reflect a number of errors. It might mean wrongly inferring an opinion when the author maintains a neutral stance, or missing subtle or implied opinions. Often, this misinterpretation goes so far as to distort or exaggerate the author's stated position. The author's view is rarely extreme in a CARS passage, but there will often be trap answer choices that take the author's views too far. Yet another common problem students run into is crediting an opinion to the wrong. For example, perhaps you understand the positions of Vales and Bookchin, but you have trouble predicting how each would react to the other's ideas. Or perhaps you're able to discern passage opinions and credit them to the right people, but encounter difficulty with applying these views to new situations and predicting how these individuals would react to new information.

Remember, for CARS questions, you should be able to point to the textual evidence–be it an adjective, phrase, or statement–that serves as direct proof for your answer selection, and anyone else reading this passage should be able to draw the same conclusion. It's natural to be affected by your own knowledge and opinions on the passage topic, but if you can remain cognizant of them, you won't be tempted to rely on them to answer Opinion questions.

5. Detail and Inference Questions

Next up are Detail and Inference questions, which are actually two sides of the same coin. **Detail** questions, as the name suggests, ask about what's going on in the passage on a surface level: how are certain words used, what does the author say about X, what does the passage assert about Y? **Inference** questions, then, ask about what's going on in the passage that's hidden under the surface: what are the unstated assumptions, what does the author *suggest* or *imply* about a topic, what can we *infer* about a topic?

Detail questions are typically some of the most manageable questions you'll see in the CARS section. The term "detail" may feel misleading if you think of details as small, unimportant facets of the passage. What *we* mean by "detail" is any surface-level information, or things mentioned explicitly by the author. For this reason, these questions fall firmly into the Foundations of Comprehension skill, and you can almost always go back to an isolated part of the text to quickly locate the relevant information you'll need to answer a Detail question. Some sample Detail questions include:

> - How is the word X used in the passage?
> - What is the meaning of the word X in the passage?
> - According to the passage, what is the cause/effect of X?
> - According to the author, why did X happen?
> - Which of the following assertions does the author make in the passage?
> - According to the passage, what is the focus of X?
> - What examples of X are given in the passage?

Note that many of these questions use the phrase "according to the passage," and that this phrase could be added to any of the other Detail questions. Although not every Detail question will include this phrasing, it is common enough that anytime you see a question that says "according to the passage," you should stop and consider that you may have a Detail question on your hands. The takeaway here is that Detail questions essentially ask, "What exactly did the author actually say about a particular subject?"

Our first word of caution is to avoid answering these questions from memory. This is one of the most common mistakes with Detail questions, and it can be easily avoided by returning to the relevant passage section to quickly confirm your answer. If you can do that, you have a good chance of answering nearly every Detail question correctly. While these questions may feel "easier," since they don't require added layers of reasoning, keep in mind that they're worth the same number of points as "harder" CARS questions, so it's important to invest the extra little bit of time and attention needed to get as many of the "easier" questions right as possible!

Detail questions sometimes specify the exact location of a given word, idea, or direct quote, which is very helpful. However, if the location isn't specified, this is where effective highlighting will pay off. If you didn't happen to highlight the word or phrase you're looking for, there are a few things you can do. First, you can continue to optimize your highlighting technique. Complete a practice passage and its questions as you normally would, with highlighting. Afterwards, take a look at all the questions associated with the passage, and then highlight the parts of the passage that answer each of the questions, paying special attention to Detail questions that require you to return to a specific part of the passage. Compare this highlighting to what you highlighted originally, and continue practicing, not necessarily until your highlighting captures *everything* that's tested, but until your highlighting captures the main ideas and allows you to quickly locate details you might need for the questions.

Another thing you can do is improve your mental outline of the passage. If you employ active reading techniques, you'll have a better understanding of the passage structure and the location of certain examples. Furthermore, you'll improve at predicting elements of the passage that are highly testable. For example, if there are quotation marks around a word or phrase, or a term is defined within the passage, there's a good chance there will be a question on it. If all else fails, notice how numbers, quotation marks, and proper nouns tend to be more salient visual features within a block of text. Use these to help you navigate to examples of specific individuals, dates, or quoted statements in the passage.

There are four general steps to effectively answering a Detail question. The first is understanding the question, which may mean translating the question into a more simplified form. What is the question really asking? Is it asking about the definition or meaning of a word in the context of the passage? Is it asking about a claim the author made? Is it asking about a cause, effect, or some other relationship? Once you understand the question, return to the relevant location of the passage. In most cases, the answer will be in the same paragraph, if not the same sentence, as the detail in question. Try to come up with a general prediction for what you expect to be in the correct answer based on the passage information, and finally, use this prediction to eliminate wrong answer choices and zero in on the correct answer.

Questions asking about the meaning of terms used in the passage can be particularly tricky because they might focus on a word that is either unfamiliar or that is used in an unusual way. However, we have some advice for these questions. First, the right answer isn't always what it seems. The most obvious definition for a specific term may not be how it's used in the passage, so context is important. In fact, be wary of answer choices that seem "too obvious." This isn't a cut-and-dried rule, though; as with all answer choices, a red flag like this should not be used as a basis for elimination. Rather, you should approach the answer choice with skepticism and look for support in the passage before eliminating it entirely. For example, the term "artifacts" in paragraph two of the sample passage isn't intended to mean historical relics excavated by archaeologists. The immediate context tells us this is describing modern technological devices used in people's homes, like TVs or central heating systems.

Our second piece of advice for questions about unfamiliar words is to use clues in close proximity to the term or phrase in question. Very likely the context clues you'll need to answer the question are close by. A good rule of thumb is to read from one or two lines above the term to one or two lines below the term. And finally, especially if context clues are helping you out, try to relate it back to the function and main idea of the paragraph it's in. This will often help lead you to the most appropriate answer choice or, at least, help you eliminate some wrong answer choices.

Next, let's explore **Inference** questions. These are questions that ask about unstated parts of the passage. Inference questions might seem leagues apart from Detail ones, but they have one big thing in common: premises. As a brief refresher, a premise is a statement that necessarily leads to a logical conclusion. In other words, if Premise A is true, Conclusion B must be true. Sometimes the premise and conclusion are made explicit, and detail questions may quiz you on these stated facts. However, sometimes these premises and conclusions are unstated, or implicit, and that's what Inference questions are all about. Specifically, as we've mentioned elsewhere, inference questions will ask you about assumptions and implications. An assumption is the unstated, underlying premise for something to be true. An inference is an often unstated conclusion that the author wants you to logically *infer* based on evidence in the passage. An implication is made when the author suggests or hints at something without stating it explicitly.

Assumptions and implications are both fair game in CARS, and for the purpose of categorizing CARS questions, we lump them together under the umbrella of Inference questions because they require similar skills. Such questions will often use the words "assume," "suggest," "imply," "infer," or some variation on these. Others may ask about conclusions that "may" or "could" be reasonably drawn. For example, Inference questions might include:

> What does X passage statement imply about Y?
> The wording of the passage suggests what about X?
> The author seems to be concerned that X will do what?
> The passage suggests that the author believes X for what reason?
> On the basis of the passage, understanding X might lead to what conclusion?
> Implicit in the passage is what assumption?
> One can infer what about X?

As with Detail questions, it's critical to return to the relevant location in the passage to answer the question. The biggest difference between Detail and Inference questions is that with Detail questions, you essentially need to go back to the passage to identify exactly what the author said. With Inference questions, you will still need to return to the passage, but your goal is to identify what the author *meant* but didn't state explicitly. Consequently, Inference questions use both the Foundations of Comprehension and Reasoning Within the Text skills. Any inferences you draw should follow logically and directly from the exact wording of the text. You should always be able to point to direct evidence in the text that *must* lead to a certain logical conclusion. Even if that conclusion is not explicitly stated, it should be one that would naturally be drawn by anyone reading the same text. In other words, based on a given sentence or paragraph or passage, what is the *only* thing one can be led to conclude? If this information from the passage is true, then what absolutely *must* be true? For this statement in the passage to be true, what underlying premise *must* be true?

When the author implies something or presents a conclusion based on some underlying assumption, all the information you need to identify the assumption, or implication can be found in the passage, usually nearby. Sometimes you'll only have to return to the passage once if the relevant passage information is mentioned in the question stem. Other times, however, you may need to reference the text for each answer choice, such as when you're asked to identify which of the answer choices are inferences that can be drawn from the passage. Either way, with Inference questions, you can typically localize the relevant text for any given inference to one or two sentences within the passage that contain all the information you need.

You may miss some assumptions and inferences, or at least not consciously consider them while initially reading through a passage. This is okay! You will have opportunities to look for these while answering Inference questions. However, with consistent practice throughout your prep and a careful reading you will learn to consider underlying assumptions and implications as you read the passage. This, in turn, will allow you to more efficiently determine whether or not the author's arguments follow sound logic. For example, let's try to identify assumptions and inferences that can be drawn from paragraph two's discussion of Vales's ideas. In this first sentence, the author uses the word "persuasive" to describe Vales's argument, from which we can infer that the author agrees with Vales's position. Then from the phrase "it takes more than efficient space heating and house design to reduce our impact on the planet," we can infer that the author believes efficient space heating and house design *do* have positive environmental impacts, just that they're not the complete answer. In the second sentence, the author suggests that well-insulated, free-running houses oriented in the right direction exemplify energy-efficient housing design, which suggests that many houses do not meet these criteria. Later in this paragraph, the author discusses everyday practices with environmental impacts (laundry practices, public transportation, sources of electricity), and thus we can infer that these factors do have a non-negligible impact on housing efficiency.

Inference questions can get particularly tricky due to common inference traps in wrong answer choices. To start, you'll want to avoid taking the author's implications too far, perhaps assuming the author is making some universal or grandiose claim beyond what's actually suggested by the passage. We would be making this logical error if we inferred from this passage that more efficient use of technology would *completely* close the energy performance gap between how we expect buildings to perform and how they actually perform, or that the total elimination of technology is the only way forward.

Another common pitfall is falling into false logic traps, like confusing a cause with an effect or an underlying assumption with a logical conclusion. Remember that if you're asked for an implication, or unstated conclusion, you'll want to identify what *must follow* based on a premise stated in the passage. If you're asked for an underlying assumption, you'll want to identify what *must precede* a certain conclusion in the text. If that assumption falls apart, then the author's assertion also falls apart. For example, when the passage states that "energy demand stems from the use of stuff," we can *infer* that the use of "stuff" has a non-negligible impact on energy consumption. Similarly, with the phrase, "when housing is constructed with ample insulation, is oriented in the right direction, and is free running," there is also an underlying *assumption* present: namely, that there exists a "right" orientation for houses that is most energy-efficient. If that's not true, then this part of the sentence falls apart, and so does the author's argument.

Another common error is drawing inferences based on situations that *could* be possible, but are not *necessary* conclusions based on passage information. An inference must be directly suggested by the passage. For example, suppose the author stated that extreme temperatures can drastically increase a building's energy consumption. We can logically infer that moderate climates tend to be associated with greater energy efficiency. We *cannot* infer that extreme cold temperatures have a greater impact on efficiency than extreme warm temperatures. *Could* this be true based on this passage assertion? Sure! *Must* it be true? No. Furthermore, just because something is possible or even likely, does not make it a necessary and logical conclusion—especially if it's based on outside knowledge. For this reason, be careful not to bring your own ideas to the table when they do not align with the author's, and try to avoid going off on an extended train of thought.

6. Function Questions

Function questions ask you how specific parts of the passage help further the author's thesis. Such questions will ask about the purpose of certain examples, statements, words, rhetorical devices, and arguments, and how they function in a paragraph or the passage as a whole. These are questions may appear as:

> What is the author's purpose for stating X?
> What is X example meant to suggest?
> The author probably mentions X for what reason?
> The passage uses X word to describe Y for what reason?
> What role does X statement play in the passage?

These questions are united by a single idea: *why* is a given component essential to the passage? To rephrase the question, what is the author trying to accomplish? You may see words and phrases like "motive," "intention," "purpose," "in order to," or "because" in questions that ask why the author made a particular rhetorical decision. The answers to some of these questions may be made explicit in the passage, requiring only the Foundations of Comprehension CARS skill, while others require you to dig deeper into the implicit, involving the Reasoning Within the Text skill. It's worthwhile to distinguish Function questions that ask about the author's own reasons for including something in the passage from Detail questions that ask for the stated explanations for an event or phenomenon in the passage. This all goes to show that it's more important to try to understand exactly what the question is asking than to rely on shortcuts to tell you what kind of question you're dealing with.

Let's consider our sample passage on the use of buildings. Suppose we were asked, "What is the author's purpose for mentioning "Cat and Vauban in Freiburg" in the final paragraph?" First, use contextual clues. Go back to the passage to locate the example that's cited, and treat it first in the context of that sentence, then in its paragraph, and then in the passage as a whole. Ask yourself, what would happen to this sentence if we removed or replaced this example? How is this example *essential* to this sentence? In this case, this an example of environmentally-friendly living models that were established forty or so years ago. Without this example, the author wouldn't have been able to make the point that a few decades ago, green living wasn't easy and required a lot of "personal commitment" on behalf of "pioneers" to achieve. To further identify the real reason behind mentioning this, let's zoom out to the paragraph level. This paragraph is essentially about how, 40 years ago, a low-impact lifestyle was considered alternative and took a great deal of personal effort, whereas today this has entered the mainstream and has been made easier. Without this example, we wouldn't have a point of reference for the author's statement that low-impact living wasn't so easy 40 years ago, so this example functions to support this claim.

Finally, let's zoom out to the passage level. A second tip for Function questions is that, ultimately, everything in the passage leads up to passage's main argument, so you can almost never go wrong by looking for answer choices that explain how an example furthers the big-picture passage thesis. This example, and this paragraph, are used by the author to show that low-impact living isn't a pipe dream, but is instead well within the realm of possibility in the mainstream. This helps the author argue that not only are individual efforts critical to reducing our collective environmental impact, but also that today this is a realistic, actionable goal for us as a society.

One potential pitfall with Function questions is being tempted by off-topic answer choices that are either not directly relevant or sound appealing but contain a crucial error. Let's go back to our sample question: What is the author's purpose for including the example of "Cat and Vauban in Freiburg?" A wrong answer choice might draw from text elsewhere in the passage, perhaps referring to Bookchin's social matrix or Vales's ideas about everyday practices like public transportation being part of the environmental impact equation. A wrong answer choice might also only slightly misinterpret the function of this example. For instance, it might state that these settlements were examples of low-impact living that took effort only at the *individual* level, when in fact it's suggested that this required social coordination at the *community* level. Keep in mind that particularly tempting answer choices may adopt language that's used in the passage, but a deeper dive reveals that part of the answer choice is too extreme or flat-out wrong.

Another potential pitfall is selecting an answer choice that's too narrow or too broad relative to the *specific* function of a passage element. With our sample question, an answer choice that's too narrow may focus too much on the nature and evolution of low-impact settlements over time. While this is certainly relevant, the author has a broader purpose in mind. An example of a choice that is too broad would be one that says this is an example of using buildings efficiently. While this may not technically be inaccurate, we're looking for an answer choice that defines the *specific* purpose of the example in mind and *directly* ties that to a bigger-picture concept. The best answer choice, then, would indicate that Cat and Vauban in Freiburg help us understand some of the history of low-impact living in order to contrast this with the feasibility of green living today, which has potential to reduce our environmental impact.

The better you're able to recognize and name rhetorical devices used throughout the passage, the better you'll be able to identify the specific functions of passage elements. For example, suppose we were asked about the function of the following text: "habits relating to how clothes are washed and dried, access to public transportation, and sourcing electricity locally." What function does this serve in the passage? Is it a counterpoint given to refute a passage argument? Is it some kind of evidence that backs up a bold claim? Is it a historical trend that the author uses to predict a future outcome? Is it a contrast meant to transition between opposing ideas? Is it a rhetorical question for the author's audience? Actually, these are examples of "local habits and practices" that the author believes could be modified to reduce individuals' environmental impact, as indicated by the statement "but one cannot ignore these lifestyle issues" and the idea that these habits are "written into larger-scale assessments of environmental impact".

One way to improve at identifying the functions of passage components is through practice. Take a sample passage, and line by line, ask yourself what purpose each sentence serves in relation to the rest of the passage. While doing so, remember that these questions aren't asking you to literally get into the author's head. Instead, they're asking you to make a reasonable, objective assessment of the "work" that each sentence does in building the overall argument. When in doubt, as we've mentioned, thinking about how the passage would change if a sentence or paragraph was removed can help illuminate its purpose, and doing so will also help you build your overall skill with passage reading and analysis, which will help on *all* types of CARS questions.

7. Support Questions

If an argument has no support or includes support that is irrelevant, defies logic, or simply isn't rooted in facts, then it's unlikely to be persuasive. CARS passages are usually full of arguments and claims, in addition to the passage's main argument, which ultimately provide fodder for **Support questions**.

Check out our sample passage on the use of buildings. The author's thesis is that action at the individual and community levels plays an important role in reducing our environmental impact through green technologies. The author supports this throughout the passage. Note, though, that other claims are found within the passage and are supported, to varying extents, by evidence, including:

"There is renewed interest in understanding how people use buildings."
"The occupants of buildings are seemingly doing something different within the built form than what the designers of the simulation programs assumed."
"When housing is constructed with ample insulation, is orientated in the right direction, and is free-running, then its energy demand stems from the use of stuff."
"Forty years ago, it took high levels of personal commitment for the pioneers of progressive initiatives at Cat and Vauban in Freiburg to live in settlements with less impact on the environment."

What ties these claims together is that they're arguable, defensible positions. The author is tasked with "proving" to us that the "energy demand stems from the use of stuff" "when houses are constructed" in the most energy-efficient way possible. Likewise, we can't simply take for granted that the Freiburg settlements took "high levels of personal commitment." However, the author may select at his or her discretion which arguments to flesh out and what level of support to provide for each claim. As you might imagine, if an author pursued *every single claim* endlessly, we could be going down rabbit holes that may or may not be critical to the thesis. All that said, how and what support the author chooses to use for each claim is completely subject to scrutiny, which is where we come in.

Support questions will ask things like:

> For which conclusion does the passage author provide the most support?
> Which of the following passage assertions is NOT clearly supported by evidence?
> What is the most serious weakness of X argument within the passage?
> What passage information provides the strongest support for X passage argument?
> According to the passage, X claim was called into question by what evidence?
> The author treats X passage information in what way?
> How could the author best clarify X passage assertion?

One common manifestation of Support questions requires you to identify claims in the passage that are *most* or *least* supported by evidence, for which you will be required to go back to the passage for each claim and rule out those that are or are not supported by evidence, respectively. You may also be asked to evaluate the evidence for a specific passage claim. In this case, you will have to locate the claim in the passage, look for evidence used directly in support of that claim, and evaluate its strength. This applies both to evidence used in support of a claim and to evidence that calls a claim into question.

Additionally, you may be asked how evidence is used or treated by the author. For example, a question might ask whether the author treats certain information as fact-based evidence, theoretical example, or irrational thought. Such questions require interpretation of what the *author* thinks of passage information based on his or her word choice and rhetorical decisions. In particular, this type of question is often seen when the author provides support for claims that may be in opposition with one another or that the author ultimately disagrees with. Additionally, questions like this are also common when the author provides evidence used to contradict certain claims. In other words, the passage may offer evidence in support of the author's claims or the claims of others, or it may provide evidence that refutes or critiques the claims of individuals or groups.

Finally, you might be asked what kind of support the author *could have* used to best support or clarify a passage assertion, or how various forms of support would *strengthen* or *weaken* passage claims.

We need two skills to address any possible variation on Support questions: first we must **recognize evidence** when we see it, and then we must **recognize how that evidence functions** to support a claim. Let's return to those passage claims we identified earlier, starting with: "There is renewed interest in understanding how people use buildings." Before we read any further, what would supporting evidence for this look like? Let's be skeptical of the idea that there's "renewed interest" in this idea, and consider what evidence might be necessary to convince us. We might be convinced if the author cited that more papers were being published on the topic, or that new coalitions had been formed to address how buildings are used. Evidence in support of a specific claim is typically nearby and, in this case, the next sentence says, "This interest is in part driven by the low-carbon agenda." Be careful here: does this provide evidence of renewed interest? Well, this provides a *cause* or *reason* for this supposed "renewed interest," but doesn't necessarily provide evidence that more people have become interested in this issue.

How about the next claim we mentioned: "The occupants of buildings are seemingly doing something different within the built form than what the designers of the simulation programs assumed." In the previous sentence, the author describes "a gulf between the energy performance of buildings as simulated at the design stage and the actual energy consumed in use," and this builds up to the claim that this energy performance gap *must* be explained by user actions. Later in this paragraph, studies are cited that report "difficulties some occupants have with building controls, and understanding the operation of heating and micro-generation technologies." Now we have some evidence that occupants quite possibly have trouble using green technologies, which could certainly result in inefficient usage and "doing something different" than what was originally intended.

To evaluate the support for an argument, we should ask ourselves whether it's directly related to the claim in question. Does the argument logically follow from this support, such that if the evidence is true, the claim is all the more likely? And is the support rooted in fact-based evidence? In the example we just used, the studies provided in support are certainly directly related and relevant to the claim about how occupants use buildings. Furthermore, they create a logical sequence, in that, if occupants in fact don't know how to use building controls, the possibility certainly follows that they might not be using the buildings as intended. Imagine if the inhabitants of a building ran around flipping the light switches on and off at random. This may be a silly example, but fabricating specific scenarios in your mind can sometimes help ground abstract logical and causal relationships in a more concrete, understandable way. Finally, the support provided here is fact-based, assuming that these studies are real, and that the author interprets them correctly. This support would be much weaker if it were based on an opinion, like if the author said something like, "no offense, but some people are just really bad at using technology." When the author cites a study that provides factual evidence, it's almost always going to be more compelling.

Now, a few words of caution. First of all, restating or paraphrasing a claim is not the same thing as evidence. For example, in paragraph two, the passage states: "To reduce our impact on the environment by moderating some small habits, everyday practices and lifestyle are important." The next sentence then states: "Technological change in the built form matters, but one cannot ignore these lifestyle issues." Is the latter sentence an example of *support* for the former? No, it's not. For one, it wouldn't be very good support because it's an opinionated claim itself. Just as importantly, however, this largely echoes the same sentiment from the prior sentence about the importance of everyday practices and lifestyle. It doesn't add any new evidence that would persuade us that the former statement is true.

As we've said before, evidence will usually be in close proximity to the claim it supports, very frequently within the same paragraph. However, this is not a hard-and-fast rule. For example, claims made in the last sentence of a paragraph may only be supported by evidence that occurs earlier in that paragraph or in the following paragraph, if at all. Big-picture, thesis-level arguments may be supported throughout the passage. There may be evidence in support of a given claim in one paragraph, and then evidence in the next paragraph provided to *refute* that claim. The moral of the story is: first look for supporting evidence immediately following a given claim, but if you don't find any, that doesn't necessarily mean evidence isn't provided. The better your understanding of the passage structure as a whole, the more likely you are to locate support effectively. Thoroughly reading and highlighting a passage before getting to the questions will prevent you from losing precious minutes scouring the passage for the information you're looking for.

Finally, when evaluating the evidence for a claim, make sure to evaluate the claim in its entirety. Just because one part of the claim is supported does not mean the entire claim is well-supported. This can be especially helpful when answering questions like, "Which of the following claims is supported by the LEAST evidence?" Sometimes there's a clear binary between arguments that are clearly supported and arguments that have no support whatsoever. Other times, a passage claim is supported insufficiently or with weak evidence, and detecting those subtleties is what will really give you an edge on the CARS section.

8. Application Questions

The Reasoning Beyond the Text skill, which tests the ability to approach new information that goes beyond the passage text and integrate it into your understanding of the passage, is challenging for many students and accounts for a full 40% of questions in the CARS section. One way this is skill is tested is through Application questions, which challenge you to take passage information and extrapolate it to new contexts.

Application questions ask you to make predictions and generalizations based on the author's positions throughout the passage, often focusing on identifying the most reasonable or likely outcome *solely* based on such positions. For example, if a CARS author posited that vegetarianism has a positive impact on the environment, it might be reasonable to conclude that the author would applaud efforts to reduce one's meat consumption, but we might not necessarily be able to conclude the author believes everyone *must* abandon meat consumption, as that might take the author's argument too far. Application questions might include:

> Which of the following answer choices exemplifies X idea from the passage?
> Which of the following answer choices would be the most effective solution for X problem in the passage?
> If the passage information is true, which of the following is the MOST reasonable example of X idea?
> The passage suggests that X individual would be LEAST likely to support which of the following ideas?
> Someone who agrees with X idea is likely to agree with what other idea?
> The author would most likely agree with which of the following ideas?

Often, Application questions are essentially asking you to identify a relationship or example that's *analogous* to an idea described in the passage, which is one of the reasons making connections between passage ideas is so critical.

The first step to solving a Reasoning Beyond the Text question is identifying that the question includes new information. Sometimes the question itself will present a new scenario, but other times it won't become clear until you look at the answer choices. As soon as you know what to look for, stop looking at the answer choices, as it's easy to get bogged down by information that seems outside the passage scope. Rather, go back to the question and re-read it if necessary. Then pause. Make sure you understand the question and translate any new information into the idea it's really getting at. Then think about what part of the passage is relevant to the question. This may require going back to the passage to find the relevant information. Once you've figured this out, craft your own answer to the question as if there were no answer choices. In other words, try to predict how the relevant part of the passage would affect the new information that's provided.

Now you're ready to look at the answer choices and apply your prediction. Simply compare your own answer to each answer choice and select the one that best matches it. If the question stem is vague or open-ended, like "Which of the following ideas would the author endorse?", then you may have to look at the answer choices first before you can make a prediction. In this case, you may need to go back to the passage for each answer choice if they each refer to different parts of the passage.

Let's try an example drawn from our sample passage about how buildings are used. We might be asked, "What type of living conditions would the author believe has the least impact on the environment?" We might be presented with four answer choices that exemplify some general principle or idea. From a careful read of the passage, we should have an idea of how the author feels about this issue. We know from the passage thesis that this author feels quite strongly that low-impact living requires a combination of efficient housing design and environmentally-conscious everyday practices. Making predictions can be very helpful for Application questions, as even a prediction that is as simple as a generalized principle can help you zero in on an "analogous" example. For this example, we want to look for an answer choice that exemplifies efficient housing design *and* environmentally-conscious everyday practices, like "A house with solar panels on its roof inhabited by a couple that chooses not to water their lawn." This is analogous to "A house with efficient housing design inhabited by people who practice an environmentally-conscious lifestyle."

One reason Application questions are so tricky is because some of these analogies will *sound* really tempting, especially if they borrow directly from passage language. For example, a wrong answer choice might describe "An old studio apartment inhabited by a single father who hand-washes all his clothes," and another might describe "A well-insulated townhouse inhabited as a co-living space by multiple families." The examples of hand-washing clothes and proper insulation are references to the passage text, but keep in mind that the entire analogy must be valid for these to be correct. If one word is off, the entire answer choice is invalidated. There's nothing in the passage that suggests an "old" apartment exemplifies efficient housing design, or that co-living is the kind of low-impact lifestyle the author is talking about. Furthermore, avoid going off of your own intuition. You may be able to convince yourself that co-living *could* be low-impact if everyone participating agrees to share resources and so forth or if you're thinking of communal housing arrangements that tend to attract people who care about the environment. However, we have to make direct connections to what the author actually says and only extrapolate within a reasonable degree. We want to make generalizations about which we can say, with confidence, the passage author would wholeheartedly endorse. We also need to be careful to recognize when the author remains neutral on an issue, which ultimately comes down to distinguishing the author's opinions from factual statements, the opinions of the others in the passage, and our own opinions.

Finally, it's worth paying some specific attention to Application questions that ask you to predict how certain actors in a passage may feel about other ideas, either those expressed elsewhere in the passage or to completely new ideas. For example, we might be asked something like, "Which of the following statements is Vales most likely to agree (or disagree) with?" The right answer choice will directly apply Vales's philosophy to a new context. Answering this question simply requires us to understand Vales's belief that individual efforts play an important role in reducing our environmental impact, and then we'll have to look for an analogous idea. In the case of "disagree" questions, of course, we'd be looking for an answer choice that most strongly contradicts Vales's beliefs. For these, common wrong answer choices might reflect other ideas in the passage, like Bookchin's beliefs, or even the author's beliefs. A wrong answer choice might also take Vales's position too far, or just slightly distort his position. Recognizing these patterns gives you a basic template and a strategic plan for approaching Application questions in the CARS section.

9. Incorporation Questions

Incorporation questions are in many ways reciprocal to Application questions, in that they ask how new information affects the passage arguments. At times, they may even invite you to question the author and to recognize potential flaws or vulnerabilities in the author's arguments. In other words, while Application questions ask you to assume that the passage information is true and valid, Incorporation questions ask you to examine each passage assertion critically. This question type asks you to analyze the author's arguments for weak spots that could either use more reinforcement, and to recognize the relationship between new pieces of information and the author's arguments. This involves determining whether a new piece of information directly supports, directly weakens, or has no effect on the author's arguments. Incorporation question stems may include things like:

> Which of the following would most directly challenge X idea from the passage?
> Assume X piece of information is true. How would this further the author's argument?
> What information could be used to verify the accuracy of the author's arguments?
> Suppose the author stated X. This is most consistent with which passage assertion?
> Which of the following best supports or contradicts X passage argument?
> Which of the following would most strengthen or weaken X passage argument?

Many questions that use verbs like "strengthen", "weaken", "agree", "disagree", "support", or "contradict", are ultimately variations on Incorporation questions. Incorporation questions may present new information in the question stem and then ask us to predict which passage assertion it affects, or how it affects a specific passage assertion. Alternatively, you may be presented with new information in the answer choices and asked which is most or least consistent with passage arguments. Regardless, Incorporation questions should be approached very similarly to Application questions. Once you recognize a Reasoning Beyond the Text question, re-read the question stem. Try to translate the new information into the general idea it represents. Then consider what part of the passage is relevant to the question and go back to that section of the text if necessary. Finally, try to make a prediction and compare each answer choice to that prediction.

Sometimes the question stem will be left vague or open-ended, such as, "Which of the following contradicts a passage assertion?" In such cases, you may need to look at the answer choices before you can make a prediction, and you may need to return to the passage for each answer choice if they each refer to different parts of the passage. With Incorporation questions in particular, you should be able to take each new piece of information, splice it into the passage, and identify whether it fits, directly contradicts, isn't clearly relevant to, or doesn't affect passage arguments. Be sure to evaluate each answer choice before moving on, unless you're squeezed for time at the end of the section.

Sometimes Incorporation questions simply ask you to identify which new piece of information is most similar to or would least change the passage thesis. Alternatively, if new information *does* affect passage arguments, how would the passage have to change in order to accommodate this new information? Once you've taken the information and spliced it into the text of the passage, does it directly support anything the author says? Does it directly contradict anything the author says? Is it even relevant?

Keep in mind that each new piece of information might provide a specific example, but your job is to consider the *idea* it represents or is most analogous to in relation to the passage, and whether that idea is in agreement with, in conflict with, or has no effect on the passage. For example, a question might ask which answer choice is consistent with a given passage assertion, and answer choices A through D might provide examples or analogies that are consistent, or inconsistent, with four different views or ideas in the passage.

Let's analyze an example, returning to our passage on the use of buildings:

Which of the following would most weaken a passage assertion?

A: Public transit options only reduce greenhouse gas emissions when a critical threshold of commuters opts in, which is unrealistic in some smaller metropolitan areas.

B: Environmentally friendly housing is more likely to have modern washing machines installed that use less water than conventional washing machines do.

C: Proper insulation is estimated to save homeowners at least twice as much in energy costs compared to lifestyle changes, like hand-washing clothes.

D: Computer algorithms do fully account for the actual lifestyle practices and behaviors of building residents in energy performance simulations.

We'll have to analyze each answer choice one-by-one because we can't make very specific predictions here. However, we can make a general prediction based on the author's primary argument. The author argues that design principles matter in reducing the environmental impact of green technology, but the collective way that individuals *use* that technology also matters. If this is the author's belief, then a statement *weakening* the author's arguments might poke holes in the idea that how individuals use green technology matters, perhaps providing evidence that users can do whatever they want with negligible effects on how energy-efficient buildings are. In other words, an answer choice that is in conflict with the passage thesis or "big picture" likely weakens passage assertions. Of course, the correct answer choice very possibly could weaken a different argument in the passage, or do so in a very different way. So we should use this prediction as a guiding principle but, as always, be open to other possibilities.

Let's take a look at the answer choices one by one. The first says that: *Public transit options only reduce greenhouse gas emissions when a critical threshold of commuters opts in, which is unrealistic in some smaller metropolitan areas.* First, let's figure out what idea this represents in relation to the passage. This answer choice gets at the idea that public transit can have a positive environmental impact, but not always, depending on how popular it is in a given area. So what does the passage say about public transportation? Public transportation is mentioned in paragraph two as one of the "local habits and practices" that affect the environmental impact of localities. We have to be very specific about what the author *literally* says. The only thing the author actually states about public transportation is that it affects environmental impact ratings. If we splice this answer choice into the passage, would it weaken this argument? Does the idea that sometimes public transit isn't particularly environmentally friendly *refute* the idea that public transportation contributes to the assessment of environmental impact? No, it doesn't. It could very well still be true that we should take public transit into account when evaluating the environmental impact of a locality because sometimes it *does* reduce greenhouse gas emissions, so it's still an example of an everyday practice that should be accounted for.

Let's check out answer choice B: *Environmentally friendly housing is more likely to have modern washing machines installed that use less water than conventional washing machines do.* Again, first let's get a sense of the idea this represents, which is that low-impact appliances, like energy-efficient washing machines, are more likely to be found in low-impact housing, thereby continuing to minimize their environmental impact. This gets at the idea of people possessing green technology, without addressing how they actually *use* it. The next step is to figure out which passage idea this is most closely related to. Paragraph two tells us that when housing design is optimized to minimize its impact, "energy demand stems from the use of stuff, the technical artifacts people use within houses, and not primarily from the material[s] it's made from." While water-conserving washing machines certainly constitute technical artifacts within the home, this doesn't refute the argument that *how* people use such technology within the home contributes to the energy performance difference of buildings. Therefore, this answer choice might be tempting if the main passage argument were misinterpreted, but it does not in fact refute any passage assertions.

How about choice C? *Proper insulation is estimated to save homeowners at least twice as much in energy costs compared to lifestyle changes, like hand-washing clothes.* In a nutshell, this answer choice suggests that housing design principles contribute more to environmental friendliness than do everyday lifestyle practices. What does the author actually say about this? The author does make reference to insulation in paragraph two, stating that, "When housing is constructed with ample insulation, is orientated in the right direction, and is free-running, then its energy demand stems from the use of stuff." In order for this new information to refute a passage assertion, the author would have had to claim that housing design features, like insulation, have a similar or smaller impact than do lifestyle practices. The author never states that housing design is unimportant, but the author also never states that it's *less* important than everyday practices and lifestyle in environmental impact. The only thing the author asserts is when housing design is optimized, *that's* when lifestyle behaviors really matter and become the major determinant of environmental impact. So if we inserted this statement into the passage, would it directly refute something the author said? No, it very well could be consistent with the author's assertions. It's also still possible that the author could find a reason to disagree with this statement, but we would need direct, textual proof to conclude that this statement refutes a passage assertion.

Finally, choice D states that: *Computer algorithms do fully account for the actual lifestyle practices and behaviors of building residents in energy performance simulations.* This answer choice basically states that when simulations make predictions about the energy performance of a building, they *do* take into account the behaviors of its occupants. What did the passage have to say about this? Paragraph one's discussion on computer simulations states that: "There is a gulf between the energy performance of buildings as simulated at the design stage and the actual energy consumed in use," and that "the occupants of buildings are seemingly doing something different...from the in-use conditions that the software algorithms model." Now, suppose we added this new statement to the passage. How would it affect this assertion? The passage assertion relies on the idea that these computer simulations are imperfect representations of actual in-use conditions by building occupants. That would certainly be weakened by the claim that these algorithms "do fully account for the actual lifestyle practices and behaviors of building residents." Clearly there's an inconsistency here, and, if this were true, the energy performance gap might not be attributable to occupant use, and the author's entire argument falls apart. Therefore, choice D is correct.

When we're given a new piece of information, we should ask ourselves, "If this is true, does it provide support for an argument that the author makes?" Alternatively, "If it is true, is one of the author's arguments exposed as flawed or no longer true?" It may help to rephrase questions that ask about information that strengthens or weakens passage claims as: "Which of the following is the author most likely to agree or disagree with?" This can help you align your thoughts with the author's beliefs and positions as you sort through potentially tricky answer choices. The better you understand major passage arguments, the better equipped you'll be to handle Reasoning Beyond the Text questions, which are some of the toughest in the CARS section.

Remember that the point of learning about CARS question types isn't to recite back a list of question types and all the ways in which they may be asked on the fly. Rather, our goal is for you to be able to take any CARS question and understand that this question is *really* asking for the main idea, or for the scenario least consistent with the author's arguments. With an understanding of the question under your belt, the next step is to go back to the passage, look for the passage arguments in question, and go from there. In other words, our goal is for insight into CARS questions to set you up for the *actions* needed to answer them.

10. Must-Knows

> AAMC CARS skills:
  – Foundations of Comprehension (30%): direct elements of the text; either basic components or inferred meaning.
  – Reasoning Within the Text (30%): relationships among claims in the passage, support for claims, function of statements/arguments.
  – Reasoning Beyond the Text (40%): how would (a) outside information affect the author's argument or (b) the author's argument generalize to other situations?

> Main Idea questions ask about major themes and the purpose of the passage.
  – What is the main idea of the passage?
  – What is the author's central thesis?
  – What is the primary purpose of the passage?
  – What title would best capture the main idea of the passage?
  – What is the most likely background or profession of the author?
  – Who is the intended audience?

> Opinion questions ask about the author's opinion, and also the opinions, attitudes, perspectives, and motivations of other people mentioned in the passage and how these are related.
  – What is the author's response to X topic within the passage?
  – Which most accurately describes the author's attitude towards X topic in the passage?
  – X assertion in the passage is least or most consistent with which point of view?

> Detail questions ask you about details, assertions, and relationships that are explicitly stated in the passage.
  – How is the word X used in the passage?
  – What is the meaning of the word X in the passage?
  – According to the passage, what is the cause of X, or what is the effect of Y?
  – According to the author, why did X happen?
  – Which of the following assertions does the author make in the passage?
  – According to the passage, what is the focus of X?
  – What examples of X are given in the passage?

> Inference questions ask about passage assertions, relationships, and assumptions that are implied, requiring an extra layer of interpretation.
  – What does X passage statement imply about Y?
  – The wording of the passage suggests what about X?
  – The author seems to be concerned that X will do what?
  – The passage suggests that the author believes X for what reason?
  – On the basis of the passage, understanding X might lead to what conclusion?
  – Implicit in the passage is what assumption?
  – One can infer what about X?

> Function questions get at why certain examples and rhetorical devices are used in the passage, largely focusing on how they ultimately further the main argument.
  – What is the author's purpose for stating X?
  – What is X example meant to suggest?
  – The author probably mentions X for what reason?
  – The passage uses X word to describe Y for what reason?
  – What role does X statement play in the passage?

> Support questions ask about support for arguments in the passage, what support is used, if any, and how well is it used to bolster passage claims.
  – For which conclusion does the passage author provide the most support?
  – Which of the following passage assertions is NOT clearly supported by evidence?
  – What is the most serious weakness of X argument within the passage?
  – What passage information provides the strongest support for X passage argument?

- According to the passage, X claim was called into question by what evidence?
- The author treats X passage information in what way?
- How could the author best clarify X passage assertion?

> Application questions require extrapolating passage information and opinions to new information.

- Which of the following answer choices exemplifies X idea from the passage?
- Which of the following answer choices would be the most effective solution for X problem in the passage?
- If the passage information is true, which of the following is the MOST reasonable example of X idea?
- The passage suggests that X individual would be LEAST likely to support which of the following ideas?
- Someone who agrees with X idea is likely to agree with what other idea?
- The author would most likely agree with which of the following ideas?

> Incorporation questions ask you to assess how new information affects your interpretation of the passage.

- Which of the following would most directly challenge X idea from the passage?
- Assume X piece of information is true. How would this further the author's argument?
- What information could be used to verify the accuracy of the author's arguments?
- Suppose the author stated X. This is most consistent with which passage assertion?
- Which of the following best supports or contradicts X passage argument?
- Which of the following would most strengthen or weaken X passage argument?

Applied Practice

The best MCAT practice is realistic, with detailed analytics to help you assess where things went wrong. For those reasons, we recommend completing practice questions in an online setting that simulates the real MCAT interface, and using the analytics provided to help you decide how to best move your studies forward.

CARS does not require knowledge of specific subject areas, but it does require development of strong test-taking skills. To ensure you are honing those skills as you work through this book, we suggest you go online after wrapping up each chapter and generate a Qbank Practice Set of 2-3 CARS passages to practice and review. While not every chapter of this book is directly applicable to CARS, regular CARS practice is key to test day success.

As a further supplement, given the importance of active learning for effective studying, we also suggest that you consult the Must-Knows at the end of each chapter of this Reasoning text as a basis for creating a study sheet. This is not a sheet to memorize in the more traditional sense of content memorization, but rather a quick reference of the most important strategies for you to refer to during and after practice in your early prep. Frequently revisiting the most important strategies for the MCAT - in both CARS and the Sciences - will help you continue to improve your performance.

This page left intentionally blank.

Answering CARS Questions

CHAPTER 7

0. Introduction

One of the most counterintuitive aspects of the CARS section is that it's difficult to predict which passages will be harder than others. Difficulty doesn't neatly correlate with the passage topic. You could see "hard" passages with "easier" questions, and easy passages with harder questions. There's no single trick to answering CARS questions, so the issue of "how to answer CARS questions" can't be answered in isolation from the reading skills needed to analyze a passage effectively. Of these skills, two of the more important ones include picking up on its main ideas and identifying its arguments. These skills build the foundation for approaching CARS questions. However, another important piece of the puzzle is familiarity with the wording of CARS questions, how to determine the task that question sets for you, and how to apply your knowledge of the passage to answer it effectively. We'll discuss those themes in this chapter, along with common wrong answer patterns and how to effectively use process of elimination.

1. Getting Started

Our goal here is not to present a one-size-fits-all formula because there simply isn't one. Instead, our goal in this chapter is to *explicitly* discuss reading comprehension and analysis skills that, as critical readers, we usually apply *implicitly* to dissect our reading material. When we're presented with new information, our brains automatically interpret it in a way that makes sense to us. Doing so is fundamental to understanding what a question is asking. In CARS, we will often need to rephrase or paraphrase the question stem in a way that guides us towards the *action* of answering the question.

As is often the case, it is helpful to discuss these techniques with a specific passage in mind. For the first part of this chapter, we will use the following passage on economic inequality:

> Amid instability in economics and social relations, it was plain for all to see that there were problems in American society. Naturally, contemporaries questioned what exactly was wrong. With rigid class formation, America seemed to have developed the very conditions that were supposed to be left behind in Europe, so observers were left scrambling for answers. People of diverse political persuasions and social

backgrounds commented on the current state of affairs. There was general consensus that indeed there was a problem—in fact, most industrialized countries of this era struggled with the "social question," namely increasing poverty and class unrest. However, the suggested remedies for the problem proved contentious among Americans. Views on what exactly had gone wrong had huge implications for the nature of economic inequality and how best to address it.

One response to the economic hard times was reactionary. A collection of economists, businessmen, and editors came to support classical liberalism and traditional economics. Liberal reformers like E.L. Godkin and William Graham Sumner believed that economic and social issues could be solved with a return to the values of classical economics, which, they argued, had been forgotten during the Civil War. Seeing a large tariff, taxes, and Reconstruction measures, liberals argued that the state needed to go back to its minimal antebellum role. Most importantly, the individual should remain the primary economic actor with no outside interference. With such biases, they stuck with the free labor view that low-paid wage labor was only a temporary condition meant for young men. In time, if they were frugal, they would be able to accumulate enough capital to start their own businesses and escape the wage system. The classical liberals maintained that if workers would only learn to save their money, economic problems could be alleviated, a view woefully inadequate for modern society.

While the liberals took their influence from traditional ideals, the New School's inspiration came from what they considered a more modern source, the German Historical School. At the core of their creed was a rejection of the liberal view that society was merely a collection of individuals. Rather, as Richard Ely articulated, society was its own organism that had different needs than its individual parts. Since society was an organism, poverty among one class inhibited the development of the whole social body. Using this logic, the New School rejected the belief that wages and profits were at odds. Alleviating poverty and economic inequality would serve as an economic stimulus, as the working class could therefore have more disposable income. With better economic conditions, workers would have no reason to strike, leading to a peaceful and prosperous society.

To advance this theory, the New School had to break the notion that wages and profits were at odds with each other. That line of thinking assumes that workers are only producers and not consumers as well. As Gunton wrote, "consumption is the economic basis of production," and "the laborer is as important a factor in the one as he is in the other." Therefore, widespread low wages result in a limited market because the working class can only consume necessities. This hurts the capitalists, because it eliminates the consumer base and prevents the expansion of markets. Gunton argued that wages did not represent a cost, but an investment. Higher wages were a temporary expense that would provide capitalists with an expanded market for their goods. This investment would eventually return to them in the form of profits.

Adapted from Leccese, S. (2017). Economic Inequality and the New School of American Economics. Religions, 8(6), 99 under CC BY 4.0.

Suppose we were asked, *Which of the following statements, if true, would most weaken the claim that "if workers would only learn to save their money, economic problems could be alleviated?"?* This question asks us to determine which answer choice would most *refute* or *weaken* the belief that economic woes would be bygones if workers would *only* learn to save their money. In other words, we need to look for an answer choice that punches a hole in that claim, indicating that workers saving their money wouldn't necessarily alleviate economic issues.

Here's another, more hypothetical, question to consider: *If a government sought to create a program to alleviate poverty, a New School economist would be LEAST likely to approve of which program?* Our approach here will largely apply to most, non-hypothetical CARS questions. Start by paraphrasing the question stem and creating an **action plan**. To answer this question, we need to identify the core of what New School economic thought says about governmental programs to alleviate poverty, and then use that as a filter to evaluate the answer choices and to pick out the one that is *least* consistent with the New School approach. Another action plan is to identify the three answer choices that describe programs that these economists would approve of. The remaining answer choice, then, would be the correct answer.

Paraphrasing question stems in an action-oriented way goes hand-in-hand with understanding the purpose of a question: what is it *really* getting at? For example, a question that asks for an appropriate title for a given CARS passage is really asking you to identify the main idea of the passage. A question that asks you about the author's profession or background is really getting at the author's perspective and motivations. Additionally, a question that asks why the author included a particular example to support an argument is really getting at how arguments are structured and supported by persuasive examples. A question that asks you what the author thinks about a given idea is getting at the author's opinions within the passage. Thus, by interpreting a question stem, you're not just understanding the literal meaning of the question; you're trying to identify what concept or skill it's testing, and what you need to do in order to figure out the answer it's looking for.

Let's return to those two questions we just discussed. First, consider *Which of the following statements would most weaken the claim that "if workers would only learn to save their money, economic problems could be alleviated"?* Clearly, this question is asking about how arguments are supported, or in this case, challenged. In fact, the question directly gives us the argument we need to evaluate, so we might be able to answer it on its own terms, without returning to the passage. However, if we want more context, we'll want to zoom in on this quote in paragraph two, so that we can focus on the content of the claim itself, identify who makes the claim, and figure out what evidence, if any, is used to support it within the passage. Then we can pick out which answer choice is *least* consistent with this claim.

Let's again consider that second question. *If a government sought to create a program to alleviate poverty, a New School economist would be LEAST likely to approve of which program?* Again, our task is to figure out what the New School economists think about how to address poverty, and then apply this to the answer choices that we're given. At this point, we may need to reflect more globally on New School economists' positions throughout the passage, meaning that we need to locate a specific position on this issue within the passage that we can use to predict their thoughts on such governmental programs. The New School is discussed in paragraphs three and four, and, in particular, their position on alleviating poverty is introduced in the third paragraph, so we'll want to focus our attention on this section of the passage. Thus, by understanding the purpose of the question at hand, we can give ourselves a concrete task and begin to formulate a strategic approach.

One reason why we focus so much on interpreting questions is that some questions are easy to misunderstand. The most classic examples of this, are questions with negative or opposite terms like "not" or "weaken" or "least." Even more confusing are questions with double negatives, such as "Which of the following is LEAST likely to weaken the author's claims?" or "Which of the following does NOT contradict the author's beliefs?" With questions like these, it can be especially helpful to translate the question in the most straightforward way possible. For example, we can remove the negative terms in both of these questions by rephrasing them in the affirmative as "Which of the following is most consistent with the author's claims?"

Suppose we're given a question with just one negative term. Let's use an example that isn't related to our CARS passage, just so that we can see this idea more clearly without distractions. For example: "Which of the following does NOT support the author's claim that the legal driving age should be lowered?" We can rephrase this by flipping how we think about the question to focus on support for the opposite of the author's claim, in which case we might look for answer choices that *do* support the idea that the legal driving age should stay the same or be raised. But we have to be careful here, because information that fails to support a claim does not necessarily advocate for the opposite position. It might just be irrelevant, or point out a flaw in the author's reasoning. For example, the author might argue that the legal driving age should be lowered because 11-year-olds can qualify for farm work licenses to operate farm machinery in some states. This would be challenged by information that the youngest age one can qualify for such a license is 13 or 14, depending on the state. As the information undermines the author's reasoning, it fails to support the author's claim, matching up with what the original wording of the question asked us about.

However, that piece of information isn't an argument that the legal driving age should stay the same or should be raised. This question is a great example, but, more generally, just remember that it can be really helpful to "translate" a question to avoid stumbling over confusing wording. It is also important to remember that paraphrasing can take you away from the original meaning of the question, so if you find yourself in a situation where none of the answer choices really fit, it can help to go back and take a look at the original phrasing, keeping an eye out for similar issues.

What do you do when you're completely stumped? Well, one thing you can do right now is to be proactive and practice identifying and working through CARS questions. You're unlikely to encounter a CARS question on your MCAT wholly unlike anything you've ever seen before. Thus, it's in your best interest to pick up on question phrasing and question types that make you more likely to misinterpret the question. Are some questions harder for you than others? Do you tend to forget the words "NOT" or "LEAST" in question stems? Noticing these patterns will allow you to practice rephrasing questions that you've been missing consistently, which is a small change you can make that will add up over the course of an entire CARS section.

In addition, sometimes a question stem will be vague, but you can **use the answer choices** to help figure out what it's asking. If you approach an intimidating question from the perspective of "How can I rule these answers in or out?", it may become more clear what the question is asking. Likewise, if the passage text is confusing or if you doubt whether you've interpreted it correctly, the way questions are asked may help you retroactively decipher the passage, or confirm your understanding of the text.

Let's briefly discuss strategies for **Roman numeral questions**. Each CARS section will have a number of questions with several answers indicated by Roman numerals, and the answer choices require you to determine which Roman numerals are correct. As you can imagine, these questions can be tricky because they require you to make multiple determinations within a single question. There's no secret trick to these questions, but we recommend addressing each Roman numeral option one-by-one, starting with the option that occurs in exactly two answer choices, and deciding if it's correct. If you're certain that it *does* satisfy the question stem, then you can eliminate the two choices that do *not* include that Roman numeral by striking them out using the strikeout tool. If you're certain that it does NOT satisfy the question stem, then strike out that Roman numeral in the question stem *and* the two answer choices that contain that Roman numeral. In either case, you've eliminated half of the answers and it is unlikely that you'd need to check more than one more numeral to get to the correct answer.

In the worst-case scenario, if you're unable to interpret or translate a question off the bat, it's okay to forge ahead, as sometimes its meaning becomes clear as you review the answer choices, or think about the passage in new ways. If you're not certain of your answer and could benefit from more time, flag that question so you can review it later. However, never leave a question blank, as there are no penalties for guessing, and there's a 25% probability that you'll get a question right by chance!

2. Working Through the Question

After understanding a question, and determining what it's looking for, the next step is to decide if you can predict the correct answer right away, if you need to return to the passage, or if you need to start by evaluating the answer choices.

Let's return to our first sample question:

Which of the following statements, if true, would most WEAKEN the claim that "if workers would only learn to save their money, economic problems could be alleviated"?

A. Investment knowledge is correlated with wealth.

B. Economic inequality has not been shown to be driven by an excess of savings.

C. Most economic crises are precipitated by excessive consumer debt.

D. Workers are not paid enough to cover their living expenses.

We're looking for a statement that, if true, would mean that workers saving their money might *not* be the antidote to economic woes. Since the quote from the passage is provided, we can evaluate this claim on its own without needing to return to the passage. By translating any CARS question stem into language that's unambiguous, and by clearly identifying what we're looking for in a correct answer choice, we can predict what the correct answer will look like, since we know exactly what we're looking for.

At this point, we just need to be able to identify a single flaw in each wrong answer choice to eliminate wrong answers. Evaluating answer choices as your first step is a necessary strategy for questions that ask "Which of the following supports or weakens some idea or claim?" It would be impossible to predict all possible examples of acceptable answer choices. That said, if you encounter a question that is clearly asking about the passage's main idea, it might be helpful to take a minute and try to frame what you think the correct answer would be in your own words before delving into the answer choices. The basic routine stays the same: read the question, interpret it, and make a reasonable **prediction** about what you're looking for in the correct answer choice. Then either move directly to the answer choices or go back to the passage if you need a refresher on what the question is asking about. As you examine the answer choices, it may also be possible that you will need to return to the passage to evaluate each in the context of the passage. Furthermore, elimination can be an effective strategy for arriving at the correct answer simply by identifying the three incorrect choices!

Let's go one by one, and remember, our goal is to eliminate three answer choices that support, or are at least consistent with, the idea that money-saving would alleviate economic problems, while the answer we're looking for punches a hole in this claim. Answer choice A says that investment knowledge correlates with wealth. Just like we did with the question stem, let's try to translate this into simpler language. This tells you something about wealthy people. It's described as a correlation, so we don't know whether being wealthy causes you to know about investments, or if knowing about investments causes you to be wealthy. So, how does this relate to the idea that low-wage workers need to learn to save money in order to solve economic problems? Well, it's kind of irrelevant. It just tells you something about what traits correlate with wealth. In that sense, it's consistent with the idea that teaching workers to save money and learn about investments could help them become wealthy, but it definitely doesn't weaken that claim, so we can eliminate choice A.

Choice B says that economic inequality is *not* driven by an excess of savings. Just like our question stem, let's see what happens when we eliminate the word "*not*." What if saving money *did* drive economic inequality? Well, that would suggest that workers saving money would *not* solve economic problems—it would create them! But remember, we removed the "*not*" from this answer choice, so if we stick to the original meaning of choice B, we would arrive at the opposite conclusion: that workers saving money would *not* drive economic inequality, and thus this *would* help solve economic problems. Thus, choice B supports the claim in question, and we can eliminate it.

Choice C says that economic crises are precipitated by excessive consumer debt. How does *debt* relate to savings? Well, it's the opposite term, so we can re-interpret this answer choice as a *lack* of savings precipitating, or causing, economic crises. The claim in the question stem states that saving money solves economic problems, which is consistent with the suggestion that *not* saving money causes economic problems. So we can eliminate choice C as well.

Before we commit to choice D, let's examine it to see if it weakens the claim in question. Choice D tells us that workers aren't paid enough to cover living expenses. What does this mean in terms of savings? Well, this tells us that workers aren't even *able* to save because every dime goes towards supporting themselves, which contradicts the claim that workers need to exhibit better financial self-regulation and learn to save more judiciously. Rather, it's not that they don't *try* to save—it's that they *can't*, even if they wanted to! Thus, choice D is our best option, as it does indeed weaken the claim that workers not learning to save is the root of economic problems.

Unlike what we saw in this question, sometimes you will need to return to the passage to retrieve more information. Reading thoroughly and highlighting strategically will help you set yourself up for this in advance, by enabling you to identify where to return to in the passage efficiently when needed. In addition to knowing where to go in the passage, the other half of the challenge is knowing when it's worth returning to the passage. Sometimes you may be able to predict the answer to questions about main ideas without returning to the passage, or a claim from the passage may be directly quoted. However, if you're asked to examine or identify examples or details from the passage, more often than not it's a good idea to quickly locate and consult the relevant paragraph.

Let's consider our second sample question:

> If a government sought to create a program to alleviate poverty, a New School economist would be LEAST likely to approve of which program?
>
> A. A monthly stipend of several hundred dollars provided to all families
>
> B. The elimination of income taxes for low-income families
>
> C. The reduction of corporate taxes to improve profits
>
> D. A requirement for companies to allow their workers to unionize and bargain collectively

Here, we're really being asked about New School economists' views on programs to alleviate poverty. Again, once we've interpreted the question and know what we're looking for, there are three things that we need to do: 1) **make a prediction**; 2) **go back to the passage if needed**; and 3) **evaluate the answer choices**. To be able to predict an answer, we need to summarize the New School economic views in the passage as they relate to this question. Then we'll want to examine each answer choice and decide if each is consistent or inconsistent with New School economic views. Returning to the passage, the New School economic philosophy is outlined in paragraphs three and four.

Paragraph three's main idea is that New School economic views were based on the idea that society is more than groups of individual people, but rather is its own organism with its own needs. New School economists believe poverty is bad for society, and that alleviating it is good for society and for the economy. Furthermore, economic problems aren't caused by wages that are too high, but rather the opposite. Increasing workers' wages gives them more money to invest in the economy as consumers, and this results in greater profits. So what would such economists think about government programs to alleviate poverty? They clearly think that alleviating poverty is good for society, and that higher wages are good for the economy because more money is being spent by workers. Let's check out those answer choices, and again recall that the correct answer choice is the one that New School economists would *least* support. So let's try to eliminate three answer choices and find one that *doesn't* boil down to helping low-wage workers out.

Turning to choice A, what would the New School economic philosophy say about a monthly stipend of several hundred dollars provided to all families? The key words here are "stipend" and "all." "All families" by definition includes low-income families. This is consistent with the New School philosophy that supplementing the pay of low-wage workers will help reduce poverty and economic inequality and is good for the economy as a whole. Thus, New School economists would probably be in support of choice A in theory. Remember, we're looking for something *inconsistent* with their beliefs, so let's eliminate choice A.

Choice B is a related idea: that income taxes ought to be eliminated for low-income families. This would relieve some of low-wage workers' financial burden, and perhaps they'd have a little extra money to spare. The result of this would be a financial benefit to the working poor, which is completely consistent with New School economic thought. Let's eliminate answer choice B as well.

Choice C would reduce taxes for corporations to stimulate profits. What exactly did New School economists propose we do to improve profits? They indicated we should increase wages and provide financial relief to the working poor, not necessarily to corporations. Unless corporate tax reductions *directly* resulted in increased wages, and there's no indication that they would, New School economists would be unlikely to support this effort. So let's keep choice C in mind as a potential answer.

Finally, choice D describes a requirement for companies to allow workers to unionize and bargain collectively. Collective bargaining would allow workers to demand higher wages, which aligns with New School logic that increasing worker wages reduces economic disparities and stimulates profits. Therefore, let's eliminate choice D and return to choice C, which describes a program that New School economists are least likely to approve, making it our correct answer.

Before we move on, though, there's a point we should make about choice C. The idea that cutting corporate taxes will reduce poverty by boosting profits might seem familiar to you if you follow American politics, because it's been a pretty influential idea over the last 30 or 40 years. However, this question is *not* asking you to take a stance on this issue. This answer choice stands out from the others just because it doesn't directly affect workers. From the point of view of the MCAT, maybe cutting corporate taxes would eventually help low-wage workers, and maybe it wouldn't. However, that's beyond our scope; it involves too many extra leaps of logic and doesn't line up with what the passage tells us about the New School economists. Therefore, this answer choice reinforces two important lessons: don't get bogged down in possible downstream implications of an answer choice and, as hard as it can be, try to keep your own personal convictions out of it.

3. CARS Questions in Practice

Becoming comfortable with CARS questions won't happen overnight. There's a misconception that CARS isn't possible to "study" for in the same way that you'd study other MCAT sections. Studying for CARS doesn't involve growing your content knowledge. Instead, studying for CARS means developing, practicing, and troubleshooting your approach so that, no matter what passages you encounter, you'll have seen enough passages to recognize common patterns and feel completely confident in your approach. This actually has some non-trivial overlap with preparing for the science sections of the MCAT, and, most importantly, these are skills that you can deliberately practice.

There are two broad categories of passage practice: **timed and untimed**. Untimed practice is especially useful for developing your approach and building familiarity with CARS questions. Note that you *can* use a clock during untimed practice if you want, just to get a sense of how you're doing timing-wise, even if you're not trying to stick to the exact pace of the MCAT itself. Timed practice may be intimidating at first, but it's valuable to mimic testing conditions as you get closer to your test date so that you can focus on applying your reasoning skills efficiently. Each time you sit down for a practice session, set discrete goals for yourself, and work on one skill at a time. Not only is this helpful if you feel like you've been hitting a plateau, but it also helps disrupt the false belief that it's impossible to work intentionally to improve on the CARS section.

When it comes to CARS questions, one of the most obvious skills you can work on is improving passage comprehension. Once you're on solid footing with the passage, your next goal might be to become more proficient with predicting what questions will ask and, subsequently, interpreting and understanding questions. Practice rephrasing question stems in ways that make sense to you. As you begin developing this skill, you might even take the time to literally write down your translation. Notice when this is and isn't helpful, making a special note of difficult questions that particularly benefit from this step. Be vigilant for questions with opposite words like *not* or *except*, and for questions that are easily misunderstood. Try different ways of rephrasing questions you have difficulty with. Once you've found a method that works for you, apply it consistently in practice so that it'll be second nature on your MCAT.

Once you understand the question, you'll then have to decide if you need to return to the passage, if you can predict an answer right away, or if you can make a beeline for the answer choices. Consider titrating this method by reading a passage and then answering all of the questions without ever returning to the passage. Then see how you did. Which questions did you *think* you needed to return to the passage for, but you didn't really need to? Were there things in the passage you overlooked, like opinions or main ideas, that could save you time by not needing to return to the passage for? What question types should you have returned to the passage for, and why? How successful would you have been at quickly locating the relevant parts of the passage to return to?

After a few rounds like this, try returning to the passage for every single question. Compare the amount of time it takes to answer questions, and how well you do on those questions, to when you forced yourself not to return to the passage. How often were you successful at returning to right parts of the passage, and how often did you end up focusing on the wrong thing? How useful was your highlighting in directing you to the relevant parts of the passage? How much actual re-reading did you have to do to answer each question? After you've tried this, titrate back down so that you limit yourself to choosing only three or four questions for which you'll return to the passage. Did you end up returning to the passage for the right questions? Do you wish you'd returned to the passage for more or fewer questions? How did this affect your timing and performance? At the end of the day, there's no right or wrong answer as to which or how many questions are worth going back to the passage for, but there is a best way for you. Importantly, the only way to identify your best plan of action is to practice and troubleshoot until you feel more comfortable identifying when (and where!) to return to the passage for information.

If you understand a question and have the information you need, can you predict the answer? This doesn't necessarily mean predicting a detailed answer, but rather approaching the answer choices armed with an idea of what you're looking for. This is particularly useful for questions that assess main ideas, or that require an understanding of main ideas or the author's views. By heading over to the answer choices with an idea of what you're looking for, you're less likely to fall for trap answers or be thrown off by misleading answer choices. Another skill you can develop is your ability to evaluate answer choices. Just like the question stem, interpreting answer choices in ways that make sense to you is essential to understanding what concept each answer choice represents and how it relates to the question at hand.

You know, at this point, that practice in CARS is crucial for both increasing your accuracy on questions as well as building your familiarity with the MCAT itself. As for the latter, ideally almost nothing on your MCAT should feel entirely unknown to you, and that's certainly true of the computer-based tools featured on the MCAT interface. Practice strategic use of the highlighting, strikeout, and flagging tools. The flagging tool is especially important with regard to analyzing how accurate you are at predicting whether you've answered a question correctly. Do you flag questions when you're less than 50% certain in your answer? More than 50%? How do your predictions correlate with the likelihood of you answering a given question correctly? Also, analyze whether you've been changing your answers as you review questions. Are you replacing wrong answer selections with correct ones, or do you second guess yourself and change correct answers to the wrong ones? Doubting your answer when there's no reason to can not only result in selecting the wrong answer choice, but it can also steal time that you could be using to review other questions.

When it comes to CARS practice, focus on **the quality of your practice and review over the quantity.** The right number of practice questions is the exact number it takes to feel confident enough in your reasoning skills to achieve your goal score. For this reason, it's extremely important to schedule review time into your prep as another necessary component of MCAT prep, and this review should include CARS. After any practice passage, perform a post-mortem: what went wrong and why? The CARS section is unique as it not's content knowledge-based, so you're really asking what reading deficiencies or reasoning flaws impacted your score. What types of questions or passages or reasoning skills tend to give you the most trouble—and why? Is it valuable for you to identify certain question types, such as those that ask about statements that strengthen or weaken passage claims, for example, so you can be on the lookout for them and troubleshoot your approach or apply special care to them during practice? Use the information you collect during review to try something different during practice when something isn't quite working. This will help you get over the hump when you feel like you've started to hit a plateau and don't know what to do next.

4. Introduction to Wrong Answer Patterns

Answering CARS questions can sometimes feel a little bit like a shot in the dark. It's tempting to think of answering CARS questions as an all-or-nothing phenomenon, but instead, we should use an approach in which we gather evidence that supports one answer choice, while collecting evidence that refutes others, ultimately increasing the likelihood that our selection is correct.

There are two ways to approach answering CARS questions: **zero in on the *correct* answer choice** by gathering evidence in the passage, making a prediction, and then looking for the answer choice best supported by the passage or identify and eliminate ***wrong* answer choices**. If you can eliminate one wrong answer choice, you've boosted your chance of getting the question correct to 33%. If you can eliminate two wrong answer choices, probability dictates you'll get these questions right about half of the time, just by luck alone. If you can eliminate three wrong answer choices, you've got the correct answer!

Eliminating wrong answer choices is particularly helpful when you're feeling stuck on a question. If you aren't quite sure what the right answer looks like, instead consider what the *wrong* answers look like. Similar to how CARS questions follow a fixed set of patterns that we can categorize into eight different question types, answer flaws in the CARS section also follow particular patterns. Generally speaking, wrong answers fall into one of three categories: (1) the wrong answer choice will very directly **contradict** something stated *explicitly* in the passage; (2) it will draw an **incorrect inference** or interpretation from *implicit* passage information; or (3) it will **improperly integrate or apply new information** to the passage.

As we proceed, keep in mind that our goal isn't to provide shortcuts or "rules" for how to go about eliminating wrong answer choices. Instead, the key point is that every wrong answer choice was written intentionally in such a way that it involves at least one error. However, we can't make sense of a question or its answer choices outside of the context of the passage. In other words, to understand why an answer choice is "extreme" or "opposite" or has "faulty logic," we *must* evaluate it in the context of the passage. If we don't thoroughly examine the context, we risk eliminating an answer choice that only *seems* extreme or like it has faulty logic. Remember, focusing your efforts on understanding the major arguments of the passage is the number one thing you can do to help you answer questions correctly. Once you've done this, identifying answer flaws will help you avoid tempting and tricky answer choices so you can feel confident in your answer.

One exception to this is if you are short on time at the end of the section, and only have a few minutes or seconds to answer any outstanding questions. In this case, you can lean on wrong answer patterns to help steer you away from choices that are unlikely to be correct. In all other cases, take the time to fully vet each answer choice before coming to a conclusion. Ultimately, only one answer choice will be right, and three answer choices will always be wrong, so choosing the correct answer choice is tantamount to eliminating the others—these are two sides of the same coin.

5. Contradiction Answer Patterns

One of the more common patterns for answer flaws in the CARS section is for the answer choice to contradict information from the passage. This is especially common for Detail questions, in which case the right answer will be *directly* supported by the passage text, and wrong answers will either be directly contradicted in the passage or not supported by any passage information. As always, let's consider a practice passage:

Monster of the Week (MOTW)-style television shows involve antagonists that appear in only one episode. Baba Yaga affords a wondrous form in a MOTW television show. An ambiguous Slavic figure, her origins stem from primeval sources in a Russian pantheon where she plays mythological and ritualistic roles of earth mother and death guardian. With her iconic huge nose, iron teeth, her mortar and pestle flying contraption, and her chicken-legged hut, she is distinctive and easily recognized. In Russian folktales such as "Baba Yaga," "The Feather of Finist the Bright Falcon," "The Tsar-Maiden," and "Vasilisa the Beautiful," she may simultaneously be known as a witch, grandmother, cannibal, examiner, and helper. Never the protagonist of tales, Baba Yaga may be both an antagonist and a helper, a threat to life and a benefactor of light. Her wonder, thus, is marked by being awful and full of awe.

Since the 19th century, Baba Yaga's presence has spread from Russia to the West. She may be thought of as a constellation of iconic features and ambiguous functions that together may coalesce and reconfigure in an array of genres, themes, modes, and media. Indeed, she has become a transcultural figure associated with a wide array of popular, global products and productions from picture books to sneakers to punk rock to video games. An International Fairy Tale Filmography (IFTF) search brings up thirteen Baba Yaga films over the past seven decades, mostly Soviet, Russian, or Eastern Bloc productions and two from the United Kingdom. This indicates that she maintains some bearing over space and time and adapts to various media and cultures.

Baba Yaga's appearances on television remain quite limited, especially outside of the film rebroadcasts and animated shows on Soviet and Russian TV; however, the Fairy Tale Teleography and Visualizations (FTTV) database does list a few Baba Yaga television shows from Western countries, including the United States and Canada. Given the small number of Western Baba Yaga television shows, it is striking that they contain a perceptible pattern; whether an anime, supernatural drama, or children's mystery episode, Baba Yaga is portrayed as an antagonist in Western MOTW shows.

MOTW programming's strict requirements specify that each "monster" only appears in one episode and does not become part of an ongoing story arc. The threat catalyzes social relations between protagonists in order to confront the monster's deformity and deviance. When Baba Yaga takes the monster position, her wondrous ambiguity lessens as her tendency for deformity and self-interest makes her yet another MOTW villain to be defeated. Regrettably, we see Baba Yaga's traditional form affiliated with Slavic folk narrative being appropriated by the Western MOTW shows to serve as a pop culture form, robbing Baba Yaga of her inherent ambiguity.

Passage adapted from: Rudy, J., & McDonald, J. (2016). Baba Yaga, Monsters of the Week, and Pop Culture's Formation of Wonder and Families through Monstrosity. Humanities, 5(2), 40 under CC BY.

A Detail question might ask us:

Which of the following are NOT cited as examples of Baba Yaga's ambiguity?

A. Helper and antagonist.

B. Deformity and deviance.

C. Earth mother and death guardian.

D. Witch and grandmother.

We know this is a Detail question because it asks us to identify examples that are provided *in* the passage. Since this is a "NOT" question, the incorrect answer choices will list examples that *are* provided in the passage, and the correct answer choice will either list examples that the author expressly tells us are *not* examples of Baba Yaga's ambiguity or ones that are simply not supported as examples of her ambiguity.

Our approach for answering a question like this one is the same approach we'd use for Detail questions in general: once we have read and understood the question, we should locate the relevant part of the passage and find information that supports or refutes each answer choice. Baba Yaga's traditionally ambiguous nature is discussed predominantly in the first paragraph, where several contrasting sets of terms are given as examples characterizing her as both a "helper and antagonist," an "earth mother and death guardian," and a "witch and grandmother." Thus, answer choices A, C, and D are all found directly in the passage and are therefore wrong. Answer choice B we know must be the correct answer then, but why? Well, the last paragraph makes reference to Baba Yaga's "deformity and deviance," but context is essential: these terms aren't used as an example of her ambiguity. Rather, they are cited as two negative aspects of Baba Yaga that Western Monster of the Week-style television shows use in order to portray her simply as a villain.

Notice how this correct answer choice is unlike the other answers. While answer choices A, C, and D list sets of contrasting terms—such as helper versus antagonist, or earth mother versus death guardian—the correct answer choice contains two similar terms. In addition, the incorrect answer choices were located in paragraph one, while the correct answer choice referred to the last paragraph. Thus, if three answer choices are similar and one is unlike the rest in a significant way, investigate that difference further and see if it provides a clue that'll help you solve the question. As long as the three answer choices actually *are* similar—meaning, as long as you haven't misinterpreted their meaning—it's quite possible that the fourth choice, the "odd man out," is the correct one. Along similar lines, if you are ever absolutely stuck between three seemingly-identical answer choices after eliminating the fourth choice right away as contradicting the passage, it's possible that you misinterpreted either the passage or the question, and that fourth choice is actually correct. After all, only one answer choice can be correct!

Another thing to keep in mind is that when two answer choices make *opposite* claims, it is possible, though not certain, that one of them may end up being correct. For example, if a question asked about Baba Yaga's characterization in Russian folklore, and one answer choice claims she has an ambiguous nature, and another answer choice says she has an entirely unambiguous nature, there is a good chance one of these is correct. However, as always, be careful to use this only to help guide your reasoning so you can investigate these answer choices more thoroughly. Your reason for selecting an answer choice shouldn't be, "Well, answer choices A and B were opposites, and B seemed wrong, so A must be correct." Rather, identifying these two "opposite" answer choices should lead you to ask yourself whether the passage asserted a position on whether Baba Yaga has an ambiguous nature. If it did, one of these answer choices may be correct. If not, you might need to take a look at the other answer choices.

Detail questions contain great examples of answer choices that directly contradict the passage text. However, wrong answer choices can also provide contradictory *interpretations* or *applications* of the passage. Here, we still need to apply the same reasoning skills. For example, consider the following question:

Which of the following would be considered a MOTW-style television show?

I. A show in which the protagonists partner with a new consultant in each episode
II. A show that discusses the life of a murderer over several episodes
III. A show that follows the day-to-day activities of a police officer, with one suspect being introduced and later arrested during each episode

A. I only

B. III only

C. I and II only

D. I and III only

As the answer choices list examples or analogies of passage concepts, this is an Application question that requires us to *apply* passage information to identify the most *analogous* example of what the passage considers a Monster of the Week-style television show. To answer this question, we need to find out exactly what elements the passage considers fundamental to a Monster of the Week-style TV show, make a prediction, and then match this prediction to the answer choice that most exemplifies these elements. The author states repeatedly—in both paragraphs one and four—that Monster of the Week-style shows feature antagonists or "monsters" that appear in only one episode. Therefore, we should look for an answer choice that provides an *antagonist* that appears just *once* per season. If an answer choice violates either of these parts—one that either does not contain an antagonist, or describes an antagonist who appears in more than one episode—then it provides an inaccurate interpretation of the passage.

The answer choices fit the pattern of this prediction: each describes some character in a show and the frequency with which that character appears in the show. Since Roman numeral three appears exactly twice in the answer choices, let's assess it first. Roman numeral three describes a show with one suspect introduced and arrested per episode. This correctly matches our prediction, so we should eliminate choices that do not have Roman numeral three. A and C are out. This leaves us with only choices B and D. Based on this, we now only need to assess Roman numeral one to determine the correct answer. Roman numeral one describes a show in which protagonists partner with a new consultant in each episode. The mention of protagonists here doesn't invalidate this answer choice, but this option does not mention any antagonist. Thus, we can eliminate Roman numeral one, making choice B the correct answer.

For the sake of being thorough, let's take a look at Roman numeral two. This one describes a show that discusses the life of a murderer over several episodes. A murderer would certainly fit the description of antagonist, but we need an antagonist that only appears in one episode. So, we can confirm that numeral two is false.

6. Faulty Logic Answer Patterns

In CARS, you will likely encounter answer choices that, on the surface, might not seem to contradict passage information, but rather reflect **faults in logical reasoning**.

As answer choices tend to be fairly concise, we need to be on the lookout for specific words that indicate logical relationships. Words or phrases like "therefore," "thus," "consequently," "as a result," "it follows that," "we can conclude that," "which demonstrates that," and so forth, indicate the conclusion of an argument, while words or phrases like "since," "because," "assuming that," "given that," "for the reason that," "as indicated by," and so on, indicate the rationale for a given conclusion.

In CARS answer choices, faulty logic may appear as conclusions that aren't grounded in passage evidence, apply passage information too broadly or too narrowly, do not present a reasonable link between a conclusion and the rationale for that conclusion, or are otherwise invalid. This also includes answer choices that misinterpret whether information supports or challenges a given assertion, as is often the case with Incorporation questions that ask how new information strengthens or weakens passage arguments. A wrong answer choice might also present a conclusion when the question asks for a claim's reasoning. Logic errors also appear as errors in causality, such as those that reverse the direction of causality, assume causation when there is none, misidentify the causal variables, or draw flawed conclusions from causal relationships.

Let's consider the following example:

> If an American boy wore Baba Yaga sneakers and perceived Baba Yaga as both a witch and a grandmother figure, the author's conclusion in the final paragraph would be:
>
> A. strengthened because the boy understands Baba Yaga's ambiguous nature.
>
> B. weakened because the boy's exposure to MOTV shows has allowed him to understand Baba Yaga's ambiguous nature.
>
> C. weakened because the boy contradicts the author's opinion that viewers perceive Baba Yaga as a villain.
>
> D. neither strengthened nor weakened because the boy is not relevant to the author's conclusion.

Notice how these answer choices have similar structures with two parts: first, we have to decide if this information strengthens, weakens, or doesn't affect the author's conclusion. Then we identify the correct rationale for this relationship. This is an Incorporation question as it requires us to incorporate new information into our interpretation of passage arguments. It's also a Support question as it asks us to analyze the support for a given conclusion, namely the author's in the final paragraph. So, to answer this question, we need to go back to the passage for two pieces of information: (1) to identify the author's conclusion in the final paragraph, and (2) to determine the author's purpose for mentioning Western cultures, "Baba Yaga sneakers," and perceptions of Baba Yaga as a "witch and grandmother." Then we need to determine the relationship between these two pieces of information.

In the final paragraph, the author concludes that Monster of the Week-style shows have reduced Baba Yaga's ambiguous aspects so she is now just seen as an antagonist. The American boy who perceives Baba Yaga as both a witch and a grandmother is meant to represent someone from a Western country who perceives Baba Yaga as an ambiguous figure. Baba Yaga sneakers are used in the second paragraph as an example of the global products Baba Yaga has inspired. But the author isn't concerned with how Baba Yaga *products* have influenced people's perceptions of Baba Yaga, only with how Monster of the Week-style *television shows* have. We don't know whether or not this boy watches Monster of the Week-style shows, so we can't really say that this either strengthens or weakens the author's argument, meaning choice D is correct.

Let's take a moment to look at answer choice B. Is this evidence in the question stem sufficient to *weaken* the author's conclusion? What exactly is the author trying to argue, and how could we poke holes in this argument? Well, if someone actually *did* watch Monster of the Week-style shows *but also* maintained a view of Baba Yaga as an ambiguous figure, this would directly conflict with the author's argument. Now, is it *possible* that this kid's perceptions of Baba Yaga were shaped by watching Monster of the Week-style shows while growing up? Sure! But we don't actually *know* that. In other words, we need to be careful not to make our own assumptions or stray from the actual information that's given to us. We have to stick to the evidence!

Here are three pieces of advice to help you avoid this type of logic error. First, make sure you know the exact reason you're choosing to select or eliminate an answer choice. Is this reason based on a gut feeling or instinct? That's not a great reason. Is the reason that you *assume* this boy has watched Monster of the Week style shows? The problem is that we don't have evidence to support that assumption. Additionally, when you've made an assumption, try to think of ANY possible exception that violates this assumption. For example, could it be possible that this American boy wears Baba Yaga sneakers, and *hasn't* watched Monster of the Week-style shows? That very well could be true, invalidating this assumption. Finally, make sure you understand what the question is actually asking. Does it require you to determine *possible* explanations or *possible* outcomes, like whether it's *possible* that this boy watched Monster of the Week-style shows growing up? More often, the question is asking about *certain* explanations and *certain* conclusions, like whether this boy *must* have watched Monster of the Week-style shows that *must* have influenced his perceptions of Baba Yaga. A particular outcome might be *possible*, but it isn't a certain conclusion that *absolutely* must be true unless it's supported by textual evidence.

Next, let's take a look at an example of the logic error that occurs when an answer choice provides a rationale or assumption when the question asks for a conclusion. Consider the question below:

What is an underlying assumption inherent to the author's argument in paragraph four?

A. The protagonists must work together to defeat the monster.

B. Western television viewers must perceive Baba Yaga as an unambiguous, dimensionless figure.

C. Each monster only makes one appearance in Monster of the Week-style shows.

D. Appropriation of traditional cultural themes has often been practiced by Western scriptwriters.

As a reminder, an assumption is an unstated premise that must be true in order for the argument based on that assumption to be true. If that assumption is flawed, then the conclusion based on that assumption must be flawed. In the fourth paragraph, the author argues that Western-style shows oversimplify Baba Yaga, reducing her to the role of villain alone. In support of this, the author says that in Monster of the Week shows, "the threat [of the monster] catalyzes social relations between protagonists in order to confront the monster's deformity and deviance." We need to look for something that's assumed by this sentence. Underlying this statement is the assumption that the protagonists must work together to defeat the monster in each episode. If this is not true, then "social relations" between protagonists are really unnecessary in order to confront the monster. Therefore, choice A is correct.

What about the wrong answers? Let's consider choice B, which states that Western television viewers must perceive Baba Yaga as an unambiguous, dimensionless figure. This statement flows from the claim made in paragraph four that Western MOTW shows "rob Baba Yaga of her inherent ambiguity"—in other words, it's a conclusion that we could draw, NOT an assumption. How do we know this is a conclusion? Let's try to spell out our thought process using some of the keywords that we discussed above. It makes more sense to say *"because* Western shows strip

Baba Yaga of her ambiguity, *therefore* viewers must perceive her as unambiguous," than it is to say "*because* viewers perceive Baba Yaga as ambiguous, *therefore* Western shows must strip her of her ambiguity."

Other wrong answer choices might simply reiterate or paraphrase direct statements from the passage, such as choice C, which states that "Each monster only makes one appearance in Monster of the Week-style shows." Assumptions are implicit, unstated premises, and since this is explicitly stated in the passage, it's not an assumption and not the answer we're looking for. Choice D is also wrong, since it's consistent with paragraph four, but is not actually an assumption of the argument made in this paragraph. To see this point, consider what would happen if the statement in choice D was incorrect. The author's more specific point about Baba Yaga could still hold, regardless of whether such patterns of cultural appropriation are common. Again, the key here is understanding the anatomy of the argument made in paragraph four, and of arguments in general.

7. Poor Fit Answer Patterns

Some answer choices are wrong because they are too extreme or do not fit the question or passage in terms of content, opinion, or tone. On one end of the spectrum are answer choices that are **too broad** or that extrapolate too far beyond the author's stated position, and at the other end of the spectrum are answer choices that are **too narrow**.

Let's demonstrate this through an example:

The author most likely includes details about Baba Yaga's physical appearance in the opening paragraph in order to:

A. help create a mental picture of Baba Yaga.

B. explain that Baba Yaga's facial features are physically unattractive.

C. describe what Baba Yaga looks like in Russian depictions only.

D. highlight features that make Baba Yaga unique.

This is a Function question, as it asks for the purpose of a passage element, specifically details about Baba Yaga's physical appearance. The answer choices describe four different possible reasons for the author's use of this description, but we want to make a prediction based on its function in the passage. Recall that Baba Yaga's appearance was introduced pretty early on, in paragraph one, which describes her "iconic huge nose, iron teeth, her mortar and pestle flying contraption, and her chicken-legged hut," followed by a clause that asserts that her appearance is "distinctive and easily recognized." Therefore, the author included this information not just to satisfy our curious imaginations, but more specifically to highlight the distinctiveness of her appearance. This is a good match for answer choice D, which is correct, but let's identify why the other answer choices are wrong.

Choice A says this description "help[s] create a mental picture of Baba Yaga." While the description certainly does create a mental picture, that wasn't the author's principal intention. After all, it wasn't the author's primary goal for us to understand the precise shape and size of her nose, or to picture the engineering work it took to create a mortar and pestle flying contraption. Therefore, this answer choice is too broad. The best answer is one that describes the *specific* and *primary* function of the passage element that in some way helps further the passage thesis. Generally speaking, choices that are too broad are often wrong because they do one of two things: (1) they aren't specific enough to address the question being asked, as we saw in the example of answer choice A, or (2) they generalize or extrapolate too far beyond what the passage actually says, putting words in the author's mouth.

Choice B states that the reason for depicting Baba Yaga's appearance is to "explain that [her] facial features are physically unattractive." This answer choice is wrong for two reasons. For one, the better answer choice is one that is more specific to the author's intended purpose, which is to illustrate the *distinctiveness,* not *attractiveness,* of Baba Yaga's features. The other reason why this is a poor answer choice is because it's too narrow in scope. While the list of features in this description does include her nose and teeth, it also includes her flying contraption and hut, so the author is clearly talking about more than attractiveness or the lack thereof. Some answer choices that are too narrow in scope present a subpoint or subargument when the question is looking for bigger-picture arguments and main ideas. For example, if we were asked for the thesis of this passage, an answer choice that solely focuses on Baba Yaga as a transcultural figure would be too narrow in scope. This isn't to say that all answer choices that appear to have a narrow scope are automatically wrong. Rather, an answer choice is wrong when it's either too broad or narrow relative to the focus of the passage, and *then* these become legitimate reasons for eliminating such answer choices.

Choice C states that the author discusses Baba Yaga's appearance in order to "describe what Baba Yaga looks like in Russian depictions only." Extreme terms like "only," "always," "never," "ideal," "exactly," and so forth are signs that you should slow down and proceed with caution. This is not a comprehensive list of all extreme language that might appear in CARS answer choices. This category includes some terms that may not initially seem extreme. For example, superlatives like "most," "worst," "kindest," or "weirdest" are considered extreme because they express the highest or lowest quality of something. For example, it's one thing to be weird, and it's quite another for something to be the absolute weird*est.* That's a pretty high bar. Other terms like "identical" might not seem extreme at first glance, but this is also a pretty rigid, inflexible term that leaves no room for *any* differences. It's one thing for the author to say two things are similar, and quite another to say two things are identical. Better answer choices are more flexible or tentative, and less rigid, often including words like "may," "might," "can," "maybe," "possibly," "probably," "usually," "often," or "perhaps." Contrast these to extreme terms like "must," "cannot," "always," or "never." Having more wiggle room makes an answer choice hard to refute, whereas if an answer choice is too rigid, it may crack under pressure if even a single exception is found that invalidates it, making extreme answer choices more vulnerable to critique.

Including an extreme term is an easy way for a CARS test-writer to turn an otherwise tempting answer choice into a definitively incorrect choice. For example, had this answer choice claimed that the author's description of Baba Yaga's appearance matches Russian depictions of her, this would more than likely be true. However, the word "only" limits this physical portrayal of Baba Yaga to Russian depictions alone, excluding the possibility that she could be portrayed in the same way in other countries. Since no evidence in the passage directly addresses whether she's depicted differently elsewhere, this answer choice is incorrect because it's too extreme. Extreme answer choices like this one are too narrow, as they focus on just a subset of all applicable situations, but extreme answer choices can also be too broad, such as an answer choice asserting that *all* depictions of Baba Yaga are *identical* to the one given in the passage. Certainly it's possible that Baba Yaga is depicted differently elsewhere, unless the passage states otherwise. As such, an excellent way to help you determine whether an answer choice is too "extreme" relative to the passage is to think of exceptions to the rule.

That last point is key: an extreme term doesn't automatically mean an answer choice is wrong. We need to apply context from the passage. An "extreme" answer choice may be correct if it aligns with the author's assertions in the passage. If the author makes what we'd otherwise call an "extreme" assertion that the huge nose, iron teeth, and other features described in the passage are *only* used in Russian depictions of Baba Yaga, then answer choice C could very well be correct. If you simply eliminate an answer choice because it contains an "extreme" term without looking for evidence to support your decision, you might end up missing the question. There's no substitute for evidence, and that's why "shortcuts" don't end up working on the MCAT. Instead, allow the presence of an extreme term to elevate your suspicion, and then investigate whether that answer choice reflects an extreme interpretation of the passage that takes its actual arguments too far.

A final example of answer choices that are a poor fit are those that don't align with the author's tone. This occurs when the author expresses an opinion in the passage (either directly or through word choice and tone) and the answer choice expresses an opinion or uses a tone that doesn't match. It can also occur when the answer choice attributes an opinion to the author where the author *didn't* express one. Sometimes this tone is opposite that of the author's, but more often it takes the author's tone to an extreme. Critically, however, we always need textual evidence we can point to in the passage to make our case about how the author really felt about a given issue.

Let's consider the following example:

Which of the following is the author most likely to agree with?

A. Baba Yaga does not have wide appeal.

B. More commercial products inspired by Baba Yaga should be made in Western countries.

C. MOTW relieves Baba Yaga of her inherent ambiguity, allowing her to assert a more powerful role as an antagonist.

D. Baba Yaga should be able to appear in more than one episode in Western television shows.

This is an overt Opinion question. Let's take a look at each answer choice. Choice A asserts that Baba Yaga does not have widespread appeal, however we know that the author *does* believe she has widespread appeal from the author's description of her as a "transcultural figure" who "maintains some bearing over space and time and adapts to various media and cultures." Thus, choice A is clearly contradictory to the author's opinion.

Choice B says that more commercial products inspired by Baba Yaga should be made in Western countries. The author does discuss the "wide array of popular, global products and productions from picture books to sneakers to punk rock to video games" that have come to be associated with Baba Yaga, but the author doesn't assert an opinion either way on whether this production should be increased in Western countries. Therefore, choice B is wrong because it attributes an opinion to the author where the author did not express one.

Choice C says "MOTW relieves Baba Yaga of her inherent ambiguity, allowing her to assert a more powerful role as an antagonist." It *is* true that Monster of the Week shows take away Baba Yaga's inherent ambiguity, according to the author's beliefs. However, pay close attention to the word choice the author uses in the passage: "*Regrettably*, we see Baba Yaga's traditional form...being *appropriated* by the Western MOTW shows...*robbing* Baba Yaga of her inherent ambiguity." The author is not happy about this. Choice C chooses to spin this as a good thing, that removing this ambiguity is somehow a "relief," allowing Baba Yaga to step into this new, powerful role. While some might view this transformation in this way, the author does not. Choice C is wrong because it does not align with the author's tone, and this is particularly important because if you miss the author's attitude toward this transformation, you miss the entire point of the passage.

Choice D, which claims "Baba Yaga should be able to appear in more than one episode in Western television shows," is ultimately the correct answer. The author doesn't make this statement *directly*, but if we understand how the author feels in the passage, we should be able to identify opinions that are consistent with, inconsistent with, or have no bearing on the author's. What exactly *does* the author say about this? Well, in the last paragraph the author claims that Western shows requiring that monsters appear in just one episode pigeonholes Baba Yaga in the antagonist role, stripping her of the level of ambiguity and nuance afforded her traditional role in Russian folklore. Thus, the author is likely to believe that if monsters were allowed to become part of an ongoing story arc, more ambiguity and nuance could be built into her character, restoring Baba Yaga to her original form. We also know the author views this as a good thing, so the author is likely to believe this "should" happen in Western television shows to restore Baba Yaga's traditional image.

There are a few question types for which you should be especially vigilant for these kinds of answer choices. As we saw in some of the examples we used, extreme answer choices tend to show up in Main Idea and Function questions, expressing an idea or function that's too broad or too narrow in focus. They also appear in answer choices that provide extreme analogies or applications of passage concepts, as in Application questions. Answer choices that do not align with the author's tone also show up in Opinion questions, and to some extent, any answer flaw can show up in almost any CARS question.

8. Irrelevant Answer Patterns

Some CARS answer choices are wrong because they're irrelevant to the question asked or to the content of the passage. We use the term "irrelevant" specifically to refer to answer choices that do not address or are not immediately relevant to the topic specified by the question as well as answer choices that are too disconnected from the passage text. In other words, an irrelevant answer choice may have *absolutely nothing* to do with the question or passage at hand, but more often it will be somewhat relevant but then veer off topic.

Consider the following example:

> If valid, which of the following statements would most weaken the author's argument in the last paragraph?
>
> A. Canadian television viewers see Baba Yaga as a complex, ambiguous character.
>
> B. Slavic fans of Baba Yaga more frequently consume films than television shows.
>
> C. Some folktales depict Baba Yaga as a trio of sisters.
>
> D. Russians recognize Baba Yaga as an earth mother and a death guardian.

This is an Incorporation question, as it asks us to evaluate how new information affects the author's argument. To answer this question, we first need to determine what argument this question is discussing, and then think about what information would weaken that argument. In the last paragraph, the author argues that Western Monster of the Week-style television shows deprive Baba Yaga of her traditional ambiguity, reducing her to a villain. This assertion would be *weakened* by evidence that in fact, these Western-style shows don't necessarily take away Baba Yaga's complexity or reduce her to just an antagonist. In fact, the correct answer to the question is choice A, precisely for this reason.

Let's turn to choice B, though. This statement is not particularly related to the author's assertion in the last paragraph. Paragraph three compares Baba Yaga's appearances on film and television, but it says nothing about general film versus TV viewership among Slavic fans. Furthermore, this isn't very relevant to the author's argument about how Western-style shows rob Baba Yaga of her enigmatic character. Therefore, this answer choice is irrelevant to the question asked. Notice too how this answer choice most closely relates to the topic of discussion in paragraph three, not the argument made in paragraph four. Unless a question is asking about the main idea or other big-picture themes and attitudes that span multiple paragraphs, the correct answer will very often be found in the part of the passage most closely related to the question, especially when the question tells you exactly where to look.

Choice C is also clearly irrelevant: there is no discussion whatsoever about viewing Baba Yaga as a trio of sisters in the passage. Choice D isn't *irrelevant*, exactly, but it clearly draws upon the language in paragraph one, so it doesn't weaken the author's argument either.

A word of caution: just because an answer choice introduces new information that's not *directly* addressed in the passage doesn't automatically mean it's wrong. For example, Application and Incorporation questions, like this one, will always ask you to analyze new information to determine whether it fits with the passage material. Notice how the correct answer, for instance, describes the perceptions of Canadian viewers. Since the passage cites Canada as an example of a Western country, this is intended to be an *example* of how *Western* viewers perceive Baba Yaga, which *is* addressed by the passage. So when you're evaluating answer choices that contain examples, analogies, or applications of passage information, try to identify what passage concepts they refer to before you judge their relevance. The flip side of this rule also holds: an answer choice may include words taken from the passage, but embed them in an irrelevant statement. In other words, when judging relevance, we have to go beyond first impressions.

9. Tempting Answer Patterns

Some answer choices are tempting for a number of different reasons, but are still incorrect. There are three common patterns these types of answer choices will follow that we'll demonstrate through the following example:

The author of this passage would most likely agree with which of the following ideas?

A. Children exposed to Slavic depictions of Baba Yaga are more likely to empathize with her character.

B. Artists should be free to reconfigure and adapt the distinctive features of transcultural figures in new media.

C. Characters should be presented in their traditional form so that audiences can appreciate their sophistication.

D. Transcultural adaptations of characters should seek to preserve their original cultural context to the extent possible.

This is clearly an Opinion question as it requires an understanding of the author's opinions, and it's also an Application question as we're asked to apply our understanding of the author's positions to new contexts.

Let's consider choice A. The author certainly contrasts depictions of Baba Yaga as an ambiguous, interesting, dynamic figure in Slavic folklore, versus an unambiguous, one-dimensional figure in Western media. However, what we're really asked is: Are children more likely to empathize with the ambiguous form, the one that's both an antagonist and helper, or with the unambiguous form, the one that's just portrayed as an antagonist? Psychology research or our intuition might tell us that we're *more* likely to empathize and relate with an antagonist who also has characteristics of a protagonist. However, we're asked specifically which ideas the *author* is most likely to agree with. It's possible the author agrees with this, but we don't really know, as the author never weighs in on this issue. There's no mention of "empathy" in the passage. The author maintains the position that preserving Baba Yaga's traditionally ambiguous character is a good thing, but never asserts an opinion on how or whether this might affect viewers' empathy towards her.

This is an excellent example of an answer choice that may be appealing based on external knowledge, commonly-held attitudes or beliefs, your own assumptions, common sense, or gut instinct, but that is beyond the scope of the passage. The correct answer should be derived from reasoning and passage evidence alone, so make sure you can identify the exact reason for selecting the answer you did, and that you can support this answer with evidence.

Choice B says, "Artists should be free to reconfigure and adapt the distinctive features of transcultural figures in new media." On the surface, this answer choice is certainly tempting, as it mimics some of the language used in the passage. Specifically, in paragraph one, Baba Yaga's features are characterized as "distinctive," and paragraph two asserts that her features may "reconfigure in an array of media" and that she "adapts to various media and cultures." However, a superficial comparison just based on similarities in word usage runs the risk of obscuring the deeper meaning present here, which requires context. We need to make sure that the *meaning* of this answer choice is consistent with the author's views in the passage. This answer choice doesn't say "Artists *have* reconfigured and adapted the distinctive features of transcultural figures in new media." It says "Artists *should* be free to reconfigure and adapt the distinctive features of transcultural figures in new media." In the passage, paragraph two tells us what artists *have* done with Baba Yaga, transforming and adapting her to various forms of media. Paragraph four, however, outlines the consequences of this, and how the author feels about these consequences. Specifically, even though Baba Yaga *has* been adapted to Western media, her traditional character has been oversimplified in Monster of the Week television shows in a way that the author disapproves of. Therefore, do you think the author thinks artists *should* have free rein to adapt such figures in this way? Probably not.

One take-away here is to avoid the temptation of selecting answer choices based on keyword similarity alone. Context and meaning are essential. In fact, question writers will take advantage of this temptation by intentionally writing attractive, incorrect answer choices that mimic the language of the passage and match key words and phrases to set up easy traps for test-takers. If an answer choice is almost identical to the passage, with only a few changed words, look at which words were changed. Do these changes distort its context or give it a different meaning? If so, that answer choice is almost certainly wrong.

Let's analyze choice C. The first part reads, "Characters should be presented in their traditional form." This aligns well with the author's main argument that Baba Yaga should be presented in her traditional form, rather than stripped of her enigmatic character. The next part of this answer choice says "...so that audiences can appreciate their sophistication." This part of the answer choice attempts to provide an explanation for the position that characters should be presented in their traditional form. However, we need to be careful about *why*, exactly, the author argued that Baba Yaga ought to be presented in her traditional form. The author's point is that Western adaptations of this character diminish her complexity and ambiguity, not her *sophistication*. As far as this passage is concerned, sophistication has nothing to do with it! This is an example of an answer choice that *sounds* appealing but is *subtly* wrong, because even if most of the statement is correct, just one or two incorrect words can invalidate the whole thing.

Here are a few things you can do to avoid selecting answer choices with this error. First, always read every single word of the question and the answer choices *carefully*. Sometimes there is a temptation, especially toward the end of the section when mental fatigue starts to set in, to skim through the answer choices rather than to read through them thoroughly. Or we might start reading a long, rambling answer choice and already have our minds made up about it before we've read the entire thing. Or something might feel a bit "off" about the answer choice, but most of it sounds good, so we pick it anyway. However, if something doesn't sit quite well with you, investigate that feeling further, because you may be onto something! Remember, though, that ultimately you should have an evidence-based reason to eliminate an answer choice. In our case, we were able to point to passage evidence and build the case that the presence of the word "sophistication" makes this answer choice wrong.

It's better to choose a relatively vague answer that's 100% correct than to choose a very specific answer choice that uses lots of keywords from the passage and is *mostly* correct. That is, if any part of an answer choice is incorrect, the entire answer is incorrect. For example, an Incorporation question might ask whether a passage argument is strengthened or weakened by new information. An answer choice might correctly identify the effect of strengthening or weakening the passage argument, but it might be coupled to an incorrect rationale for this, making the entire answer choice wrong.

Finally, choice D is correct. Although it uses slightly different wording, it extends the author's point that it would have been desirable to preserve Baba Yaga's ambiguities in transcultural adaptations.

10. CARS Elimination Strategies

Elimination is an effective approach in the CARS section, in circumstances where you're not sure what the correct answer looks like, if you're torn between two answer choices, or even if you want to make *sure* you've identified the right answer.

In addition to its general usefulness, elimination is especially suited to certain types of questions. These include, but aren't limited to: **NOT, EXCEPT, or LEAST questions; two-part answer choices;** and **Roman numeral questions**. If a question asks, "Which of the following is LEAST supported by evidence from the passage?", the best approach is to return to the passage for each answer choice, looking for evidence that rules out each of the three wrong answers. For "two-part" answer choices, a common pattern in the CARS passage is that each choice will contain some conclusion, followed by its explanation. For example, suppose a question asks if new information strengthens passage arguments. Two answer choices might begin with "Yes," followed by their explanations, and two answer choices might begin with "No," followed by their explanations. If you know the correct conclusion is "Yes," you can eliminate both "No" answer choices. Likewise, even if you're not sure what the correct conclusion is, you may still be able to eliminate answer choices based on flawed explanations. On Roman numeral questions, if you can rule out one or more Roman numerals, you can eliminate all of the corresponding answer choices that contain that Roman numeral. Conversely, if you know one or more Roman numerals *must* be true, you can readily eliminate any answer choices that lack that Roman numeral.

When eliminating wrong answer choices, the goal is to have a **specific reason** for eliminating each wrong answer choice, as well as a reason for selecting the one that we believe is correct. By "reason," we mean something more objective than "it just didn't feel right" or "it had too many 'tempting' keywords, so it's probably wrong." The reason should hold up to scrutiny, to the point that there is no universe in which *this* particular answer choice is the right answer to *this* particular question. The reason for this is that CARS questions (like every other question on the MCAT, for that matter) *must* be written in a way such that there exists an objective explanation for why the wrong choices are wrong and why the right answer is right. In other words, wrong answer choices are *always* wrong for a reason. Practically speaking, you might have trouble seeing that reason in the heat of the moment, and it might not be realistic to engage with every single question at this level of depth when you're taking a timed test, but when you go back to review practice materials, we really do recommend analyzing why every single wrong answer choice is wrong. This can be time-consuming, but it will pay serious dividends in terms of building up your expertise and instincts when it comes to taking the real thing.

The patterns of incorrect answer choices that we discussed above form a solid foundation for implementing process of elimination on the MCAT. Another common pattern is that when two answer choices are so similar that they basically say the same thing, they can't both be right, so more often than not, they'll both be wrong. For example, consider the following question, which we can view as a standalone (i.e., independent of any passage):

The author would most likely view curriculum reform in public education as:

A. a fraud.

B. an act of deceit.

C. a failure.

D. a moderate success.

Let's just take a look at choices A and B. Choice A says "a fraud" and choice B says "an act of deceit." Fraud and deceit are synonymous, so it's unlikely that one of these is correct and the other is not. However, note that choice C characterizes this attempt as "a failure." While "fraud," and "deceit" are compatible with "failure," they don't actually mean the same thing. Something can fail because it's bad, even if it's not deceitful. The trick of eliminating synonymous answers can be useful, but you do have to be careful, because two similar-sounding answer choices can have subtle distinctions that might actually make a difference. For example, "failure" is not quite the same thing as "catastrophe," and "success" and "prosperity" aren't complete equivalents.

Furthermore, when two answer choices are opposites, there is a good chance that one of them is the correct answer. If a statement is false, then the opposite of that statement is often true. For example, choice C and choice D in this question are opposites: C says curriculum reform was a "failure," and choice D calls it a "success" (although a moderate one). Although it's possible for something to be neither a failure nor a success, and it's also always possible that the author just didn't weigh in on the issue, these answer choices point to two opposite opinions, so we would be well-served to investigate if either of them corresponds to the author's point of view. Once you're confident that an answer choice contradicts the passage, doesn't address the question, or results from some kind of logical error, strike it out using the strikethrough feature, and move on to the remaining answer choices. Using elimination, you'll find that you will often be able to narrow it down to two answer choices, which is where things start to get trickier.

11. What to Do When You Feel "Stuck"

MCAT students often experience a pattern of almost narrowing a question down to two answer choices...and then getting stuck. When you find yourself stuck between two answer choices, ask yourself these four questions:

> Do you understand the question and its relationship to the passage?
> Which answer choice is best supported by passage evidence?
> Which answer choice is the best *fit* with the scope of the passage and question?
> Can you find any non-obvious flaws that allow you to eliminate one of the two choices?

Turning to the first question we mentioned, sometimes it's helpful to take a step back and get a fresh perspective on a question to make sure you're not missing anything. First, **re-read the question**. If you're spending a lot of time on the answer choices, it's easy to forget what was asked. This will be especially helpful for NOT, EXCEPT, and LEAST questions. Make sure you understand what the question is asking, and can break it down into its parts and paraphrase it in your own words. Do you know what passage *concept* the question is asking about? Is it really asking about main ideas, or opinions, or assumptions, or about the purpose of a passage element, or about something else? Next, do you understand the answer choices you're debating between? Check that you can paraphrase them and that you know what passage concept each refers to.

It can be easy to get stuck on long, wordy questions and answer choices, and waste a lot of time re-reading to try to sort out their meaning, which typically just results in more confusion. To help with this, use your **highlighter** tool to keep you focused on the important parts of the question, and use your **strikethrough** tool to help you ignore answer choices that you've already eliminated. Another advantage to this is that, if you're struggling to understand a question and decide to flag it and come back to it later, you've in a way bookmarked your progress on that question and can start right back up where you left off.

Being stuck between answer choices may also indicate an issue with passage comprehension. If you don't fully understand parts of a passage, it can be hard to interpret exactly what the questions and answer choices mean and how they're relevant to the passage. It's sort of like trying to answer a set of CARS questions without the passage! In the setting of a real exam, it's not exactly practical to re-read entire passages, but if you can identify these issues in practice, then you can focus your efforts on passage comprehension and hopefully stave off these issues when you take your actual MCAT. Furthermore, you may find that moving on to other questions associated with the same passage will help illuminate the meaning of that passage and perhaps influence you to think about it a little bit differently. This fresh perspective may come in handy when you decide to go back to that troubling question.

In addition to considering question and passage comprehension, the second question you should ask yourself is which answer choice is best **supported by evidence** in the passage? Since you've already done the work of eliminating one or more answer choices, searching for passage evidence will be a more efficient process by this point. Do you have all the information you need to answer the question? Have you missed a critical piece of information in the passage, or perhaps focused on the wrong thing? Was your interpretation of that part of the passage correct the first time, and have you spent sufficient time thinking about the relevant evidence?

Remember that in the CARS section, clues to the correct answer *must* be somewhere within the passage. If the question stem references a specific paragraph or part of the passage, they've made your work a little easier by telling you exactly where to look—and this also means you *will* need information from that part of the passage. For each answer choice, whether or not you're told where to look, go back to the passage to forage for evidence, no matter how confident you feel that you remember the relevant content and context. During practice, try to figure out how accurate you are at correctly identifying the relevant parts of the passage by comparing the parts of the passage that you *thought* were important to the parts of the passage that ended up *being* important. If you did identify the right part but still got the question wrong, did you interpret that part of the passage correctly? If not, could spending more time analyzing the evidence have made a difference? Were there any other clues in the passage you missed?

Sometimes you'll find passage evidence that appears to support two answer choices to a question. When this happens, the first thing you should do is question the strength of the support. Is there *more* support for one over the other, or more *straightforward* support? Does support for one answer choice require more leaps in logic, or are there any exceptions or conditions where this support does *not* lead to the conclusion in one of the answer choices? If one answer choice is well-supported, while the other one may or may *not* be true, go with the answer choice that is more clearly supported. Sometimes an answer choice may or may not be true, or it might seem plausible based on intuition, but if the question asks for a conclusion that *must* be drawn from the passage, or a position that we know the author *must* support, then we have to stick to answer choices that are firmly rooted in passage evidence.

The third question you should ask when you're stuck is: which answer choice is the **better fit**? Is there one that fits better within the passage's scope, or that's more closely related to the main thesis? Does one of them more directly answer the question? When you can't mentally "prove" one answer right or wrong, you can resort to using what's called "fuzzy logic." In contrast to standard logic, which divides statements into a strict binary of true and false, fuzzy logic uses degrees of truth that fall somewhere in between, particularly when the information you're given is vague or uncertain. Fuzzy logic has important applications in artificial intelligence, but we can also adapt these principles to the MCAT. In other words, when you're stuck between two answer choices and have exhausted your options for exploring them further, you might not have enough evidence to determine which is certainly true and which is certainly false. Using MCAT "fuzzy logic," you can find the more *likely* answer by identifying which best matches the style and tone of the author's arguments. This is by no means a guarantee, but if you're torn between two answer choices, choose the one that has the closest "feel" and fit to the opinions and themes of the passage. Along similar lines, you can apply heuristics like eliminating "extreme" answer choices in situations like this. Such strategies won't work *all* the time, but might tip the scales to something better than a 50-50 shot.

This leads us into our final question: which answer choice is **flawed**? Since identifying the right answer and identifying the wrong answers are two sides of the same coin, we've already dealt with this to some extent, but if trying to find the *best* choice isn't working, it may help to put on a critical lenses and try to find non-obvious flaws. Some possible flaws to look for in this context include statements that are correct on their own, but don't answer the question, or subtly exaggerate or over-extrapolate the author's opinion, even without using typical examples of "extreme language," or sound good but have one crucial detail that invalidates them.

This also brings up an interesting possibility: what if both of the remaining answer choices are flawed? In such a case, it's likely that you already eliminated the correct answer choice, so you may want to take a step back and re-evaluate. This happens surprisingly often, because the correct answer choice might have some wording that initially seems random or out of nowhere, even if the underlying logic is a good fit. Remember how we said that a gut feeling isn't a good reason for eliminating an answer choice? Part of the reason why we emphasize this point is that such immediate reactions can lead to eliminating correct, but non-obvious answers. So don't let this possibility psych you out, but be aware of the possibility, and try not to view eliminating an answer choice as a final, irrevocable decision to the point that you force yourself to pick between two wrong answers.

Ultimately, though, your goal is to minimize the amount of guesswork that goes into choosing between answer choices. During CARS practice, focus on identifying your reasons for determining which is the best answer choice, and compare your reasoning to the explanation. You can also use CARS practice to keep track of questions that you're able to narrow down to two answer choices. Then see how often you end up selecting the right one, make note of any trends or patterns you notice, and observe your progress over time.

12. Testing Tools and Review

Finally, let's discuss the interface features that you can use strategically to steer clear of wrong answer choices. These include the strikethrough and highlight features, the flagging tool, and the navigation and review panels.

First things first: make sure you're taking full advantage of the **highlight** and **strikethrough** tools. These two functions can be used on any of the passage, question, or answer choice text. We recommend using the highlighter tool to create an effective outline of the passage text. For questions, use the highlighter sparingly and consistently. Reserve highlighting for cases where you don't want to miss a key term or phrase in a question stem or answer choice. For example, you may decide to highlight the words "not," "except," or "least" when they occur in the prompt to remind you to select the answer choice that is *unlike* the first part of the question stem. But if you use this strategy, do so consistently. You might also choose to highlight terms that keep you centered on the main focus of a question or answer choice. For instance, a long, wordy CARS question might present a new example where the entire point is to resemble the concept of, let's say, "democracy" from the passage. If you can highlight a word or two in the question stem that reminds you to think of "democracy," you'll be better able to narrow down your answer choices without veering off track. Finally, highlighting can also be a useful visual strategy if it helps remind you of the content of a question and its answer choices when you flag it to review later. Of course, highlighting the question and answer choice text is optional, as you'll need to weigh these potential benefits with the time it takes to physically highlight each word or phrase.

The strikethrough function is even more important for eliminating incorrect answer choices. You can use this on any text, but it's most useful for eliminating wrong answer choices, especially when you choose to flag a question that you plan to return to later, and you want to keep track of your cognitive progress. Strike through any answer choice that you feel confident cannot be the right answer. Additionally, try to strike through at least two answer choices if possible. It may be that you cannot eliminate a second answer choice with 100% certainty, but if the remaining two answer choices are much more likely to be correct, then you should strike through this answer choice. Furthermore, any time there is reasonable doubt, leave that answer choice so that it's still in consideration. Finally, you don't need to use the strikethrough feature on every single question. Use the strikethrough feature for questions that are highly conceptual, long, confusing, tricky, or anywhere else you need to use process of elimination, and make sure to use it when you choose to flag a question for review so you can pick back up where you left off when you come back.

Flagging questions is another feature that can come in handy when you're having trouble eliminating answer choices. The challenge is identifying *which* questions to flag. If you feel like you're not making progress but still need more time on a CARS question, it's okay to take a step back, choose the answer choice that feels like a better fit, **flag the question**, and move on. That said, for the CARS section, you should always plan to return to a flagged question *before* you've moved on to the next passage, rather than at the end of the entire section. You can do this by finding the flagged question in the Navigation Panel at any point during the section. When you return to the question, you'll be better equipped to jump right back in if you've saved your progress by striking out clearly wrong answer choices.

Of course, you may not have time to return to flagged questions if you're always pushing the time limit in the CARS section. Some people like to consider all their options thoroughly and waver back and forth and back and forth before making a final decision. While being thorough is a meticulous approach, learning when to be decisive is a strategic one. Make sure you're fighting the right battles, knowing when to make a decision and move on when necessary, and knowing when to take your time when you're on the cusp of a revelation. Try to recognize and stop yourself when you're stuck in a repetitive cognitive loop in your head ("well, A might be right because of this, but B might be right because of that, but A could still be right because of this…"). Flag questions for review when you're stuck and either a fresh perspective or more time is likely to help you get the right answer. However, it can be hard to know which questions may benefit from more time. After all, when you don't know how to solve a question, it's natural for the solution to seem completely out-of-reach. Don't make the mistake of simply flagging all "hard" questions, but rather, flag "hard" questions when you are stuck between two answer choices and feel like a breakthrough is possible. You may see a question in a completely new light when you take a breather and come back to it.

At the end of the CARS section, you'll be brought to the Review screen. If you have any remaining flagged questions, then you can use any extra time to review them. There are a few things to keep in mind when choosing the order in which to review flagged questions. First, your memory of more recent passages will be better, so if you only have time to review one or two questions, choose ones near the end of the section. Second, try to review flagged questions in order, either in the forward or reverse direction they are asked. This way, you'll keep better track of which you've reviewed, you'll navigate through them more efficiently, and multiple flagged questions belonging to the same passage will be reviewed in sequence. Finally, some flagged questions will be higher-priority than others. In other words, some questions will benefit from more time to review, while some questions may be either too difficult or too time-intensive to return to. To prioritize more manageable flagged questions over others, jot their numbers down on your wet-erase board as you proceed through the exam. Come review time, you can navigate directly to those questions first to maximize your chances of success.

As you review, re-read the question, skim your highlighted passage outline, and ignore stricken-through answer choices at first. Evaluate the remaining answer choices, but if you start to think about the question in a significantly different way, you may need to reconsider answer choices you'd previously eliminated. One of the reasons we review questions is so we can change incorrect answer selections into correct ones, but changing answer choices purely out of doubt will often lead to the wrong answer, especially if you've forgotten relevant information from the passage. Maintain the same standards as usual for selecting and eliminating answer choices, making sure that you have a good reason for each decision you make. You might want to have *higher* standards than usual for the answer you choose, since reviewing flagged questions at the end of a section is an especially high-stress setting, and the temptation to switch to an answer choice that just "sounds good" can be powerful. Sometimes a good reason for changing an answer choice will come in the form of passage information you'd glossed over, hints from other questions associated with the same passage, or some new connection you've made. Certainly pay attention to your instinct and "gut feeling," but get in the habit of acting rationally and purposefully as much as possible, and then you'll feel much more confident on the real thing.

13. Must-Knows

> Key steps to answering CARS questions:
  - Paraphrase the question.
  - Make a prediction about what you're looking for in an answer choice.
  - Create an action plan (i.e., passage research, process of elimination).
  - Execute that plan.
> Two major approaches (two sides of the same coin):
  - Zero in on the correct answer.
  - Eliminate the incorrect answers.
> Some tips:
  - To avoid misinterpreting the question (esp. "least," "weaken," "not" etc.), consider using highlighting too.
  - For confusing questions, using the answer choices can help.
  - For Roman numeral questions: begin by evaluating the numeral that occurs in exactly two answer choices.
> Ways to improve CARS question skills:
  - Regular practice (timed and untimed).
  - Hone passage comprehension skills.
  - As you practice, experiment with different ways to tweak your process.
  - Focus on quality of your CARS review over quantity (number of practice tests completed).
> Contradiction Answer Patterns: answer choice contradicts something stated explicitly in the passage:
  - These answer choices often function as being the opposite of correct.
  - To identify these choices, carefully reference the passages.
  - If two answer choices contradict each other, one may be right.
> Faulty Logic Answer Patterns: answer choice draws an incorrect inference/interpretation from implicit passage information (i.e., faults in logical reasoning):
  - Draw conclusions that are not grounded in passage evidence.
  - Applies passage information too broadly or too narrowly.
  - Beware of unreasonable links between a conclusion and evidence.
> Poor Fit Answer Patterns: answer choice mismatches the passage information or tone in some way.
  - Choice may not fit the tone, or be too broad, narrow, or extreme.
  - Remember that "too extreme" has to be understood relative to the author's opinion.
> Patterns in tempting answer choices—they may:
  - Contain keywords that match passage wording, but have logical problems or refer to the wrong part of passage.
  - Appeal to external knowledge, not information explicitly given in passage.
  - Be mostly appealing, but contain a crucial problem (remember that ≥1% wrong = 100% wrong).
> Strategies for elimination:
  - Always have a specific reason for eliminating answer choices (not just gut feelings).
  - If two answer choices are so similar as to be equivalent, both can't be right, so both must be wrong.
  - Incorrect answer choices must be inconsistent with the passage in some way.
> If you feel stuck…
  - Reread the question.
  - Use highlighter/strikethrough tool to focus on key parts of the question.
  - Ask: Which choice has better evidence in the passage? Which choice is the better fit? Which choice is flawed?
  - If you're going back and forth between two choices that both feel wrong, revisit eliminated choices.

Applied Practice

The best MCAT practice is realistic, with detailed analytics to help you assess where things went wrong. For those reasons, we recommend completing practice questions in an online setting that simulates the real MCAT interface, and using the analytics provided to help you decide how to best move your studies forward.

CARS does not require knowledge of specific subject areas, but it does require development of strong test-taking skills. To ensure you are honing those skills as you work through this book, we suggest you go online after wrapping up each chapter and generate a Qbank Practice Set of 2-3 CARS passages to practice and review. While not every chapter of this book is directly applicable to CARS, regular CARS practice is key to test day success.

As a further supplement, given the importance of active learning for effective studying, we also suggest that you consult the Must-Knows at the end of each chapter of this Reasoning text as a basis for creating a study sheet. This is not a sheet to memorize in the more traditional sense of content memorization, but rather a quick reference of the most important strategies for you to refer to during and after practice in your early prep. Frequently revisiting the most important strategies for the MCAT - in both CARS and the Sciences - will help you continue to improve your performance.

This page left intentionally blank.

How to Study MCAT Science

1. How Does the MCAT Test Science?

Moving from CARS to MCAT science, we need to explore how the MCAT tests science, as the best way to optimize our studying will include carefully targeting our process to match what the test expects.

The most important thing to understand about how the MCAT tests science is that it is not a memorization-based exam. The MCAT's main goal is to assess how well you can **apply your knowledge**. In other words, the MCAT uses science as a language, of sorts, to test your ability to apply information and think critically. You still have to have a deep understanding of that language in order to do well, though. This is what brings us to this discussion of how best to study science for the MCAT.

MCAT tests science primarily through passage-based questions. Each science section contains 59 questions, but only 15 of them are stand-alone, or discrete. The remaining 44 questions (nearly 75%) are associated with passages. Some passages present primary research with real experiments, while others give you some background information about a content area you've studied.

The AAMC has defined four skill categories that the MCAT is designed to test, as well as the approximate frequency of each on any given test. These skills, called Scientific Inquiry and Reasoning Skills, are:

> Skill 1, *Knowledge of Scientific Concepts and Principles*, corresponds to questions that ask you to recall factual knowledge. These questions account for roughly 35% of MCAT science questions.

> Skill 2, *Scientific Reasoning and Problem Solving*, includes questions that ask you to apply your knowledge in a specific context, most commonly introduced in a passage. These questions make up a full 45% percent of the science portion of the MCAT.

> Skill 3, *Reasoning about the Design and Execution of Research,* is comprised of questions that ask about aspects of study design and how studies are carried out. This category makes up 10% of the questions on the MCAT.

> Skill 4, *Data-Based and Statistical Reasoning*, includes questions that require you to interpret research findings. This category comprises 10% of questions.

Additionally, the AAMC has also defined a set of 10 **Foundational Concepts**, with various subdivisions, to arrange the vast amount of science knowledge you need to master. For instance, Foundational Concept 1 is "Biomolecules have unique properties that determine how they contribute to the structure and function of cells, and how they participate in the processes necessary to maintain life." Within this larger concept, Content Category 1A then corresponds to "Structure and function of proteins and their constituent amino acids." Most MCAT students, including those who are very successful, don't become familiar with these categories, but these categories are worth paying some attention to for a couple reasons.

First, when you take a practice exam as part of your course, these **content categories** will be part of the breakdown of your results. This will allow you to target your studying to focus on content areas that need more work. Second, it's worth spending some time browsing through the full descriptions of the content categories, which you can access on the official AAMC website by searching for "what's on the MCAT." The reason why this is useful is that the AAMC directly tells you what they care about in connection to various content categories and why. For instance, the description of content category 1A, which deals with proteins and amino acids, includes four full paragraphs, in which they tell you that they care about "protein behaviors which originate from the unique chemistry of amino acids themselves", and give you some examples of what they mean by this. Reading through the full description of the foundational concepts can provide you with a useful sense of what the MCAT tends to care about, which will help build your intuition for the kinds of questions they're likely to ask and the thought process that they tend to reward.

Now that we've oriented ourselves to what the MCAT expects in terms of science content, we can discuss practical tips to study in a way that aligns with those expectations. Most fundamentally, the goal is to engage actively with the science material and to prioritize building a solid conceptual foundation upon which you can then layer details.

2. Effectively Engaging with Content

When studying MCAT science, it's a good idea to pause and reflect on how you've studied science in the past, and what has and hasn't worked for you. Everyone's different, but some common experiences include taking extensive notes in lectures and/or from textbooks or slides, turning those notes into flashcards, rehearsing that factual information either by yourself or with a study group, and then hoping to see familiar questions on the test. Some of these study habits translate better to the MCAT than others, though.

A common pitfall is acquiring information passively. For example, if we're studying amino acids, we might decide to associate "alanine" with "nonpolar" and "glutamic acid" with "acidic and negatively charged." There's nothing wrong with making that association. In fact, this is necessary knowledge for the MCAT, but there are two problems if we stop here. First, random associations are hard to remember over the long term. We need some kind of conceptual scaffolding to solidify this information. Second, to be blunt, so what? We don't pose this question sarcastically. As the MCAT is mostly interested in how you can apply your knowledge, you should study MCAT science in a way that anticipates questions that go beyond the purely factual. Thinking about "**so what?**" automatically gives you a preview of how this information is going to be tested.

The next question is how to translate this goal of being more "**active**" into a concrete set of steps. One useful habit is to ask questions while studying. As we just suggested, "so what?" is a great question (and the AAMC content outline that we discussed above, with its description of the foundational concepts, is a good place to turn to for ideas about "so what?"), and another great question is "**how does this actually work?**" If you run into a roadblock where you don't really see why something you're studying works the way it does, it's time to reach out for help, such as from a fellow student, a tutor, or (if you're a Blueprint course student) at our office hours sessions.

Two other tools that help with active engagement are taking questions instead of notes and making study sheets. "**Taking questions**" means that during lecture or studying, you periodically pause and jot down a question. You don't write down what the material says, you write down a question for which the material is the answer. That is, say you're watching a lecture on amino acids, and the video says "we should remember that proline is unique because it is the only amino acid whose side chain connects to its own amino backbone." Instead of jotting down that proline is unique because it connects to its own backbone, you would write down "Proline unique because _____." Then, later on when reviewing, see if you can answer the questions you jotted down. If you can't remember, review the video. A couple days later, return to your questions and answer them again. Finally, a few weeks later, you could do a comprehensive review by trying to answer the questions you took from all of the lectures or chapters you've done over that period. Whether you're watching a video or reading a chapter, as you take notes, focus on new information, not knowledge you already have. The end goal of this process is not to have the nicest set of notes, it's to have the information in your head, because your notes aren't going to take the MCAT—you are.

Next, we recommend making **study sheets**. A study sheet is a single sheet of paper on which you summarize a particular topic (say, a chart of all 20 amino acids). Once you have everything in one place, copy the sheet but leave some information out. Then, quiz yourself—can you fill in the missing information? A couple days later, blank out more information and quiz yourself again. Repeat this process until you're staring at a blank sheet of paper with a title at the top, and see if you can, purely from memory, recreate the entire study sheet. An example of successive stages of an amino acids study sheet is below:

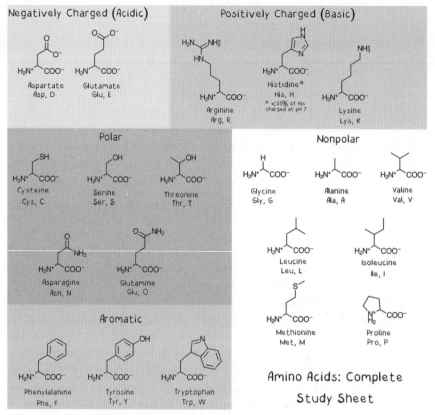

Figure 1. Amino acid study sheet: complete

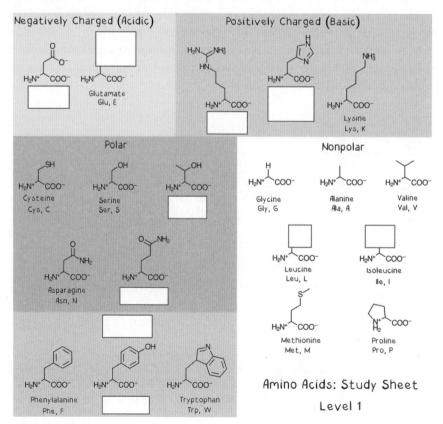

Figure 2. Amino acid study sheet: level 1

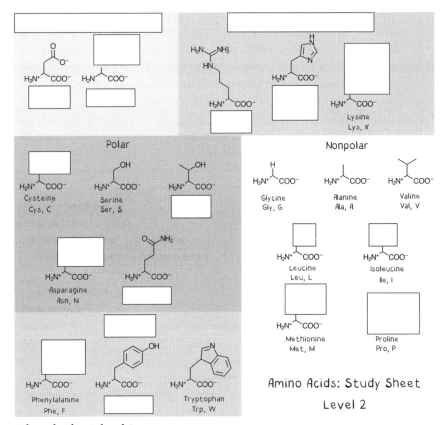

Figure 3. Amino acid study sheet: level 2

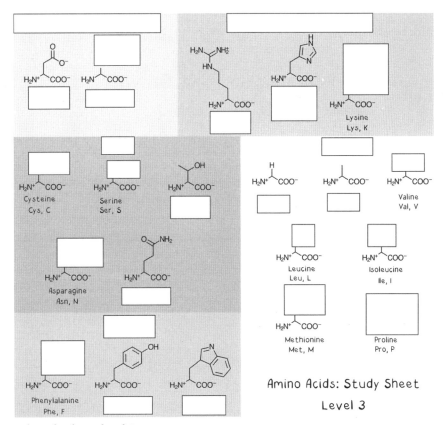

Figure 4. Amino acid study sheet: level 3

There's definitely room for variations in the study sheet themes, too. For example, you could organize the information as a flowchart, which can be especially helpful for things like metabolic pathways, physiological processes, or as a way to model content-related decision-making in problem-solving contexts (as in Figure 5 below). Alternatively, Venn diagrams are useful for when you have to learn the similarities and differences between two categories (like, for instance, metabolism in prokaryotes, as in Figure 6).

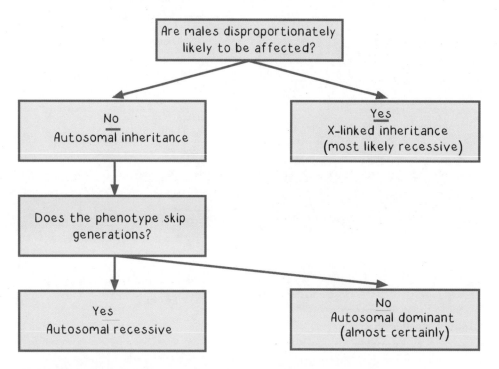

Figure 5. Flowchart for types of inheritance

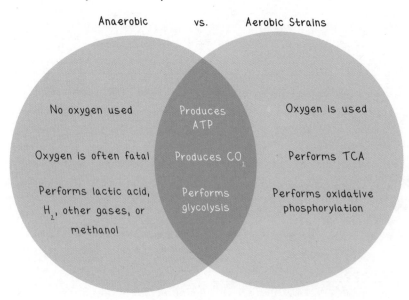

Figure 6. Venn-diagram for metabolism in prokaryotes

Diagrams and pictures, more generally, can be an excellent way to learn and remember content. We urge you to get creative in terms of finding ways to visualize information that is often presented conceptually rather than visually. As an example, consider the gases that are diatomic under standard conditions: hydrogen, nitrogen, fluorine, oxygen, iodine, chlorine, and bromine. As you can see, these form a nice L-shape on the periodic table, which is a cool visual way to organize this information. **Mnemonics** can help too, such as *have no fear of ice cold beer* in this case, which has a nice rhythm and rhyme to it that can help you remember this information about diatomic gases.

1 H 1.0																	2 He 4.0
3 Li 6.9	4 Be 9.0											5 B 10.8	6 C 12.0	7 N 14.0	8 O 16.0	9 F 19.0	10 Ne 20.2
11 Na 23.0	12 Mg 24.3											13 Al 27.0	14 Si 28.1	15 P 31.0	16 S 32.1	17 Cl 35.5	18 Ar 40.0
19 K 39.2	20 Ca 40.1	21 Sc 45.0	22 Ti 47.8	23 V 50.9	24 Cr 52.0	25 Mn 54.9	26 Fe 55.9	27 Co 58.9	28 Ni 58.7	29 Cu 63.6	30 Zn 65.4	31 Ga 69.7	32 Ge 72.6	33 As 74.9	34 Se 79.0	35 Br 79.9	36 Kr 83.8
37 Rb 85.5	38 Sr 87.6	39 Y 88.9	40 Zr 91.2	41 Nb 92.9	42 Mo 95.9	43 Tc (98)	44 Ru 101.0	45 Rh 102.9	46 Pd 106.4	47 Ag 107.8	48 Cd 112.4	49 In 114.8	50 Sn 118.7	51 Sb 121.7	52 Te 127.6	53 I 126.9	54 Xe 131.2
55 Cs 132.9	56 Ba 137.3	57 La 138.9	72 Hf 178.5	73 Ta 180.1	74 W 183.9	75 Re 186.2	76 Os 190.2	77 Ir 192.2	78 Pt 195.1	79 Au 197.0	80 Hg 200.6	81 Tl 204.4	82 Pb 207.2	83 Bi 209.0	84 Po (209)	85 At (210)	86 Rn (222)
87 Fr 223.0	88 Ra 226.0	89 Ac 227.0	104 Rf (261)	105 Db (262)	106 Sg (263)	107 Bh (262)	108 Hs (265)	109 Mt (266)	110 Ds (281)	111 Rg (272)	112 Uub (285)	113 Uut (284)	3 Uuq (289)	115 Uup (288)	116 Uuh (292)		

58 Ce 140.1	59 Pr 141.0	60 Nd 144.2	61 Pm (145)	62 Sm 150.4	63 Eu 153.0	64 Gd 157.3	65 Tb 158.9	66 Dy 162.5	67 Ho 164.9	68 Er 167.3	69 Tm 168.9	70 Vb 173.0	71 Lu 175.0
90 Th 232.4	91 Pa 231.4	92 U 238.0	93 Np (237)	94 Pu (240)	95 Am (243)	96 Cm (247)	97 Bk (248)	98 Cf (251)	99 Es (252)	100 Fm (257)	101 Md (257)	102 No (259)	103 Lr (262)

Figure 7. Diatomic gases on the periodic table

Kinesthetics can also be a useful tool for working with complex concepts. The right-hand rules for magnetism, which you should absolutely learn through actual hand movements, are a great example. An example from biology would be physically working through the steps of mitosis and meiosis, even with improvised equipment like pieces of paper, pens, and pencils. For organic chemistry, we recommend considering investing in a molecular model kit, or even build your own by improvising with items of candy, like marshmallows and jellybeans connected by toothpicks (although this would lead to the danger of eating your study supplies). Using a model will help you directly visualize the structure of organic molecules, and you can even rehearse reaction mechanisms by having one molecule "attack" another.

One of the most common questions students ask is about **mnemonics**. On one hand, they absolutely can be useful. There's some information that you just have to memorize, that there is no way to study it from a deeper, conceptual point of view. A great example of this is the mnemonic SNoW DRoP for different blotting techniques, where Southern, northern, and western blotting are used to visualize DNA, RNA, and protein, respectively.

However, mnemonics can sometimes get in your way. Here's an example: the intermediate steps of glycolysis can be remembered as *Goodness Gracious, Father Franklin Did Go By Picking Pumpkins (to) Prepare Pies*, which stands for glucose, glucose 6-phosphate, fructose 6-phosphate, fructose 1,6-bisphosphate, dihydroxyacetone phosphate, glyceraldehyde 3-phosphate, 1,3-bisphosphoglycerate, 3-phosphoglycerate, 2-phosphoglycerate, phosphoenolpyruvate, and pyruvate. Although glycolysis is absolutely core knowledge, and there's no doubt that it's tested regularly on the MCAT, the problem with this mnemonic is that it doesn't really prepare you for *how* the MCAT tests glycolysis. You could memorize this but still get every single question on glycolysis wrong, as the MCAT will never just ask you "which comes first: glyceraldehyde 3-phosphate or 3-phosphoglycerate?" What's more, this mnemonic gives you no insight into what's actually happening in these steps, which ones are more important than others, or how any of them fit into the bigger picture of metabolism. This mnemonic does contain important information, so it's not useless, but memorizing a mnemonic does not mean that you "know" glycolysis and can apply it the way the MCAT expects you to. Instead, you must pair the use of mnemonics with other study techniques and practice that encourage you to look for connections and applications of this content.

Another frequently asked question is "what about flashcards?" Our advice for **flashcards** is similar to our advice for mnemonics. Flashcards can be fine, but if used incorrectly, they can encourage over-reliance on passive rehearsal as a learning strategy. If you use flashcards, we would encourage you to phrase them as actively as possible and to also incorporate other ways of studying, like study sheets or flow charts. Blueprint's digital flash cards employ a proven learning science technique to ensure that the content you review sticks. If you prefer to make your own flash cards, that is fine too. Just be sure not to equate making or working through flash cards with being productive since you won't have to only recall facts for test day.

Study groups, in contrast, are a habit that translates well into MCAT prep, and we do recommend finding some people who are taking the test at about the same time you are, and forming a study group with them. One of the best ways to cement your own grasp of a topic and help ensure you remember it is to teach that topic to someone else. You can divide up content areas, with each person responsible for doing a teach-back of specific topics. Additionally, it can be very helpful to review practice exams in a group.

As soon as you learn something, your brain immediately starts to forget it. The good news is that every time you re-learn something, the memory loss happens more slowly. After re-learning something for a third or fourth time, it can really stick. The process of repeating content after certain intervals of time is called **spaced repetition**. In our MCAT course, we build spaced repetition into the study plan, flash cards, and, most importantly, the practice questions and full-length exams that you'll be doing. However, we also encourage you to be proactive about re-reviewing areas that might be particularly challenging for you personally.

3. Detail-Heavy Content

Although the MCAT is a test of critical thinking and your ability to apply knowledge, it's still true that you have to know a lot to succeed. The MCAT covers roughly 11 semester-long courses worth of content: two semesters of physics, two semesters of general chemistry, two semesters of organic chemistry, one semester of biochemistry, two semesters of biology, and one semester each of psychology and sociology. Of course, not everything from these courses is tested equally on the MCAT, but there are still several content areas where you have to master a lot of dense factual material. How can you best approach this task?

Step one is to have a good toolkit of **study techniques**, as discussed above. Step two, then, is to **build connections**. An interesting quirk of human cognition is that we remember information much better when it's part of a narrative that we're invested in. Since for the MCAT we don't get to choose the scientific facts, or statements, that we study, our task is to figure out how to turn a statement like "the committed step of glycolysis is when phosphofructokinase-1 catalyzes the conversion of fructose 1-phosphate to fructose 1,6-bisphosphate, consuming one equivalent of ATP" from a boring "blah blah blah" kind of statement into an engaging statement.

So, how do we do that? Here's an idea that might sound a little silly at first, but bear with us: *everything's a story*. Therefore, when we study biochemistry, for instance, we're learning the story of glycolysis, the story of the citric acid cycle, the story of beta-oxidation, and so on. These stories all have a starting point (that is, the reactants) and an end-point (the products), and they all fit into the larger story of how we as humans manage to extract energy from the environment to live. So, if we view the factual biochemical steps of glycolysis as part of a narrative, we'll be more likely to remember it.

When you're studying you always want to be alert to possible connections between the material that you're studying and anything else of interest—either connections with other elements of the outside world, like interesting facts about science or clinical implications, or connections with other areas of MCAT science. Building connections with other areas of MCAT science is important because you're getting a double return on your energy investment, as it allows you to better understand both topics. Some examples from biochemistry include how amino acids and acid-base chemistry go hand in hand, as do carbohydrates and stereochemistry, and metabolic pathways and physiology. You can even find connections between physics and biology, as studying fluid dynamics pays huge dividends in terms of understanding the circulatory system. This list isn't exhaustive, but hopefully it gives you a sense of how to think about building these connections, which we'll also point out often as we go.

Studying for the MCAT takes daily consistent practice over a period of time. You're not going to thoroughly master glycolysis in a day, no matter how smart you are. Mastery of the MCAT builds bit by bit, by reading a chapter or watching a video, and then do practice questions, re-review your notes, do some more practice questions, review those questions and your notes, and so on. So even when it gets daunting, remember that mastery of this material isn't something that you achieve in a day, it's something that you achieve by persisting throughout your entire MCAT path.

4. Equations

One of the most frequently asked questions about the MCAT is "What **equations** do we have to know?" The short answer to that question is "the equations that are included in your MCAT textbooks and course materials," because there's a reason for the inclusion of every equation in your materials. The more interesting question, though, is how to study equations for the MCAT.

There are two basic facts about the MCAT that shape how equations are tested. First, **there's no calculator**. This puts some hard limits on how complex the math can get and how precise they expect your answers to be. Second, **time is limited** for math-based questions. On each science section, you have 95 minutes to do 59 questions, which yields slightly over one and a half minutes per question. However, we have to account for the 10 passages in each science section. A brisk but not unrealistic estimate would be three minutes to read each passage before moving on to the questions. This estimate yields a total of 65 minutes to do 59 questions, which is much closer to one minute per question. Keeping in mind that many questions will require consulting the passage, meaning less leeway.

Working smart is the key to getting through calculation questions without **wasting time**. The first thing you should do after reading a calculation question is to take a few seconds to think about what is being asked and how you can solve for that value. Before writing down an equation and doing math, you must think about the problem and make a conscious choice to do calculations. One of the biggest mistakes students make is jumping straight into calculations without carefully considering the question beforehand. One of the many problems with this is that if you try to solve a problem this way, and then your answer doesn't match any of the answer choices, you won't have a good sense of why: Was it a math error? Was it a problem setup error? Both? If your honest answer is "I have no idea because I didn't really understand the question," there's no way that you can troubleshoot your solution in the limited time you have to do so.

Another way to think about equations is that they're like scalpels and solving a math-based problem on the MCAT is like performing surgery. When a patient rolls into the trauma bay, the surgeon doesn't just grab the nearest thing that has a sharp edge and start hacking away—instead, even in an emergency case, the first step is to find out what happened to the patient, give some thought to the problem, and pick the right tool for the job. Taking a moment to consider exactly what a question is asking and whether or not you really need to do calculations to solve it is analogous to a surgeon choosing the right tool. You might be surprised to hear this, but not every MCAT question that looks like it requires math actually does. Often, calculation questions on the MCAT can be answered with some basic rounding or, even better, application of what you know about the content at hand. In other words, **think twice, cut once**.

With this in mind, let's circle back to the original question: how to study equations for the MCAT? Since studying an equation is like learning how to use a **tool**, questions to ask when you encounter a new equation include: What's it for? What kind of problem does it solve? What information does it give us?

Keep in mind that equations are just extremely condensed ways of expressing statements about how the world works. F = ma says that force equals mass times acceleration, which means that if you increase either mass or acceleration, you increase force linearly, and vice versa. Taking some time to paraphrase equations in plain English can be very useful. While you're doing so, always try to figure out what happens if you change a certain variable—does that cause other variables to increase or decrease? If so, is that increase or decrease linear or exponential? This is good intellectual hygiene in general, but it's also directly useful for the MCAT in particular, because the MCAT often asks about proportional relationships, where you don't have to calculate a precise answer, but just know how one variable is related to another.

Another useful tip is to always study **units**. As a simple example, an important equation governing waves is $v = \lambda f$, or velocity equals wavelength times frequency. Velocity has base SI units of meters per second, so we need to make sure that the units on the other side of the equation also work out to meters per second or some equivalent units, because otherwise they couldn't be equal. Wavelength has units of distance, as exemplified by meters, and frequency is defined in terms of hertz, or 1 divided by seconds. Therefore, substituting these values into the equation yields:

$$v = \lambda f$$

$$\frac{m}{s} = m \left(\frac{1}{s}\right)$$

$$\frac{m}{s} = \frac{m}{s}$$

This is a simple example, but we could use this process to check our work. When initially learning equations, make sure you know the units associated with each variable - and more importantly, understand how those units relate to and interact with the units of the other variables. Finally, we can also apply this concept to MCAT questions, because if we see a question where the answer choices are all in meters per second, then we know that our problem setup has to result in us calculating meters per second. Many students swear by the method of always watching out for units and matching their problem setup to the units in the answer choices, and we endorse it too.

5. Practice and the Lessons Learned Journal

Realistic and extensive practice makes for good MCAT prep, which means that you'll spend a lot of time learning and studying science through doing practice questions. You'll get some right, but you'll be unsure on others and also get some wrong. A useful tool to incorporate into your review is a **lessons learned journal**, or **LLJ**.

An LLJ is a tool that enables you to methodically reflect on questions that you either got wrong or weren't completely sure of, identify action points for improvement, execute those action points, and track your progress through regular review. Doing this systematically and regularly is one of the single biggest predictors of MCAT success, because it's a form of review that is completely individualized to you and your patterns of thought.

Strategy and test-taking process will form a large proportion of the lessons you record in your LLJ, but, especially when you're just getting started taking practice tests, it's normal to encounter a lot of questions where you just didn't know the content. It's entirely understandable to feel discouraged by this, but making the most out of your practice material means finding a way to translate that experience into actionable steps that you can take to improve your knowledge and skill set.

The first thing you want to do with a question that you got wrong or weren't sure about is to figure out how to get it right. A few questions can help you do so: What knowledge did the question require? How could you identify what the question required based on its wording? Where did that knowledge come from? Was it the passage or outside content knowledge? How did you have to use that knowledge? It might be the case that the problem with the question had nothing to do with your science knowledge—that is, you had the right knowledge, but didn't see what the question was asking for, or made a mistake in applying that information—and we'll talk more about how to handle those issues separately—but what if it really does just boil down to not having known something?

Perhaps not surprisingly, you'll write it down in a Lessons Learned Journal. But there are some ways to do this that are more productive than others. Let's say you missed a question on amino acids because you thought that asparagine was nonpolar. Because of this, you mistakenly believed that substituting an alanine for asparagine would not make any meaningful difference to a protein's properties. You might be tempted to write down "amino acids" as something to review. However, that is too broad to be very helpful. Amino acids make up a large segment of content, and if you return to this later, you might not remember what the problem actually was, and just see a reminder to study this incredibly general area. Going to the other extreme and writing down "Asparagine = polar" would lead to the opposite problem. That is a true fact, but if you accumulate a list of facts with no context, that will also be hard to study productively when you return to it a few days or weeks later.

A productive middle ground would be something like: "AA properties → protein function, see study sheet [asparagine = polar]." There are three things happening here: First, by making a note to review how amino acid properties are linked to protein function, you have localized the problem in a way that is at least somewhat general (i.e., it gets at the underlying issue on a level deeper than just this one specific question). However, it is still specific enough to be practically actionable. Second, we're making a note to connect this question to an amino acid study sheet, which gives us a natural follow-up action step. Finally, we're also making a note of the specific piece of knowledge we missed, but in a context that will make more sense when we come back to review.

There's no single, one-size-fits-all template for writing down lessons in your LLJ, but hopefully this example gives you a sense of more productive ways to approach this task. Don't hesitate to get creative and experiment with what you personally find useful. Since practice is a major, but often under-recognized, aspect of how you study MCAT content, it's worth investing some energy in figuring out ways to make the most of it.

6. Prioritization and Stress Management

Studying the tremendous amount of content you must master for the MCAT can be daunting. Stress management is a very important aspect of MCAT success, but here we'll limit our discussion to strategies related to the earlier stages of the study process.

It may be easier said than done, but cultivating **confidence** from day one of MCAT prep pays huge dividends. Whether you're taking the MCAT for the first time or retaking it, you've still accomplished a tremendous amount so far in your academic life, and as intimidating as the MCAT is, succeeding on it is a very doable task. More specifically, if you've taken the prerequisite courses for the MCAT, you've already studied much of the subject matter in more depth than the exam requires. For instance, standard biochemistry classes test the material in much more detail than you're likely to see on the MCAT. A similar point holds true for general chemistry and physics, for which college coursework also tends to require more complicated math, uses "uglier" numbers, and asks for more precise answers than you'll see on the MCAT. The only major exception to this generalization is physiology, as the MCAT doesn't list physiology as a prerequisite course, but does test more human physiology than you might run into in a standard general biology course. However, self-teaching some physiology is completely doable. Psychology and sociology are also somewhat exceptional in that it's pretty common for people to take the MCAT before taking those prerequisite courses. However, self-teaching enough of these subjects is also completely doable. Nonetheless, MCAT prep builds on a foundation that you've already developed, so let this help feed your confidence.

A common pitfall in MCAT prep is to be perfectionistic about the first few content areas, to the point that you fall behind in your schedule and then have to rush through later content areas or even push back the test. To counteract this, focus on **progress, not perfection**. Remember how we talked about spaced repetition and the role of practice as a way to study MCAT science? Well, this means that you'll see content areas multiple times, and have several opportunities to refine your knowledge. Therefore, while it would be ideal to ace every content question as you go and never forget anything, in reality, it's OK to feel less than 100% confident and still move on. The first round of content review basically builds a scaffolding that you then build on based on practice and more review. Remember to always keep an eye out for the big picture, for how content areas fit together, and know that you can continue touching up the details as you move forward.

MCAT prep is a **marathon, not a sprint**. We seriously recommend taking regular **days off** (ideally from all of your formal obligations, but at least from MCAT prep, if you can't totally get away from school and/or work). To some degree, your brain keeps on consolidating content unconsciously even when you're not specifically studying, but even more importantly, seven days a week of MCAT prep is a recipe for burnout, which will hinder your performance.

Some other lifestyle steps that help set the stage for good MCAT prep include **regular exercise**, which research shows has serious cognitive benefits (after all, our brain is part of our body), and regularly getting enough **sleep**, which for most adults means at least seven hours. **Eating well** is also an important part of the equation. A lot of different ideas exist about what the best diet is, and there's no way that we're going to solve this question for once and for all in an MCAT book, but a good place to start would be to limit your intake of high-sugar, refined-carbohydrate foods, to consume a balanced diet with a good amount of protein, and to avoid excessive caffeine and alcohol. In a nutshell, try to notice how your dietary choices affect your energy levels and focus, and eat accordingly. Now, we get it, all of these items are more easily said than done, and we've all been in situations where we end up blowing off stress in less than healthy ways. Even so, the more you can try to set the foundation for good lifestyle habits, the better off you'll be as you study.

7. Must-Knows

> Main goal of MCAT science: application of knowledge:
  - Skill 1: Knowledge of Scientific Concepts and Principles: factual knowledge (~35% of questions).
  - Skill 2: Scientific Reasoning and Problem Solving: knowledge application in a specific context, usually a passage (~45% of questions).
  - Skill 3: Reasoning about the Design and Execution of Research: aspects of study design and how studies are carried out (~10% of questions).
  - Skill 4: Data-Based and Statistical Reasoning: interpretation of research findings (~10% of questions).
  - AAMC also specifies Foundational Concepts and content categories (e.g., category 1A = proteins and amino acids).

> Effectively engage with science content:
  - Avoid passive acquisition of information (focusing solely on associating concepts with each other).
  - Ask questions like "so what?" to zero in on how mechanisms and topics actually work.
  - Take questions instead of notes when watching/reading material.
  - Make study sheets in stages, with progressively more content that you need to fill in.
  - Organize information as flowcharts, Venn diagrams, diagrams/pictures etc.
  - Utilize kinesthetic learning as appropriate (e.g., right-hand rules for magnetism).
  - Mnemonics: can be helpful for rote learning, but be careful—students often love mnemonics, but they promote a dry, information-based approach that doesn't always match up with how the MCAT tests science. Don't confuse memorizing a mnemonic with real understanding of a topic.
  - Flashcards can be helpful, but again be careful of limitations in terms of rote approach.
  - Study groups—highly useful!
  - Spaced repetition: review materials at intervals.
  - When studying detail-heavy content: build connections, tell stories, and engage directly.

> How to go about studying equations:
  - Lack of calculator limits how complex math can be and how precise calculations must be.
  - On quantitative questions, avoid wasting effort by working smartly (and study equations with that in mind).
  - Equations are like tools: invest some thought into picking the right one for the task, and, when studying, analyze what a specific equation is good for, how it can be used, etc.
  - Always study units, since equations are condensed statements about reality.
  - Paraphrase in plain language the relationships encoded in an equation (direct/inverse, linear/nonlinear).

> When reviewing practice questions that you get wrong:
  - Analyze what it would take to get it right.
  - Distill that lesson into an entry in your Lessons Learned Journal (LLJ).

> Prioritization and stress management:
  - Cultivate confidence.
  - Remember, MCAT prep is a marathon, not a sprint.
  - Focus on progress, not perfection.
  - Lifestyle steps: regular exercise, sleep, eating well, etc.

Applied Practice

The best MCAT practice is realistic, with detailed analytics to help you assess where things went wrong. For those reasons, we recommend completing practice questions in an online setting that simulates the real MCAT interface, and using the analytics provided to help you decide how to best move your studies forward.

CARS does not require knowledge of specific subject areas, but it does require development of strong test-taking skills. To ensure you are honing those skills as you work through this book, we suggest you go online after wrapping up each chapter and generate a Qbank Practice Set of 2-3 CARS passages to practice and review. While not every chapter of this book is directly applicable to CARS, regular CARS practice is key to test day success.

As a further supplement, given the importance of active learning for effective studying, we also suggest that you consult the Must-Knows at the end of each chapter of this Reasoning text as a basis for creating a study sheet. This is not a sheet to memorize in the more traditional sense of content memorization, but rather a quick reference of the most important strategies for you to refer to during and after practice in your early prep. Frequently revisiting the most important strategies for the MCAT - in both CARS and the Sciences - will help you continue to improve your performance.

This page left intentionally blank.

This page left intentionally blank.

How to Read a Science Passage

1. Science Passage Fundamentals

What makes the MCAT notoriously tough to crack isn't just the vast amount of content knowledge required, but the fact that this information is tested in the context of dense, complex passages. The MCAT is ultimately a test of critical reasoning, which is why it places a lot of emphasis on analysis and interpretation.

Most undergraduate exams are devoid of anything that looks remotely like an MCAT passage, since (for instance) your organic chemistry professor was likely most interested in making sure you could recognize the structure of glyceraldehyde and determine how many chiral centers it possesses. Maybe they were worried about whether or not you could write down multi-step pathways with perfectly drawn electron-pushing arrows. The MCAT, however, is interested in how you can apply information about glyceraldehyde's structure and functional groups to make a quick prediction about how it will react with another molecule, or what effect manipulating certain experimental conditions might have on its biological activity. Even though science passages might feel new or intimidating, they actually tend to boil down to a similar template, and, with practice, you'll start to notice patterns that will help you interpret them.

An important caveat before beginning is that, as with CARS, there is no perfectly tailored one-size-fits-all approach to passage analysis. We all bring different backgrounds and sets of expertise to the MCAT, meaning our eyes are going to track across passages a little differently, and a philosophy major might scrutinize a passage in a slightly different way than an engineering major might. In this chapter, we discuss reading skills that we know work, but there will be some trial-and-error involved in troubleshooting and adapting these approaches so they work for you.

You'll have access to three key tools to use at your discretion on MCAT passages: a wet-erase booklet, a highlighter tool, and your eyes.

First, you'll want to put those **eyes** to good use and actually read the passage. In other words, you really ought to read the *entire* passage from top to bottom, and in order. Broadly speaking, skimming or jumping straight to the questions first tends to lead to more cognitive errors and wrong answers, and doing so can also be a more time-consuming process, counterintuitively. Stop to reflect periodically, after a few sentences or after an entire paragraph, to consider the main points. What do you want to take away from this particular paragraph, what's its significance in the larger context of the passage as a whole, and what parts are essential to highlight to create a visual outline of the passage that you can return to later?

As you read, the **highlighter** tool is your best friend. You'll want to highlight key words or phrases that help capture the main idea and any important points in a given paragraph, which will develop into an outline of the passage. Taking this approach has three important benefits. First, you will know exactly where to return to if the passage asks you about why horseradish peroxidase was applied in step 6B of the methods. Second, you can step back and reflect on the function of each paragraph and how it contributes to the structure of the arguments within the passage as a whole. Third, highlighting helps you keep moving and actively engaged.

Let's consider the following example passage:

Phenylketonuria (PKU) is a recessive disorder characterized by the inability to metabolize phenylalanine. Figure 1 shows the classic form of PKU, in which mutations in the gene coding for the liver enzyme phenylalanine hydroxylase (PAH) cause phenylalanine to accumulate. The alteration is found on the short arm of chromosome 12 and the excess phenylalanine is converted through a transaminase pathway with glutamate (Figure 2). The resulting phenylpyruvate can be detected in the urine of PKU patients. Untreated PKU can lead to brain damage.

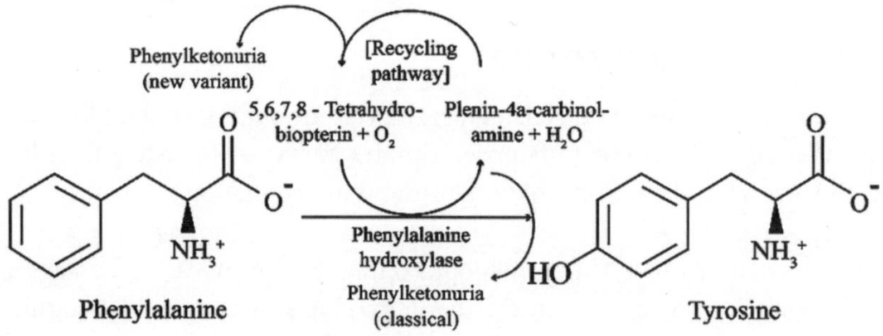

Figure 1. Deficiency of PAH (classic PKU) or BH4 reductase (variant PKU)

A variant form of PKU occurs when PAH is normal, but there is a defect in the enzyme dihydrobiopterin reductase (DHR). DHR is responsible for the regeneration of 5,6,7,8-tetrahydrobiopterin from q-dihydrobiopterin, where the former is an important cofactor in amino acid metabolism. Tetrahydrobiopterin serves as a co-factor both for PAH and for the production of L-DOPA, a dopamine precursor, from tyrosine and 5-hydroxy-L-tryptophan.

Standard treatment for PKU is to put the patient on a diet low in phenylalanine. In addition, it is suggested that those with PKU supplement their diet with large neutral amino acids (LNAAs).

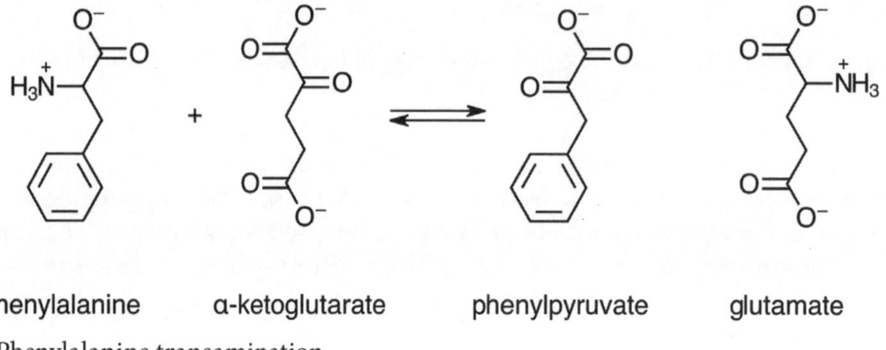

phenylalanine   α-ketoglutarate   phenylpyruvate   glutamate

Figure 2. Phenylalanine transamination

The first paragraph gives us some background information about this disorder, which is defined as an inability to metabolize the amino acid phenylalanine. It's unlikely that the MCAT is going to ask you to define PKU, as this is stated explicitly, but you may be asked about the molecular mechanisms governing the disease, or what the implications are for affected individuals, or even something about amino acid chemistry.

We're told that this metabolic deficiency is caused by mutations in a specific enzyme, phenylalanine hydroxylase. More specifically, this mutation occurs at a particular location on chromosome 12. Notice how we begin more broadly and then narrow down to the specific focus of this passage, as with this enzyme. So what happens if PAH isn't functioning normally? Well, we're told that the body accumulates too *much* phenylalanine. Thus, a buildup of a substrate or precursor molecule (phenylalanine) occurs, and we can assume that the job of PAH or phenylalanine *hydroxylase* is to hydroxylate phenylalanine, or in some way break it down or convert it to some other substance. The passage mentions Figure 1, so it's a good idea to go there next.

There's a lot going on in this figure. We don't need to account for every single atom, arrow, and label at this point, but this appears to corroborate the idea that this enzyme, PAH, converts phenylalanine into something else, specifically into tyrosine, another amino acid. It therefore makes sense to expect phenylalanine to buildup when this enzyme is is non-functional.

Towards the end of the first paragraph, we're told that the body shunts this extra phenylalanine down this transaminase pathway. We now encounter a mention of Figure 2, so let's check that out. Here we have phenylalanine plus another reactant, which can be converted into phenylpyruvate and another amino acid, glutamine. When reading the passage, we probably don't need to worry about the specific functional groups and reaction mechanisms. We can return to it if needed for a question, but it's unlikely that the detailed information in this figure is required to understand the rest of the passage. Therefore, we can use this figure to visually confirm what we're reading—that phenylalanine can be shunted down this alternative transaminase pathway to react with some other glutamate-like compound, to generate phenylpyruvate and glutamine.

At this point, it's worth mentally asking yourself why we should care about all these biochemical details in the broader scope of the passage as a whole. PKU is a problem because phenylalanine builds up in affected individuals, so this transamination reaction, as complicated as it might seem, essentially just diverts this excess phenylalanine down another pathway. The metabolic product of this pathway, phenylpyruvate, can be measured in urine, suggesting that a clinical test for PKU might exist.

Next, let's discuss what to highlight here. As we were reading, we made connections between the text, figures, and big picture. Overall, this first paragraph introduces us to PKU and points to the impairment of this specific enzyme, PAH, as causing a buildup of phenylalanine, so let's highlight words that capture this idea. Consider the highlighted paragraph below.

> Phenylketonuria (PKU) is a recessive disorder characterized by the inability to metabolize phenylalanine. Figure 1 shows the classic form of PKU, in which mutations in the gene coding for the liver enzyme phenylalanine hydroxylase (PAH) cause an accumulation of phenylalanine. The alteration is found on the short arm of chromosome 12 and the excess phenylalanine is converted through a transaminase pathway with glutamate (Figure 2). The resulting phenylpyruvate can be detected in the urine of PKU patients. Untreated PKU can lead to brain damage.

Note how sparse this highlighting is. For instance, would we want to highlight chromosome 12? Probably not, for a couple reasons. For one, numbers are more visually distinct and often will jump out at you in a block of text anyway, so highlighting might be overkill. Second, it could be worth highlighting chromosome 12 if that were an essential bit to this passage. However, the focus of the passage is on the enzyme, rather than chromosome 12. If we were asked about chromosome 12, we could probably discern that we should return to the beginning of the passage to find the information we need. Phenylpyruvate, however, is worth highlighting, since it's an important compound in this transaminase pathway, but you could also highlight "transaminase pathway." Again, the goal is to limit our highlighting to a small number of words or short phrases that give us a roadmap. The highlighting doesn't have to be (and in fact, shouldn't be) totally comprehensive of every passage detail. You can go back for those if you need them.

So, we've utilized two of the passage analysis tools available to us on the MCAT: our eyes and the highlighter tool. What about the **wet erase booklet**? The problem with the booklet is that (a), you do not have much space on any given page for jotting down notes with one of those wet erase markers, and (b) wet erase isn't easily erasable.

More generally, **note-taking** isn't actually all that helpful on the MCAT. First of all, it's quite time-consuming. Second, copying down parts of the passage word-for-word doesn't contribute to your understanding, and it steals time and brainpower that could be used to analyze the concepts presented in the passage. Even if you *are* analyzing, and *then* writing notes in your own words, this adds an extra step once you get to the questions, in that your attention will be constantly shifting between the passage, your notes, and the questions. Alternatively, you might find yourself not even referencing your notes once you reach the questions.

Notes can be helpful in limited circumstances. When working through a math problem or chemical reaction, your wet erase booklet can be a huge help. When working through a passage like this one, it may be helpful to jot down a concise biochemical pathway, especially if that helps you keep acronyms straight. For example, you might write Phe to represent phenylalanine, and then draw an arrow to Tyr for tyrosine, and write PAH under that arrow. Then you might draw another arrow to PP for phenylpyruvate and perhaps write transaminase to remind you that this represents the transaminase pathway, as shown below. If this is helpful to you, great! Otherwise, you have Figures 1 and 2 at your disposal, and referring back to those will be a fast and accurate way to derive information about these pathways.

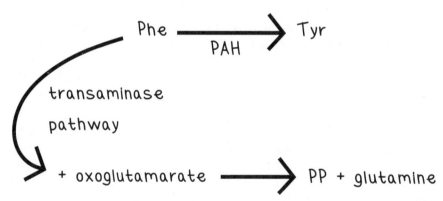

Figure 3. Sample note-taking

There are some misconceptions about shortcuts or special tricks for MCAT passage comprehension. Some approaches, like highlighting, are absolutely effective, but others are less so. As we've discussed, note-taking is great for studying, but it is a time thief on MCAT passages. A similarly ill-advised technique is skipping over the passage and navigating directly to the questions first. This might seem like a shortcut, but it's likely to put you at a disadvantage. Specifically, without the context of the passage as a whole, you'll likely end up re-reading sections of the passage more often and those wrong answers will be even more difficult to eliminate. It's also inefficient to skip around between passages or skip between questions, as this increases the risk both of accidentally leaving questions blank, and of biasing yourself against certain passages that may not be as hard as they appear at first glance. Furthermore, skipping around just requires extra clicks, which translates to extra time.

In general, defaulting to speed-reading or **skimming** passages isn't the most strategic approach either. It may appear to save time in the short run, but the time spent re-reading parts of the passage or just plain guessing on questions outweighs that benefit. That said, there are times where it is appropriate to skim a passage. One example is if you're under a time crunch where it's unlikely that you'll be able to get to all the remaining passages or questions with the few minutes left in a section. This approach involves reading the first and last sentences of each paragraph, and focusing on the most important features, like the results of experiment-based passages. Skimming can also help if a certain sentence, or even a whole paragraph, just doesn't click. That is, you read through it, but just don't feel like you *get* it. That's obviously not *ideal,* but it can happen to the best of us.

Let's move on to the second paragraph of this passage about PKU. We see some stuff about PAH, and DHR, and a bunch of reactions. What if all you can get out of it is *chemistry soup*? You've got two choices now: try to read it again or move on. The choice is less obvious than it may seem at first glance. In an ideal world, trying again would be appealing, since you want to have a reasonable sense of what this paragraph is saying. However, there's a risk of getting bogged down. That is, you might not be spending your time efficiently, but, just as importantly, you might find yourself focusing too much on small details, to the point of losing sight of the overall structure of the passage. There's also the risk of getting trapped in a negative mental spiral.

In cases like this, the best move is to move on. We want to see this not as giving up, but as a strategic choice to extract the most essential information. After all, we can always come back to the paragraph if a question asks about it, and in that case the question itself might give us some insight into how to tackle the information. What's more, it's always possible that the section you're bogged down in won't be asked about at all, so getting stuck reading and re-reading it would just waste time. It's really common for students to feel bad about moving on without understanding every word, perhaps based on anxieties that they should have studied harder or that everyone else probably understood it. In reality though, for virtually every MCAT student, mentally summarizing as best as possible and then moving on in cases like this is a smart move. For instance, we might summarize this paragraph in our heads as "PKU can also occur if DHR doesn't work." Not the *best* summary, maybe, but it's enough to allow us to move on, and that can sometimes be much more productive than refusing to continue unless we feel totally confident in what we've just read.

2. Passage Analysis

The science sections contain 10 passages, but they tend to be significantly shorter than CARS passages, and usually contain one or more figures or tables.

On the Bio/Biochem and Chem/Phys sections, there are three types of passages you'll see:

> **Textbook-style passages** should be pretty familiar; they provide information and describe scientific phenomena in a matter-of-fact manner.
> **Primary research-based passages** describe an experiment or research study, ultimately presenting results in the form of text and/or figures for you to interpret.
> **Lab manual-style passages** describe some experimental procedure, often containing unknown solutions or molecules. These passages look like they were drawn straight from a lab manual, so there tends to be a focus on the methods. Unlike primary research-type passages, though, they tend to confirm already established scientific facts, rather than developing new research findings.

Regardless of the type of passage, the first step is always to determine what information is most important, and thus, deserving of more of our attention. It's vital to capture the main ideas as you read. To do this, make sure that you stop to reflect periodically. We recommend pausing at the end of each paragraph to ask yourself what the purpose of the paragraph was. Then, using the highlighter tool, mark the words that capture that idea in order to create a rough outline of the passage. We also recommend highlighting proper nouns and important terms, like names of people, terms that are defined, and so forth. Numbers are important to note, but these don't necessarily need to be highlighted since they tend to stand out on their own in a block of text, and you'll want to highlight sparingly.

Other key elements to make note of are **opinions** and varying **perspectives** presented in passages. This is surprising for many students, but, just as with CARS passages, science passages can involve examining the views of several scientists of schools of thought. Keep an eye out for emphasis words like "should," "ought," "must," "better," "worse," and so on. Picking up on cues about opinions can be particularly challenging in science passages since scientists are typically expected to present their research findings objectively. No scientific journal would publish an article saying something like "So-and-so proposed XYZ to explain the onset of type 2 diabetes, but that theory was total garbage, so the aim of this study was to do it right." Instead, they might say something like "The putative mechanism through which XYZ contributes to the onset of type 2 diabetes has limitations, because _____." This sounds nicer, but it means that you have to be on the lookout for words like "limitations" or "putative" (which means "reputed, but not necessarily accurate") that scientists use to politely express disagreement.

Another example of subtle opinions in science passages is how scientists use words like "traditional." If the beginning of a passage says something like "Scientists have traditionally thought that....", you might initially think that "traditionally" introduces a well-accepted train of thought. However, wording like this is actually more commonly used to present an explanation that the author thinks is out of date, and in fact, it's likely that the author is about to present some new findings that she thinks are a major improvement on the "traditional" viewpoint. Additionally, always look for comparisons and contrasts. Contrasts might present as conflicting views, such as two different theories or opposing effects of various drugs or biological molecules. Unfortunately though, there's no master list of all the words and relationships that you need to keep an eye out for. Scientists learn to write this way through practice, so we too must practice reading this way. As you practice, keep these examples in mind and, with time, you'll get better at picking up on these hints.

Even more important to science passages are **cause-and-effect-like relationships**. This includes actual cause-and-effect relationships in experiments, such as when an independent variable is manipulated and a dependent variable is measured. Correlations that a passage establishes are also worth noting, but remember that correlation does not equal causality. Experiment-based science passages will often contain results in the form of text, figures, or both, and these figures are essential to understanding the outcome of the experiment. Results are prime MCAT question material and often where any correlation or causation will be found, so be sure to do a brief analysis of figures looking for these trends.

Now that we've covered some of what's important in an MCAT science passage, it's time to talk about what's not so important. To do this, let's examine a paragraph from our PKU passage.

> A variant form of PKU occurs when PAH is normal, but there is a defect in the enzyme dihydrobiopterin reductase (DHR). DHR is responsible for the regeneration of 5,6,7,8-tetrahydrobiopterin from q-dihydrobiopterin, where the former is an important cofactor in amino acid metabolism. Tetrahydrobiopterin serves as a co-factor both for PAH and for the production of L-DOPA, a dopamine precursor, from tyrosine and 5-hydroxy-L-tryptophan.

The first sentence tells us that some cases of PKU are caused by a defective DHR enzyme. This sentence also mentions PAH which we already know is the other possible cause of PKU. We can already tell that this paragraph is going to be a big bowl of alphabet soup, which can be intimidating at first. However, you don't need to know anything ahead of time about this enzyme, but if you can identify an important causal relationship in this paragraph (i.e., that defective DHR has an effect on PAH), you'll be able to do the same thing with any other acronyms thrown at you on your MCAT.

Next, we're focusing on DHR. DHR regenerates 5,6,7,8-tetra- molecule from the q-dihydro- molecule (that DHR takes the dihydro molecule and converts it into that tetrahydro molecule), which we're told is important for amino acid metabolism. How do we know what's important here? Let's see where this passage is headed next. The next sentence refers back to the tetrahydro molecule, telling us that it facilitates PAH function and helps synthesize a dopamine precursor. Therefore, we're interested in the tetrahydro product of DHR activity, as this molecule is important for amino acid metabolism, PAH function, and L-DOPA production, so let's highlight the list of these three functions. Review the sample highlighting below:

> A variant form of PKU occurs when PAH is normal, but there is a defect in the enzyme dihydrobiopterin reductase (DHR). DHR is responsible for the regeneration of 5,6,7,8-tetrahydrobiopterin from q-dihydrobiopterin, where the former is an important cofactor in amino acid metabolism. Tetrahydrobiopterin serves as a co-factor both for PAH and for the production of L-DOPA, a dopamine precursor, from tyrosine and 5-hydroxy-L-tryptophan.

This paragraph is a good example of a situation where it may be helpful to jot down a concise biochemical pathway on your wet-erase booklet. For example, you might draw an arrow from Q-D for Q-dihydrobiopterin to THB for tetrahydrobiopterin, and write DHR under the arrow for the enzyme that catalyzes this reaction. You could even show that THB is important for amino acid metabolism, as a cofactor for PAH, and L-DOPA production, as shown below.

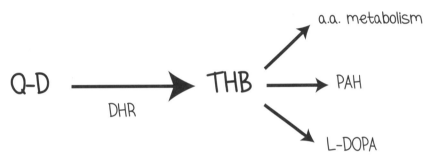

Figure 4. Sample note-taking

In general, we don't want to be *too* concerned with the exact names of compounds if they're called by their acronyms for the rest of the passage, but sometimes their names can give us hints to their function. For example, notice the similarity between "dihydrobiopterin reductase" and its substrate "q-dihydrobiopterin" and product "tetrahydrobiopterin." The "tetra" compound has four numbers in its prefix, which tells us about the positioning and numbering of hydrogen substituents in its structure. Additionally, it's worth recognizing the amino acids tyrosine and tryptophan are both mentioned here. Notice that, even in the midst of these unfamiliar enzymes and pathways, there are lots of concepts you *will* be familiar with from your content review, like the relationship between terms like "di" and "tetra" and the number of substituents on a molecule.

As a final note, remember that it's critical to actively engage when reading science passages on the MCAT to maximize your effectiveness within the time constraints. Using your highlighter to create a visual roadmap of the passage is a great example of an active process that will keep you focused on the task of identifying the passage's main ideas. Engage with the passage by contextualizing the presented information using your own knowledge. If you're finding it hard to maintain focus by the time you've reached the third or fourth passage and you're relatively early in your prep, don't fret! That's normal. As you complete a passage or two at a time and build up to full section tests and full-length exams, you'll see a noticeable difference in your ability to concentrate. If you zone out or miss more questions near the end of a section, consider taking a micro-break after five or six passages. Just pause, take three long, slow, deep breaths, and then hopefully you'll feel refreshed enough to power through the remaining passages.

3. Textbook-Style Passages

Textbook-style passages are like what you'd expect to see in an advanced textbook. Such passages start with a broad description of an MCAT-relevant subject and then focus more narrowly on a topic that will build on your MCAT content knowledge. In such passages, expect to see figures that display molecular structures or pathways, but, unlike other types of science passages, you won't have to worry about interpreting experimental results.

Let's examine this passage on the Krebs, or citric acid, cycle together:

In preparation for the Krebs cycle, decarboxylation of pyruvate occurs after pyruvate enters the mitochondrial matrix. During decarboxylation, pyruvate is converted to acetyl-CoA by a complex of three enzymes, commonly called E1, E2, and E3. The three enzymes together are called the pyruvate dehydrogenase complex (PDC).

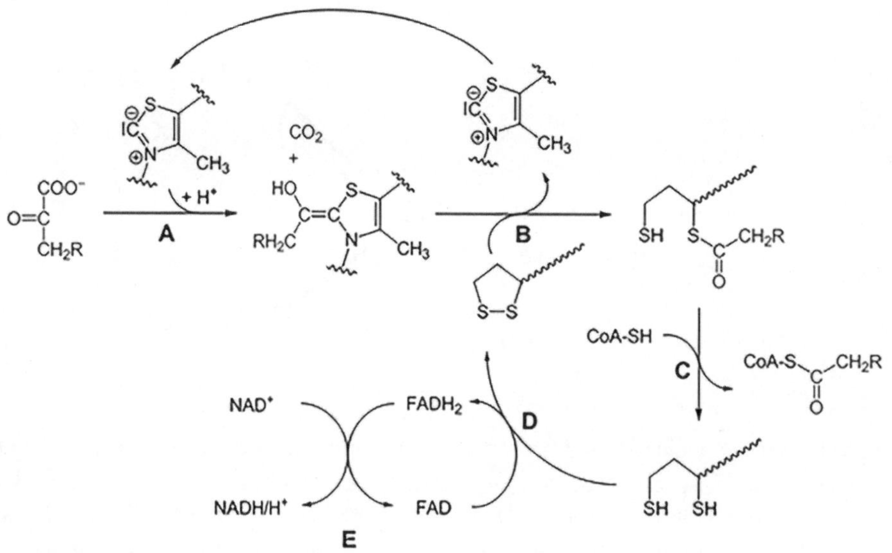

Figure 1. Enzymatic mechanism of pyruvate dehydrogenase complex

E1 contains a thiazolium ring that exists in zwitterion form. Pyruvate is added to the ring and loses CO_2. It then transfers to a lipoate on a long lysine residue arm. The lipoate is reduced and the ring is broken as an S-C bond forms. The arm then translocates the intermediate to the E2 active site on the complex. This is where the intermediate is transferred to a coenzyme A molecule. Acetyl-CoA is produced and released from the complex. The lysine arm then transfers the dihydrolipoate to E3, where it is oxidized to prepare for the next pyruvate molecule.

Pyruvate dehydrogenase is regulated by two enzymes: pyruvate dehydrogenase kinase (PDK), which can phosphorylate and deactivate E1, and pyruvate dehydrogenase phosphatase (PDP), which activates E1 by dephosphorylating it. The activity of PDK and PDP is regulated by the concentrations of ATP, ADP, NADH, NAD⁺, acetyl-CoA, and coenzyme A. The products of the reaction in Figure 1 activate PDK and the substrates inhibit PDK.

Textbook-style passages are the closest thing in the science section you'll see to CARS passages, where information is presented on a particular topic. The key difference is that in textbook-style science passages, there's an expectation that you bring in a foundation of MCAT-appropriate scientific knowledge. Such passages will start off broadly, typically with something you'll recognize, like the Krebs (or citric acid) cycle in this case.

With textbook-based passages, aim to capture the paragraph's main ideas by predicting where the passage is headed. For example, we're zooming in on the Krebs cycle to examine pyruvate, and how this molecule undergoes decarboxylation. Based on the next sentence, we confirm that we're focusing on this decarboxylation process. The Krebs cycle is relevant, as is the location in the mitochondrial matrix, but what's really necessary to understand here is the actual mechanism of this process. Specifically, we're told that prior to the Krebs cycle, pyruvate is the substrate molecule that's converted into acetyl-CoA, and the enzymes that catalyze this are E1, E2, and E3, which form a complex called the PDC. Thus, the main idea here is that in this particular step, one molecule (pyruvate) is converted into another molecule (acetyl-CoA) by three enzymes contained within this PDC complex.

The first paragraph makes it clear that decarboxylation is an important term. If it's already familiar to you, then so much the better, but if not, it's still possible to make an educated guess based on the etymology. "De" usually means "removal," and "carboxyl" refers to a carboxylic acid, or -COOH group, but even if we don't remember that, the name itself suggests some kind of carbon-based functional group. Let's consult Figure 1. Typically, we'll want to try to make sense of figures in the context of the text we've read while still moving efficiently through the passage. In textbook-style passages, figures will often depict a chemical or biological process described in the preceding paragraphs. If the title of a figure is mentioned in the passage, that's usually a good time to glance at the figure to corroborate or expand upon what you've read. When looking at figures, obtain just enough information to make sense of the passage as a whole, and then move on, since we can always come back for details.

The caption here tells us that we're looking at the PDC complex's activity, which is the complex that catalyzes pyruvate decarboxylation via the E1, E2, and E3 enzymes. Unfortunately, none of the molecules or enzymes are labeled with their names here, but this is fairly common. Since this figure's pretty complicated, it is a good idea to quickly locate the precursor or substrate molecules, and any end products or notable features. This helps us quickly orient ourselves to the figure when/if it comes up in a question. We start with step A, so the molecule to the left of this arrow must be pyruvate, our precursor. There's a ring structure added onto pyruvate while, at the same time, a molecule of carbon dioxide is released. That release of CO_2 is the decarboxylation this reaction refers to. Thus, we can follow arrow A to arrows B, C, and D. There are some products that branch off at some of these steps, but there's also some recycling going on, which makes this figure particularly complex. Recall that the goal of this process is to generate acetyl-CoA from pyruvate, so, even if it's difficult to recognize immediately where acetyl-CoA is in this figure, we can probably figure it out or narrow it down by studying this more closely. That said, we don't recommend spending more than 10 or 15 seconds on a figure like this, especially since the passage text hasn't elaborated on any of these steps in depth at this point.

Next, the text becomes more technical, but again, keep in mind the larger picture and don't let new terminology or complex reaction mechanisms distract from your primary goal. First, note that the E1 enzyme has a ring structure, and is a zwitterion (a molecule with both negatively and positively charged parts).

Next, the passage states that E1 catalyzes the process by which pyruvate loses a carbon dioxide molecule, which we can see in Step A of Figure 1, and that pyruvate is then transferred onto this lipoate group thanks to a lysine residue. Since we might not be exactly sure what that means, let's check out Figure 1 again. Sure enough, in Step B, we see pyruvate being attached to a molecule with a long carbon-chain. Lipoate sounds like the term lipid, which, in fatty acid form, has a long chain of carbon atoms, so that makes sense! You also might recognize that the amino acid lysine has a positive charge, so when this is mentioned in the passage, you'll want to take note of distinctive properties like this, as there's a good chance such properties relate to its function. Since lysine is an amino acid, and enzymes are typically proteins, this likely refers to a part of this enzyme. Next, that lipoate group is reduced, meaning it gains bonds to hydrogen atoms, and the ring breaks as a sulfur-carbon bond forms. We see this in Step B again, where one of the sulfur atoms gains a bond to hydrogen and the other gains a bond to carbon, breaking the ring.

Then we move on to the E2 enzyme. The passage tells us E2 catalyzes the transfer of a coenzyme A molecule, which we see in step C, with the release of acetyl CoA. So, this is a product that exits this reaction sequence. In the big picture here, recall that the goal of this entire enzymatic machine is to convert pyruvate into acetyl-CoA. Through a complicated series of steps, we've accomplished that!

Next, that lysine arm on the enzyme transfers this lipid-like molecule over to E3 where oxidation occurs, reversing the reduction step that occurred earlier to reform the bonds between the two sulfur atoms. We already obtained our acetyl-CoA product, so E3 is essentially responsible for housekeeping, recycling a molecule necessary to repeat this reaction sequence. As it happens, this is a common trend in biochemistry: our body uses reverse processes to recycle compounds necessary for a given metabolic pathway.

This text is highly detailed, but *not* something we should memorize. Instead, this is exactly the kind of text that you could read through relatively quickly, highlighting landmarks for important enzymes and critical steps so you can come back and analyze the exact catalytic step you need to answer a question. The big picture here is that pyruvate is shuttled between these three enzymes, gaining a functional group here, losing a functional group there, and so on. Ultimately, the end point is that we gain some acetyl-CoA and recycle necessary components to repeat the cycle with the next pyruvate molecule. Therefore, it's absolutely worth highlighting E1, E2, and E3, as these are important landmarks, and then anything else you might need to refer back to quickly. If you're asked about specific reaction steps, or the structures of any one of these enzymes, now you'll know exactly where to look.

Finally, our last paragraph is about enzyme regulation. Enzymes regulate in two basic directions, up or down. We're told that the first enzyme in the PDC pathway, E1, is deactivated by PDK and activated by PDP, which add or remove a phosphate group, respectively. Furthermore, these regulatory enzymes sense concentrations of relevant biomolecules in the surrounding mitochondrial soup, such as ATP, ADP, NADH, and coenzyme A. In the vast majority of biochemical processes, the downstream products of a process inhibit it via negative feedback, and the upstream substrates promote it. Accordingly, the passage tells us that the products of pyruvate decarboxylation (e.g., compounds like acetyl-coA) activate the regulatory enzyme PDK and thereby *inhibit* the complex, whereas substrates, like coenzyme A, inhibit PDK and thereby *stimulate* the complex. It also makes sense that when energy is high in the cell and ATP levels are high, we wouldn't necessarily want the Krebs cycle running at full speed. So ATP tends to inhibit this process, whereas ADP stimulates it. Remember though, we can always come back to analyze which biomolecules activate or deactivate what, so in real time this part can be skimmed in the interest of capturing the big picture.

4. Primary Research Passages

A common passage type you'll encounter on the biology and chemistry sections will present a core scientific concept in the context of a research study or experiment. In this way, the MCAT can test you on the content you know, on new scientific information, *and* on the design and execution of the research, all at the same time. One of the particular challenges with primary research-based passages is interpreting the results of experiments.

Let's work through this passage about protein adsorption:

> Protein adsorption is the process by which protein molecules adhere to and accumulate on a solid surface. The properties of adsorbed layers are highly dependent on the size, net charge, and structure of constituent proteins. These factors influence surface affinity, protein packing and orientation, and the water content (solvation) of the layer.

> Quantification of protein layer solvation throughout the adsorption process is an important step as this directly links to the performance of artificial nanomaterials. Researchers measured weight-%-solvation during the adsorption and desorption processes of human milk lysozyme (a globular "rigid" protein), bovine serum albumin (a globular "soft" protein), and α-synuclein (an unfolded "soft" protein). Tests were

done on both hydrophilic and hydrophobic surfaces. The bulk protein solutions were injected until surface saturation was reached and each protein formed a monolayer on both surfaces.

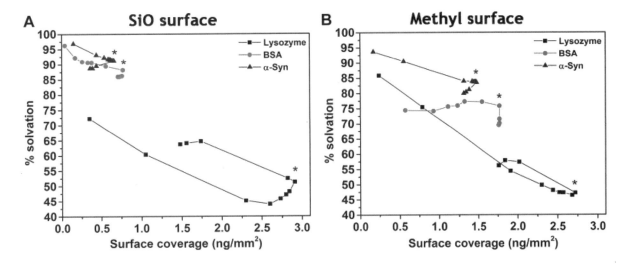

Figure 1. Evolution of the adsorbed layer hydration throughout the protein incubation and buffer rinsing process (Note: * Indicates when the solution was replaced by a protein-free solution, i.e., rinsing starts from that point.)

The combination of the complementary techniques, dual polarization interferometry (DPI), and quartz crystal microbalance with dissipation monitoring (QCM-D) provided data on protein mass coverage. DPI monitors the protein "dry" mass using a direct measurement of thickness and refractive index (RI), whereas QCM-D measures the protein mass and the water associated with the layer. These techniques were used to optically characterize adsorption of all three proteins on hydrophilic and hydrophobic sensor chips. Measurements were taken during incubation of protein and during rinsing, for all three proteins on both surfaces.

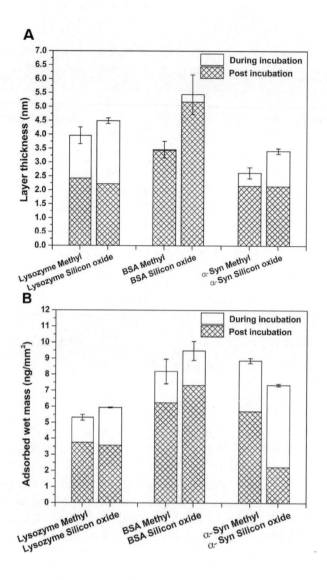

Figure 2. Adsorbed mass sensed by both DPI (A) and QCM-D (B) of all three proteins on both surfaces (Note: % Values represent the percentage of mass remaining post incubation, data is expressed as mean ± SD)

Adapted from Ouberai MM, Xu K, Welland ME. (2014). Effect of the interplay between protein and surface on the properties of adsorbed protein layers. Biomaterials, 35(24) under CC BY 3.0

Even if you're not sure what protein adsorption is, the passage tells us that it's the process by which protein molecules adhere to and accumulate on a solid surface. This is the general scientific concept that the successive research study builds upon. Primary research-based passages have a common structure: background, purpose or hypothesis, methods, and results. This first paragraph is background-focused—it tells us what general concept the study will be based on, explains protein adsorption, and details some of the factors that affect it. Let's not spend too much time here, but if a question asks us about factors affecting protein adsorption, this is where we'll want to go.

The next paragraph mentions protein layer solvation (the surrounding of proteins by water molecules), not just as something biophysically interesting, but also very practically relevant to how nanomaterials work. Then the passage states that the researchers measured weight-%-solvation as a series of proteins were adsorbed and desorbed. These statements capture the purpose of this study. Sometimes you'll see a hypothesis stating the scientists' predictions, but more often the passage will simply state the purpose, aim, or question that the researchers intend to address, which here appears to be understanding the solvation properties of these three proteins and how this relates, in some way, to development of nanomaterials.

This sentence actually starts to introduce the experimental method as well: the researchers measured weight-%-solvation of three proteins (a rigid folded protein, a soft folded protein, and an unfolded soft protein). Given these descriptions, we can begin to think about the rationale behind why these specific proteins might have been chosen. Highlighting lists like these can be helpful for visualizing the structure of the paragraph. Remember, we're examining the proteins' ability to adsorb to a solid surface, and the next sentence tells us the researchers tested this on both hydrophobic and hydrophilic surfaces, saturating these surfaces until covered by a single layer of protein. For primary research passages, we aren't too concerned with memorizing the details of the experimental procedures, so it's okay to just quickly identify the major aspects of these procedures that are essential to understanding the results. The number of milliliters of solution used or the exact surface area are details you can return to later.

Next, let's check out the figure and align it with what we've just read. When a passage mentions a figure within the text, it is often a good idea to review the figure at that point. However, if the text does not directly reference the figure the best strategy is to view the figures sequentially, as they occur, in the text. First, let's gather information from the caption. We're looking at how proteins adsorbed to these surfaces.

Now let's look at the basic architecture of this figure. We have two graphs, one for each of two surfaces, a silicon oxide surface and a methyl surface. How can we relate this to what we've just read? Well, we were told these three proteins were tested on a hydrophilic and a hydrophobic surface. Methyl groups are hydrophobic, and given the oxygen atom, silicon oxide must be hydrophilic. So, we don't really care about silicon oxide or methyl specifically, but rather we care about the properties they represent. Within each graph, we have our three proteins of interest, lysozyme, bovine serum albumin, and alpha-synuclein, which we know differ in whether they are folded or unfolded and rigid or soft.

Let's check out our axes next. Surface coverage is on the x-axis, and functions as an independent variable. We're interested in how % protein solvation on the y-axis depends on that coverage. Now let's scan for major trends that jump out. In general, the two softer proteins, albumin and alpha-synuclein, show a higher percent solvation, particularly on the hydrophilic surface. However, for all three proteins, percent solvation appears to drop as surface coverage increases. In other words, the more crowded and protein-packed the surface is, the less these proteins are solvated.

The next paragraph introduces a second experiment and its methods. If the devices and techniques mentioned in this paragraph sound intimidating, the good news is that this is a great example of a technical-sounding paragraph that boils down to a few predictable elements. We've really just got two techniques that are used, DPI and QCM-D, with the goal of detecting protein mass coverage. Notice how these complicated procedures and expensive technologies are just tools that the researchers use to find answers. As always, don't let the details bog you down. Stay focused on the big picture: what they are trying to figure out. Later in the passage we get some more information about these techniques. DPI tells us about dry protein mass and QCM-D tells us about wet protein mass. We can connect both of these methods back to the idea of protein solvation, so let's highlight these techniques and what we measure from them. This is then followed by a few more sentences about the methods, but we've already highlighted the techniques so, if a question asks, we'll know where to come back for this information.

Let's take a look at Figure 2 and square this away with what we just read. We're looking at adsorbed protein mass, without water as measured by DPI in Figure 2A, and with water as measured by QCM-D in Figure 2B. Looking next at our axes, we're looking at protein adsorption as a function of surface type (the hydrophobic methyl surface versus hydrophilic silicon oxide surface) and also as a function of protein type. The most confusing element here is probably the distinction between the incubation and post-incubation periods. We may want to refer back to the last paragraph to understand this distinction. During incubation, proteins were allowed to adhere to the solid surface, and then post-incubation, rinsing occured. The purpose of rinsing is that it removes any proteins that are not firmly adhered to the surface so that we only measure those that are truly adsorbed. This means we really want to pay attention to protein adsorption levels post-incubation. At this point, we can certainly try to identify major trends—for example, note that lysozyme has relatively high adsorbed dry mass but low wet mass, which fits with the lower solvation levels we saw for lysozyme in Figure 1. However, once you understand the figure anatomy and know *how* to interpret it, we don't suggest spending *too* much time here, as we can always come back to this figure later to analyze specific trends of interest. For reference, below is the passage with suggested highlighting. Take a moment to carefully review how the points we've been making translate into highlighting.

Protein adsorption is the process by which protein molecules adhere to and accumulate on a solid surface. The properties of adsorbed layers are highly dependent on the size, net charge, and structure of constituent proteins. These factors influence surface affinity, protein packing and orientation, and the water content (solvation) of the layer.

Quantification of protein layer solvation throughout the adsorption process is an important step as this directly links to the performance of artificial nanomaterials. Researchers measured weight-%-solvation during the adsorption and desorption processes of human milk lysozyme (a globular "rigid" protein), bovine serum albumin (a globular "soft" protein), and α-synuclein (an unfolded "soft" protein). Tests were done on both hydrophilic and hydrophobic surfaces. The bulk protein solutions were injected until surface saturation was reached and each protein formed a monolayer on both surfaces.

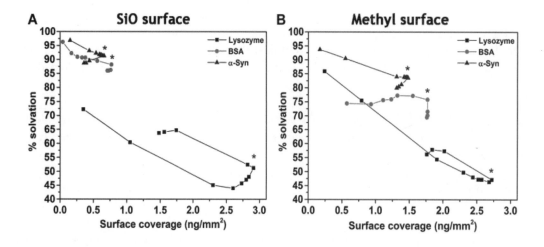

Figure 1. Evolution of the adsorbed layer hydration throughout the protein incubation and buffer rinsing process (Note: * Indicates when the solution was replaced by a protein-free solution, i.e., rinsing starts from that point.)

The combination of the complementary techniques, dual polarization interferometry (DPI) and quartz crystal microbalance with dissipation monitoring (QCM-D) provided data on protein mass coverage. DPI monitors the protein 'dry' mass using a direct measurement of thickness and refractive index (RI), whereas QCM-D measures the protein mass and the water associated with the layer. These techniques were used to optically characterize adsorption of all three proteins on hydrophilic and hydrophobic sensor chips. Measurements were taken during incubation of protein and during rinsing, for all three proteins on both surfaces.

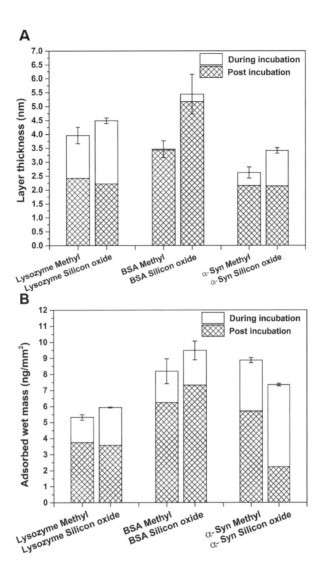

Figure 2. Adsorbed mass sensed by both DPI (A) and QCM-D (B) of all three proteins on both surfaces (Note: % Values represent the percentage of mass remaining post incubation, data is expressed as mean ± SD)

Adapted from Ouberai MM, Xu K, Welland ME. (2014). Effect of the interplay between protein and surface on the properties of adsorbed protein layers. Biomaterials, 35(24) under CC BY 3.0

To recap, with primary research-based passages, focus on recognizing the basic structure of background, purpose, methods, and results. It's okay to get the gist of the methods without getting too far into the weeds, as your attention should generally be more focused on the results, which may be in the form of text, figures, or both. Interpreting research findings means integrating this information with what you know about the purpose and methods from earlier in the passage, as well as analyzing figures for major trends. With figures, it's important to spend enough time on them to understand the anatomy of the figure, what the manipulated variables and measured outcomes are, and *how* to interpret it for specific trends that you can examine in further depth later. You'll want to get enough information out of the figure to understand how it fits into the passage as a whole without spending too much time poring over every single data point. The time to analyze individual data points on a figure in detail is if a question asks about it. When that happens, the question will point you in the direction of the data that you need to analyze. Then, you can pull the necessary information out of the figure more efficiently than if you started from scratch with the goal of completely analyzing all the data in the figure.

5. Lab Manual Passages

In addition to textbook-style and primary research-based passages, in the Chemical and Physical Foundations and Biological and Biochemical Foundations sections, you'll also encounter passages that look like they were drawn directly out of a lab manual. Lab manual-type passages are similar to primary research passages, in that both will typically contain some combination of background, purpose or hypothesis, methods, and results. However, the ways in which these are presented and tested will differ. Whereas the methods in a primary research passage are largely a means to an end, a lab manual-style passage will ask you to reflect on the methods more often or in more depth. Lab manual passages may contain unknowns, solutions or chemicals, or a molecule with an unknown function. In fact, one of the primary distinctions between lab manual and primary research style passages is that lab manual passages are typically not contributing new research findings to the existing body of knowledge. Rather, they are simply confirming something that is known or using existing knowledge to study unknowns. However, like with primary research passages, any results provided are prime targets for questions, and these results may be presented in text, figures, or both. One of your primary aims with these types of passages is to figure out the *why*: why did the researchers conduct their experiments in the way that they did?

Let's read through the following passage on lactate dehydrogenase:

> Lactate dehydrogenase (LDH) is an enzyme that catalyzes the interconversion of lactate and pyruvate, regenerating NAD^+ for glycolysis via anaerobic respiration. Its activity is closely regulated by the relative concentrations of its substrates, as well as by other small molecules. Oxalate, an organic acid found in plants, is predicted to be an LDH inhibitor.
>
> To determine the inhibitor type of oxalate, LDH activity was measured in the presence or absence of oxalate. LDH was incubated with NAD^+ and lactate using a series of oxalate concentrations to determine the IC_{50} concentration (Figure 1).

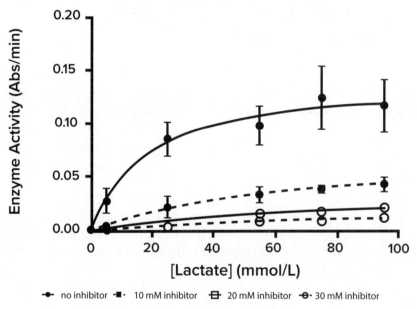

Figure 1. Determination of the IC_{50} concentration for oxalate inhibition of LDH

> Based on the IC_{50} value determined, a series of oxalate concentrations were chosen to measure the K_m and V_{max} values for LDH. Enzyme dilutions were prepared in cuvettes to which NAD^+ and varying concentrations of lactate plus 10 µL of buffer or inhibitor were added. NADH levels were monitored by

spectrometry, and changes in absorbance per unit time were used to calculate enzyme activity according to the equation:

Equation 1 $\qquad\qquad A_{340\,nm}$ for NADH = 6220 $(M \bullet cm)^{-1}$

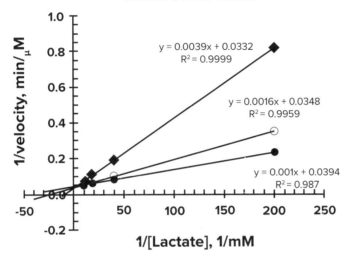

Figure 2. Lineweaver-Burk plot of LDH enzymatic activity in the presence of oxalate

Almost everything you need to know about LDH is clearly stated because this passage isn't really testing your knowledge of LDH. Instead, it's testing your knowledge and understanding of enzyme function and inhibition. LDH just happens to be a good example of this. In reality any enzyme, its substrates, or inhibitors could be used in its place, so don't worry if you happen to encounter an unfamiliar enzyme. In fact, the less familiar the example, the less background content knowledge you'll be expected to bring to the table! We know this is a lab manual passage because it describes a series of steps taken to conduct a simple experiment. However, it's perfectly fine to start out without identifying the type of passage this is, as many principles will apply to all science passages.

For example, we start out with some background information, and at this point we're mostly concerned with identifying main ideas, as usual. We start broadly with a mention of LDH and its role in the cell, and then we quickly focus on its regulation by other substrates, specifically oxalate, a putative inhibitor of LDH. Now, there's some background information here you might be familiar with by the time you take your MCAT (for example, you might recognize the roles of lactate and pyruvate in cellular respiration) but, for now, you know where in the passage you need to go for this sort of background biochemistry.

Next, we're told that presumably *somebody* measured the activity of LDH to figure out what kind of inhibitor oxalate is. Now we start to see the a familiar passage structure: beginning with background, moving on to purpose, methods, and, finally, results. For example, the short phrase "to determine inhibitor type" tells us the purpose of this experiment. Now we're getting into methods territory, and since this is more narrowly focused on a simple experiment rather than a novel research question, we can be sure that this is a lab manual-style passage. So, methods are important! First, we're told that the enzyme is incubated with lactate, which we know is its substrate, and NAD⁺, which we might be familiar with even though it hasn't been described in the passage yet. In this case, NAD⁺ is just a cofactor that's necessary for this reaction. This detail is certainly important for this procedure, but not as necessary for our understanding of the passage as a whole. Instead, the key aspect of experimental step is what's being manipulated or changed. In this case, that's the inhibitor, oxalate. As you can imagine, if the concentration of inhibitor is zero, then LDH is going to be operating full throttle, right? If we add a little bit of inhibitor, it'll work slightly less well. A little bit more, and it'll work even less well. From this, we can create a dose-dependent relationship, or a dose-response curve. This can then be used to determine the IC_{50} concentration, which is the inhibitor concentration at which the enzyme works half as well as it would in the absence of an inhibitor.

Let's go ahead and examine Figure 1 to corroborate this. First, the caption tells us that this graph displays how the IC_{50} concentration of oxalate was determined. Next, we want to check out the axes. The x-axis shows the concentration of lactate, and the y-axis shows LDH enzyme activity. Essentially, what this is showing is how LDH activity varies as a function of substrate concentration. As you might expect, enzyme activity increases as the substrate concentration is increased, up to a point. The other variable that's changed here is oxalate concentration, which is important. Based on the key, as oxalate concentration is increased, LDH activity drops way down. Let's see if we can determine the IC_{50} value. When there is no inhibitor present, LDH activity is roughly 0.12, which we see on the right side of the graph at 100 millimolar lactate. To find the IC_{50}, we need to look for the oxalate concentration that translates to half that activity, or around 0.06. The next line down, representing an oxalate concentration of 10 millimolar, is pretty close, so there's a good chance our true IC_{50} value is somewhere around there. In general, for a figure like this, we recommend getting just enough information out of it so that you have what you need to understand the rest of the passage and you can come back to it later to answer specific questions, like the approximate IC_{50} concentration.

Next, we're given part two of this experiment. Using this IC_{50} concentration, we're again going to use different oxalate concentrations to figure out two really critical pieces of information about LDH: its K_m and V_{max}. From your understanding of enzymes, you should know that V_{max} tells us the maximum velocity of the enzyme, or how fast it can convert its substrate into product, given arbitrarily high levels of substrate. K_m is slightly less straightforward. This value tells us the amount of substrate required to reach *half* the maximum velocity. It's really a measure of enzyme affinity for its substrate.

Next up are even more methods, including enzyme dilutions, more NAD^+, more lactate, and either buffer or inhibitor. Why add buffer? This is exactly the kind of question the MCAT might ask you. Basically, we need a control condition to give us the normal activity level to compare to our experimental findings. Therefore, some samples received just some buffer solution instead of inhibitor solution to control for the volume added to the samples. Then NADH levels were monitored—since NAD^+ is probably being consumed and NADH being generated in this process. Thus, the rate of NADH generation is a good approximation for the rate of LDH activity. Conveniently, we can apparently measure NADH production by spectrometry, so now we have a method for measuring LDH activity. Don't sweat too much over this equation, as we can come back to it if needed.

What are the key takeaways here? We're interested in what's manipulated in the experiment by the researchers and the outcomes measured. So in this experiment, we're varying the concentrations of substrate and measuring NADH levels as a proxy for what we *really* care about: LDH activity.

Now onto our final figure. Figure 1 gave us a result that we used to inform the set-up of part 2 of this experiment, and it's the results in Figure 2 that we are really interested in. Note how this passage doesn't reveal the results in text form. Instead, it shows you the data and requires you to put in the elbow grease. Therefore, familiarity with enzyme concepts and interpreting graphs like this one will help you derive meaning from such figures both accurately and efficiently.

The caption tells us that this is a Lineweaver-Burk plot, which we know is a specialized way of displaying enzyme function. Be careful though, this isn't just enzyme activity as a function of lactate concentration. Rather, it's the inverse of enzyme activity over the inverse of lactate concentration! This means that the farther we drift away from the 0 mark on either axis in the positive direction, the smaller our values get. So the basic trend here is that as lactate concentration goes *down*, enzyme activity also goes *down*. The opposite is also true: as lactate concentration increases, so must enzyme activity. This makes logical sense, but interesting here is how this relationship changes with inhibitor concentration.

This is where your relevant content knowledge comes in handy. Lineweaver-Burk plots are so useful because we can determine maximum enzyme velocity from the inverse of the y-intercept on this graph, and we can determine the K_m value from the *negative* inverse of the x-intercept. Notice how when the inhibitor concentration changes, V_{max} stays the same. But what happens on the x-axis is that the negative 1 over K_m value gets closer and closer to zero. In other words, as we get closer to the 0 mark on this axis, the K_m value gets bigger and bigger. This means that the oxalate inhibitor causes V_{max} to stay the same, but the K_m value, or substrate concentration required to reach half V_{max}, increases. This indicates that we're dealing with a competitive inhibitor.

Consider the highlighted version of the passage below to see how we translated those goals into action (in the form of highlighting):

Lactate dehydrogenase (LDH) is an enzyme that catalyzes the interconversion of lactate and pyruvate, regenerating NAD^+ for glycolysis via anaerobic respiration. Its activity is closely regulated by the relative concentrations of its substrates, as well as by other small molecules. Oxalate, an organic acid found in plants, is predicted to be an LDH inhibitor.

To determine the inhibitor type of oxalate, LDH activity was measured in the presence or absence of oxalate. LDH was incubated with NAD^+ and lactate using a series of oxalate concentrations to determine the IC_{50} concentration (Figure 1).

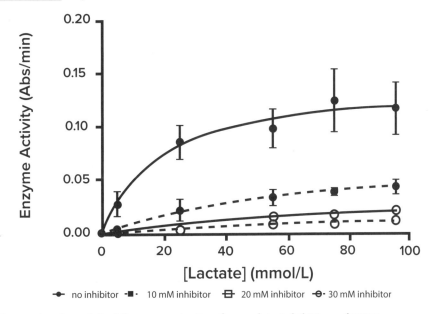

Figure 1. Determination of the IC_{50} concentration for oxalate inhibition of LDH

Based on the IC_{50} value determined, a series of oxalate concentrations were chosen to measure the K_m and V_{max} values for LDH. Enzyme dilutions were prepared in cuvettes to which NAD^+ and varying concentrations of lactate plus 10 μL of buffer or inhibitor were added. NADH levels were monitored by spectrometry, and changes in absorbance per unit time were used to calculate enzyme activity according to the equation:

Equation 1 $$A_{340\,nm} \text{ for NADH} = 6220 \ (M \bullet cm)^{-1}$$

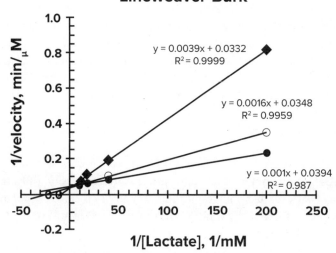

Figure 2. Lineweaver-Burk plot of LDH enzymatic activity in the presence of oxalate

Lab manual passages certainly share some similarities with primary research-based passages, but the key for lab manual passages is to critically engage with the methods *and* the results. You can then draw upon your relevant content knowledge to help you get to the right answers with greater accuracy and speed.

6. Study Strategies

It may take some practice before you feel like an expert at deciphering MCAT science passages. Even as you start to feel more comfortable with recognizing their patterns and quirks, there are always ways to work on reading passages more efficiently.

Instead of looking for outside reading material to improve your passage comprehension, we recommend going to the source itself: real MCAT-like passages. Regular passage practice is one of the best uses of your time as an MCAT student. Regular exposure to MCAT passages will make them less intimidating, and you'll start to detect the patterns and characteristics that are frequently testable. Also, there is no better way to practice applying your content knowledge than in the way you'll be tested on the actual MCAT.

Nailing the pacing of a science section on your MCAT doesn't happen overnight through brute force. Instead, it happens through consistent practice and review geared towards becoming more efficient and skilled at passage analysis. Remember, acing the MCAT isn't about finding shortcuts—it's about knowing what to look for in passages and what to avoid in order to use your time most effectively. Building the endurance required to push through this almost eight hour test also isn't something that happens overnight. Timed practice is something that will allow you to, over time, increase your stamina from just one or two passages all the way to a full length MCAT test.

Another way that you can use passage practice to your advantage is to troubleshoot your technique. We've discussed some approaches that tend to be effective, but ultimately going through the motions yourself will give you an opportunity to experiment with your approach until you find a rhythm that works for you. The goal here isn't to restrict you to a one-size-fits-all mold, but rather give you some tools that are at your disposal to help you feel confident and as ready as you've ever been on your exam date.

If you really want to make the most out of your passage practice, or if you feel like you keep hitting a plateau, you might want to break out some more advanced approaches. This will require a combination of analytics and reflection. Full-length analytics will tell you which questions you missed, which passages they were associated with, the types of question, passage, or content that are trickier for you, and what impact timing and endurance might be having on your performance. Not only can you look for patterns like whether you missed more questions on electrochemistry or spent too much time on passages, but if you're *not* doing this kind of review, you might be missing out on the benefits of data-driven strategic planning in your MCAT prep!

No computer algorithm is going to be quite enough to tell you *why* you missed particular questions, which is where *you* come in. Diving deeper into your full-length means reviewing questions you missed, passages you had trouble with, and in many cases questions that you did get right or that you guessed on. It means looking for trends impacting your performance, literally making note of these, and then creating discrete, tangible goals for your studying *and* your next full-length or practice opportunity. In this way, if you're hit a plateau you'll have at least a few ideas of what changes to make for next time.

You can also try incorporating some more advanced approaches to take your passage comprehension skills to the next level, like trying to make predictions as you read. What's this passage going to be about? What will the next paragraph be about? Are we zooming in or zooming out? Are we going to see results in the next paragraph or are we going to learn about new methods for a second experiment? If this is the hypothesis, what kind of experiment could we perform to test this? If these are the methods, what results can we expect to confirm or refute the hypothesis? What are the figures going to look like? Why is the author making these arguments, and what might the author think about this idea?

You can even start to go further by reading a passage and predicting the types of questions you'll see. Maybe one on the purpose of the experiment, one about why a particular step was included in the methods, another about the purpose of the control group, and definitely one or two questions about the major trends in the figure. You can go even further by predicting answer choices based on the questions you encounter. There might be one that ties in the main idea, one that states the opposite of the correct answer, one that is mostly correct but part of it gets a little too extreme or out of context, and maybe one that relates to something else described in the passage that doesn't quite answer the question.

Another thing you can do is to sit down with a coffee or morning drink of choice and thoroughly analyze a passage under untimed conditions. What's the flow of an MCAT science passage? Are there parts that tend to be more confusing than others? This is your chance to work through those challenges, be it technical language or a confusing figure with data all over the place. If you had an hour to fully dissect a passage and mull over each of the questions, how many questions do you think you could get right? Now, what if you could have your MCAT review resources open at the same time so that now you have access to the essential science information you need? This may help you differentiate between content deficits and cognitive reasoning errors, and also help you learn how to apply your content knowledge more effectively so that you can be the MCAT passage wizard you're meant to be.

7. Must-Knows

> Three major tools available to read passages:
  - Wet-erase booklet: Don't overuse it, but can be useful for certain passage types (alphabet soup, causal relationships, etc.).
  - Highlighter: Useful for creating passage outline, but don't over-highlight.
  - Eyes: As with CARS passages, attention and focus are key.
> Three main types of science passages:
  - Textbook-style passages: Provide information and describe scientific phenomena in a matter-of-fact manner.
  - Primary research-based passages: Describe an experiment or research study and ultimately present results in the form of text and/or figures for you to interpret; often contain new knowledge.
  - Lab manual-style passages: describe some experimental procedure, often containing unknown solutions or molecules, and tend to focus on methods and established facts.
> Things to pay attention to when reading passages:
  - Opinions (even in science sections), perspectives, viewpoints.
  - Comparisons and contrasts.
  - Cause-and-effect relationships.
  - Terms that you already know.
> Things not to agonize over:
  - Every single detail, especially in experimental methods.
  - Precise meaning of newly-introduced or unfamiliar acronyms.
> Key elements of practice:
  - Consistency and regularity.
  - Identifying action points for improvement.
  - Active reading, and predicting where the passage will go.
  - Becoming familiar with the structure and logical flow of passages.

Applied Practice

The best MCAT practice is realistic, with detailed analytics to help you assess where things went wrong. For those reasons, we recommend completing practice questions in an online setting that simulates the real MCAT interface, and using the analytics provided to help you decide how to best move your studies forward.

CARS does not require knowledge of specific subject areas, but it does require development of strong test-taking skills. To ensure you are honing those skills as you work through this book, we suggest you go online after wrapping up each chapter and generate a Qbank Practice Set of 2-3 CARS passages to practice and review. While not every chapter of this book is directly applicable to CARS, regular CARS practice is key to test day success.

As a further supplement, given the importance of active learning for effective studying, we also suggest that you consult the Must-Knows at the end of each chapter of this Reasoning text as a basis for creating a study sheet. This is not a sheet to memorize in the more traditional sense of content memorization, but rather a quick reference of the most important strategies for you to refer to during and after practice in your early prep. Frequently revisiting the most important strategies for the MCAT - in both CARS and the Sciences - will help you continue to improve your performance.

This page left intentionally blank.

Pacing in Science

CHAPTER 10

1. MCAT Timing

The MCAT is fundamentally about applying complex scientific knowledge in new contexts, or in light of new information. Even the time constraints on the test serve this purpose. That is, the test isn't strictly timed to pick out the fastest students, but it is timed in a way that forces you to be both strategic and efficient in order to be successful. There's no secret ingredient or "trick" to mastering MCAT timing. Instead, the idea is that you first develop the baseline content knowledge and reasoning skills to be able to answer any MCAT question, and then, as strategy and critical thinking become second nature, you'll learn to become more efficient at doing so. As we covered earlier in this book (Chapter 1), the MCAT has three science sections, each of which lasts 95 minutes. Considering that each of these sections has 15 discretes and 44 passage-based questions, on test day you'll have about a minute per discrete question and an average of eight minutes to complete each of the ten passages and associated questions. It's no mystery, then, that **pacing** strategies are a major factor in being successful on the MCAT.

Of course, this is only an average. Some passages will be tougher to get through and some questions will take more than a minute to answer. Ultimately, how you split your time will depend heavily on the strategies you will have, by test day, practiced and honed to a perfect fit. Some students prefer digesting passages thoroughly, and then breezing through the questions, while others would rather skim the passage and go back later, leaving more time to spend on the questions. Most students end up usually somewhere in the middle: you'll have time to read and comprehend the main ideas of the passage, but also have some time available to return to the passage, as needed, while answering questions.

Spending **too much time** on the passage can be a sign of difficulty focusing. Your goal with reading shouldn't be to memorize or even necessarily understand every single detail — you can come back to those later if you need to. Instead, focus on the big picture and the major arguments. On the other end of the spectrum, skimming the passage or going straight to the questions before reading is likely to result in falling victim to trap answers, and can end up being *more* time-intensive in the long run. An approximately even split between time spent on the passage and time spent on questions is a proven approach that works better than more extreme methods do.

These points have a few practical consequences. First of all, the goal here isn't to perfect your timing on a given passage or question down to the millisecond. In fact, obsessing over the clock on your MCAT can detract from what you're there to do: think critically about science. Rather, through practice, you should get a feel for the appropriate pacing and start adopting it into your full length practice. This also means that there's more value in focusing on your average pacing across passages rather than getting worked up about any one passage, since some passages will be longer than others, have more questions, or require more calculations. Instead of checking the clock after every passage, **check the clock after two or three passages**, or after 15 questions or so. That way you can take a pulse on your pacing without triggering a sweat-inducing panic just a few questions into a section. At roughly 30 minutes in you should be at about question 20, after 60 minutes in you should be at about question 40, and after 90 minutes or so you should be done.

A final point here is that improvements in timing on the MCAT can help boost anyone's score, even if completing a section in time isn't an issue for you. If you had even just a few more minutes at the end of a section to review flagged questions or serve as a safety net for a super hard section, you might feel less anxious during your exam. Importantly, this often translates into more questions answered correctly and a higher score. For many students, timing improvements are the investment that returns the most immediate score boost on their MCAT. For example, rushing through the last two passages and guessing on the last eight questions might mean that you miss out on some easy points tucked into those passages. In other words, becoming more efficient and practiced with MCAT pacing carries a lot of potential for points towards your overall score. Don't let the clock get in between what you know and the score you're capable of on your MCAT!

2. Pacing and Time Management Skills

Timing on the MCAT is less about racing the clock, and more about sticking to your pacing. Starting your pacing off strong at the beginning of your MCAT will help you move confidently through each question without worrying about running out of time. A rush of adrenaline, however, can make it tempting to race through the first passage you hit, and this can lead to mistakes. The good news is that you don't have to troubleshoot your pacing anew on the day of your test. Use section tests and full-length practice tests to gauge what the right pace "feels" like to you — don't sprint full throttle, but keep up a tempo and rhythm that sets you up for success.

There isn't a single defined "strategy" that will magically add time to the clock during your exam. What's more, there are some approaches that on the surface appear to be shortcuts, but in reality tend to consume even more time, or worse, result in more errors. For example, skipping seemingly "difficult" passages and saving them for later seems logical. Let's consider a few pitfalls of this approach though. First of all, it's surprisingly common for passages on difficult subjects, or passages that seem dense and intimidating, to have easy questions, and vice versa. By setting a tough-looking passage aside and moving on to greener pastures first, you've already convinced yourself that this is a "hard" passage, and studies have shown that any influence that makes you believe you won't be successful at something can actually become a self-fulfilling prophecy.

It also takes some time to navigate back and forth between passages, and an even bigger concern is that you might accidentally skip over a question and leave it unanswered. At the end of the day, your goal should be to complete every single passage and every question, so, if you're consistently running out of time with this strategy, it's probably time to consider that the act of skipping around is taking up too much time. Furthermore, sometimes starting off with a difficult passage and getting it out of the way will get your brain warmed up, which can make successive passages seem comparatively easy, especially as the day wears on and you get closer to the end of your MCAT.

The same is true for questions: skipping around between questions makes even less sense because (a) it's easy to accidentally leave a question unanswered, and (b) if it's associated with a passage, you'll have to get back in the right mental framework and remind yourself what that passage is even about if you return to that question later. Let's be honest, if there were one particular shortcut that were especially effective for zipping through MCAT questions, everyone would be using it.

Another common problem students run into is allowing the timer to become a source of distraction and anxiety. It can help to use the toggle button to hide the timer on your screen, and, instead, commit to checking the clock only at certain intervals. If you make a habit of checking the clock after, say, your first two passages, then you still have time to modulate your pacing without needing to feel anxious or rushed. Two passages in a row should take, on average, about 16 minutes or so to complete, so you can expect to still have an hour and 19 minutes left at that point. If you're behind, you can pick up the pace some, and if you're ahead, you can relax a little more. If you check your timing too soon or too often, however, this may cause unnecessary stress — so try to strike a balance that works for you.

If you've taken the time to hone your strategy for pacing, then you shouldn't have any surprises on test day. However, in case you do end up running short on time in a section, there are a few things you can do. Depending on how much time remains, you may want to use a more efficient approach to reading passages. Ultimately, your number one priority is to leave no questions blank, since there's no penalty for guessing. By practicing and implementing time management skills, hopefully you won't even have to worry about running out of time on your MCAT!

3. Passage Speed-Reading

It's a good idea to have a backup plan in case you end up running short on time in a section. Your Plan A should always be to work confidently through each passage and question at a steady pace, leaving some time at the end for reviewing flagged questions. However, we are all human and sometimes even the best laid plans don't quite work out. So, this is a good place to talk about Plan B, the "break glass in case of fire" plan. If you find yourself in a situation where you have very little time and plenty of questions still to answer, it may be time to give speed reading a shot.

There are several tiers of speed-reading that you can implement depending on how much time remains in your section. If you have about 30 seconds remaining, your best bet is to go through and just select an answer choice for every single unanswered question, as there are no penalties for wrong answers, and there's still a 25% probability you'll guess correctly by chance. If you can, try to eliminate any obviously wrong answer choices, as that will increase your chances of being correct.

If you have several minutes remaining, however, you may have time to read through some discrete questions or even skim through a passage. When you skim through a passage, you have to make very quick choices about which information to process and which information to ignore. The goal in this situation is to understand the highest level points of the passage and have some general indications of where things are in the passage so you can come back while answering questions.

The precise details of how you approach speed-reading will vary to some extent based on the passage type. Textbook-style passages usually give you factual information about some scientific phenomenon. For textbook-style passages, if absolutely necessary, skim by reading the first and last sentence of each paragraph, and pay special attention to the last paragraph or conclusion. Briefly note any figures or tables, as there will likely be some questions on these, but don't dive too far deep into the analysis just yet. Primary research-based passages usually describe some experiment or research study, usually following a structure that includes the background, a hypothesis or purpose, the methods, and results. A disproportionate number of questions will require you to use critical reasoning to interpret the results and figures, so it makes sense to focus any time you have on those parts of the passage when skimming. Don't dwell too long on the figures, but try to glean the major trends before moving on. Lab manual passages describe some kind of experimental set-up, often being conducted by students in a classroom lab setting. For such passages, it's still important to spend most of your time on tables, figures, and results, but you'll also see questions on methods. So, for these passages, it's worth it to spend a little more time relating the methodological procedures to the results.

Psychology and sociology passages are somewhat distinct and generally can be treated as a kind of hybrid between textbook-style and primary research-based passages. Again, focus on big-picture ideas and any relevant figures and experimental results.

As a demonstration of speed-reading, let's take a look at this Chemical and Physical Foundations passage on protein-carbohydrate interactions:

Protein-carbohydrate interactions are involved in a myriad of biological processes such as bacterial cell adhesion and the immune response, and a greater understanding of these interactions could enable new therapeutics in fighting infection and inflammation. While polar amino acid side chains can hydrogen bond with carbohydrate hydroxyl moieties, the role of hydrophobic aliphatic and aromatic side chains in engaging carbohydrates is unclear. Specifically, it is unknown whether the hydrophobic effect or CH-π interactions, involving the interaction of aromatic π electrons with carbohydrate C-H bonds, predominates. Utilizing a database that details which amino acid residues are in the vicinity of specific monosaccharides (including both D-glucose and D-galactose in pyranose form), researchers determined the average frequency of specific residues around carbohydrates in general (see Figure 1).

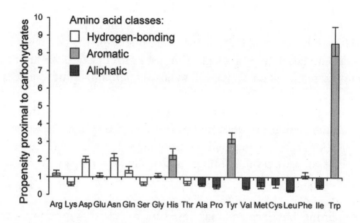

Figure 1. Propensity scores for amino acids (at pH 7.5) in proximity to carbohydrates

The two surfaces of the carbohydrate rings (α and β faces, see Figure 2) were examined for amino acid hydrophobicity, including aromatic and aliphatic groups, around the saccharide molecule and whether particular carbohydrate C-H bonds are more prone to engage with particular residues (see Figure 3).

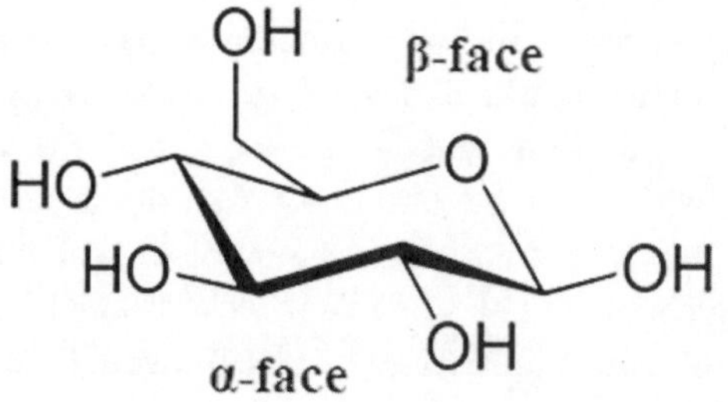

OH   β-face

HO

HO   OH

OH

α-face

Figure 2. Faces of D-glucose

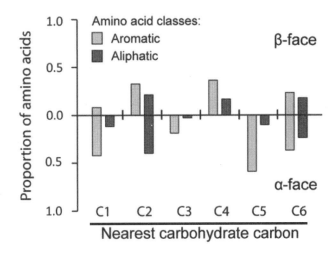

Figure 3. Proportion of aromatic and aliphatic amino acids at particular carbons for D-glucose

Adapted from Hudson, K. L., Bartlett, G. J., Diehl, R. C., Agirre, J., Gallagher, T., Kiessling, L. L., and Woolfson, D. N. (2015). Carbohydrate-aromatic interactions in proteins. J. Am. Chem. Soc, 137(48) under CC-BY.

This looks like a primary research-based passage. We see a few figures here with what appear to be experimental results. Just skimming the beginning, we see a bit of background information that has something to do with how amino acids interact with carbohydrates, which maybe we didn't read in detail because we really want to get to the meat of this experiment. Then the end of this paragraph briefly describes the methods, which tell us that the researchers investigated which types of amino acids were present near carbohydrates in these types of interactions. So now we have something we can use to interpret Figure 1. Again, we're not going to dive deep here, but we see different types of amino acids on the x-axis, categorized by class, and on the y-axis we see how often they're found near carbohydrates. Clearly, what jumps out here is the tryptophan residue. We're looking for trends, so we should probably make note that the three light grey bars for these *aromatic* amino acids really jump out. So maybe aromatic amino acids tend to hang out near carbohydrates? Let's keep moving.

Next, we take a look at the upcoming chunk of text, which tells us the researchers did something else, something to do with seeing which types of carbohydrate bonds attract which types of amino acids on either face of a carbohydrate. We can use this information to briefly look at Figure 2, which is a molecular structure that we can probably return to if needed. Next up, Figure 3 contains some more experimental results. We're looking at aromatic versus aliphatic amino acids and whether they tend to localize to the alpha or beta face of the carbohydrate. We know enough about *how* to interpret this figure that we can come back to it later for the answers we're looking for.

Regardless of how fast we read a passage, it's still valuable to read actively, with the goal of identifying the bigger picture. Think to yourself "What's the point of everything I'm reading?" At the end of the day, we don't really care about the exact database these scientists used, or even the exact identity of the carbohydrate that was used for this experiment. We're concerned with the major questions being addressed in this study, and how well the experimental results answer them.

Even in the case of speed reading in a time crunch, we want to locate a few key things in the passage and at least get the gist and highlight some key terms. First, we'll want to identify where the background information is. In this case, that's definitely paragraph one. We can quickly see that this passage is dealing with protein-carbohydrate interactions and, if we need further detail, we'll know where to go. Next, we'll want to find the purpose of the study. In this case, it seems like we are trying to determine whether hydrophobic or aromatic amino acids have greater impact on protein-carbohydrate interactions. We'll also want to do a quick glance over the methods, highlighting anything that sticks out. Finally, we always want to at least give a quick glance at any included figures and try to spot any major trends.

Regardless of whether we're poring through this passage word by word, or skimming it in the 3 minutes that remain on this section, we should still be able to identify what question or questions the experimenters are asking, and what the results have to say about it. Then, we can go ahead and move on to the questions following the passage.

4. Spending Your Time Wisely

An important skill to develop is knowing whether you're spending your time wisely during the science sections. This is a pretty ambitious topic, so let's be a bit more specific. First, we'll cover common pitfalls when reading that can either take up precious time, or take less time but end up resulting in more wrong answers, and then we'll talk about how active reading methods can help circumvent these issues. Then we'll talk about when shortcuts work and when they don't, and when to return to the passage.

If you don't know your science, knowing how to highlight or read passages efficiently won't be a ton of help. But once you've got your content down solid, learning how to be an efficient and effective test-taker can help you maximize the value you get from all that knowledge. Some of the biggest time drains on science passages involve over-using the highlighter function or taking extensive notes. The **highlighter** function is there for a reason, and feel free to use it, but use it judiciously. If you're spending a lot of time toying with the highlighter function, or if you're highlighting entire lines of a passage, then there's a good chance that time will add up over the course of 10 passages per section.

Also, remember that taking handwritten **notes** on every passage often consumes valuable time that could otherwise be spent analyzing the major points of the passage or moving on to the questions. Consider doing a time trial where you take notes on a set of passages, and then don't take notes on another set. Doing this can help you assess whether this investment of time is valuable for you getting more points, but, spoiler alert, for most students it isn't! Keep in mind that, at most testing centers, any notes you'll take on your official MCAT will be on a wet-erase board rather than paper. That can add extra challenges, such as having to worry about your marker working, or being forced to flip between pages of your wet-erase board if you run out of space on a given page. Although it can be useful to jot down acronyms or biochemical pathways at times, most note-taking will simply eat up mental resources and time that could be spent getting you points.

It's relatively easy to identify when highlighting or taking notes is cutting into test-taking time, but it's more difficult to learn to put the plug in another prevalent time drain: **re-reading**. This may be due to any number of factors, such as obsessing over the clock or worrying about previous or future sections, but the biggest cause is simply losing focus. This is where active reading strategies come into play. Remember that we're reading a passage not to get through all the words on the page, but to derive meaning from the text. Every sentence, and even every word, has a purpose, and so we should be reading through each and every passage with a single question in mind: what's the point? Taking this approach, we should be able to identify the major takeaways of each paragraph, and highlight the words that capture these ideas, or at least remind us of them. We can go back for details later.

When faced with extremely dense, science-heavy passages, you might be tempted to re-read sentences or even paragraphs if, even with active reading, you feel like it just didn't make sense. In these cases, it's important to remember that if a passage or question is difficult for you, it is also difficult for many, or even all, of your peers. It is easy to get into your head and think that if you had only studied harder, you would have understood this passage. Remember, though, you don't need to understand every detail of every passage to get a great MCAT score, and the test writers didn't intend for you to try. Ultimately, they are testing your ability to quickly extract essential information from a situation and figure out your next move. This is a crucial skill for physicians! Honing this skill now will not only get you a great MCAT score but also help you be ahead of the game in medical school and as a physician. Therefore, rather than getting stuck reading the same purpose statement or paragraph multiple times, move through these dense, scary passages actively, just like we've recommended as a general approach. As you do this, try to identify what you *do* find familiar in the passage text. Maybe in a passage with long enzyme names, you can use parts of those names to predict the enzymes' functions, or maybe the passage mentions certain amino acids, or pH dependency, or other concepts that you know inside and out from your MCAT prep and can use as clues in this otherwise difficult-to-comprehend passage. With practice, you'll learn to limit re-reading while gathering the most important points from a passage and be able to move confidently to the questions.

Once you've gotten through the passage and moved on to the questions, it's crucial that you remain alert and avoid answer choices designed to trap you. For example, you may be tempted to select an answer choice that "sounds good" because it contains certain keywords you recognize from the passage. Perhaps an answer choice is kind of complicated and you don't fully understand it, so you're tempted choose this answer because it sounds technical. Instead, use your strategies. Eliminate answer choices that contain obvious flaws. Give more weight to answer choices that relate to the major arguments of a passage. If you don't know the answer and don't have much time, select an answer choice that doesn't seem totally out of the ballpark, flag the question, and move on. After all, if you do end up running out of time in the section, spending more time on a question that you were already having trouble with wouldn't have been a good idea anyway. It would likely just eat up time that could be used for later questions, and who knows — some of those might be easy points. If you *do* end up with some time remaining, you can easily navigate back to your flagged question and give it some more thought.

Using what time you have to get a basic understanding of the passage can also help use time effectively when you get to the questions. Consider this question:

> Which class of intermolecular interaction predominates in the carbohydrate-protein complex shown in Figure 1?
>
> A. Hydrophobic effect
>
> B. Ionic interactions
>
> C. π-system interactions
>
> D. Hydrogen bonding

Perhaps the first point to keep in mind about this question is that you should absolutely consult Figure 1. It turns out that the amino acids that occur most frequently near carbohydrate molecules are tryptophan, tyrosine, and histidine, which are all aromatic amino acids. Tryptophan and tyrosine are both hydrophobic, but histidine is positively charged, so it's unlikely that the hydrophobic or charged nature of these amino acids is mediating their favorable interactions with carbohydrates. Rather, since these three amino acids have an aromatic side chain in common, it must be the electron-rich pi system of aromatic rings that interacts with the hydrogen of the carbon-hydrogen bonds in carbohydrates. Thus, choice C is correct.

Here's a less obvious example:

> If a student is looking to extrapolate from the results of the experiment, which of the following would they most likely predict about the amino acid distribution around D-galactose?
>
> A. The proportion of amino acid residues around C2 on the α face will have a higher aromatic component than for D-glucose.
>
> B. The proportion of amino acid residues around C3 on the β face will have a higher aliphatic component than for D-glucose.
>
> C. The proportion of amino acid residues around C4 on the α face will have a higher aliphatic component than for D-glucose.
>
> D. The proportion of amino acid residues around C4 on the β face will have a lower aromatic component than for D-glucose.

This question requires us to interpret the results of this experiment, and then apply them more broadly to the real world. To answer this question, then, we need to understand the results of this experiment. In particular, this question asks about the amino acid distribution around a carbohydrate, D-galactose. Hopefully we've read the passage in at least enough depth to be able to identify Figure 3 as where we should turn to. It turns out that from this figure, aromatic amino acids alternate between preferring the α and β faces, starting with the alpha face on carbon 1, then the beta face on carbon 2, etc. It turns out that these are the locations where the C-H axial bonds tend to be positioned, so these must be where aromatic amino acids like to hang out. There isn't as much of a distinct trend for aliphatic amino acids.

Now we need to apply this "rule" to a new molecule: D-galactose. D-galactose isn't given to us in this passage, unfortunately, but its structure is quite similar to that of glucose, except that the positioning of the hydroxyl group is reversed on carbon 4. Looking at these answer choices, there's a good chance we can eliminate answer choices A and B, as these sugars do not differ on carbons 2 or 3. However, on carbon 4 the C-H bond is in the axial position on glucose, facing the β surface, but in the equatorial position on galactose, facing the α surface. We said that aromatic amino acids really like hanging out around axial C-H bonds, and since we've lost that on the β surface of galactose, there's a strong possibility that aromatic amino acids are less likely to hang out near its β surface at carbon-4, which best matches answer choice D.

The key takeaway from these examples is that an important aspect of time management is knowing when to return to the passage, and then doing so efficiently.

5. Time-Intensive Questions and Flagging

What do we do about really **time-intensive questions**? We need to have both a way of identifying such questions, as well as a strategy for handling them. Most of the time, you'll want to take a stab at time-intensive questions when you first see them. Coming back later is sure to add more time, as you'll have to get back into the right frame of mind, and maybe even repeat work if the question is calculation-based. On one hand, your goal should be to try every question as you come across it, but quick and easy questions are worth exactly as many points as multi-step, monster questions. In other words, you don't want to spend all your time trying to solve one or two difficult calculation questions when there might be several more quick points just ahead.

Instead, if you've already spent multiple minutes on one question, consider **eliminating** any clearly wrong answer choices, **selecting** the best answer, **flagging** the question so you can come back to it later, and **moving on**. There's no hard and fast rule about when to move on, as sometimes you may be *just* on the verge of a breakthrough, while on other questions you might be going down a math-based rabbit hole without much clear direction, or even possibly going down the wrong cognitive route. If there's a sunk cost, spending more time on that question may just add to that sunk cost rather than help you focus on other questions, even if your spidey senses tell you that you're "so close" to a breakthrough. When reviewing practice tests, keep an eye out for questions where you notice you may have spent a lot of time pursuing a futile path, as this may help you identify situations where you're more prone to this in the future. You may notice, for example, that you consistently struggle with this on specific types of questions or calculations. Give yourself a rule that you can apply during practice and on the MCAT. Perhaps you decide that if you feel like you're spending too long on a question, you'll give yourself another 20 or 30 seconds before flagging it and moving on. You may also decide that, at the point that you start thinking about moving on, you'll shift your focus to using estimation, or determining the more likely answer, even if you need to flag it for later review. If possible, set yourself up to be able to come back to the question and pick up where you left off. Consider jotting down the question number and something to remember it by on your wet-erase board.

The ability to **flag questions** on your MCAT is a great tool to help manage your time, and will help you make the most efficient use of your time when reviewing. The key is to avoid overusing the tool. Always make sure you select an answer choice before moving on from a question, so that no questions are left unanswered by the time you reach the end. With practice and efficient test-taking strategy, you should have some amount of time left at the end of a given section to review any flagged questions. As you learn more about your own quirks and habits through taking full-length practice tests, you might also want to flag questions that fit criteria specific to you. For example, if you tend to make calculation errors on problems that involve negative exponents, flagging questions that include negative exponents might make sense, so you can easily navigate back to them to triple-check your work if you have a few minutes to spare. In general, aim to keep flagged questions under 25% or so of all questions in a given section, as flagging more than 15 questions in a science section will start to get unwieldy. For any top-priority questions—in other words, questions you are almost certain to answer correctly with just a bit more time—consider jotting down their numbers on your wet-erase board so you can prioritize those during review.

Speaking of review, it's important to emphasize that the minutes you have remaining at the end of the exam, assuming that you do have some time left, can seem very high-stress. It's easy to feel like this is your last chance to correct any errors you may have made in the exam, and this can make it really, really tempting to change lots of answers as you go through your flagged questions. Sometimes, changing your answer is a good thing. For example, if you didn't have a chance to complete a multi-step calculation the first time around, and in the final minutes you do, of course you should change your answer to the correct one if needed! However, students often fall into the trap of changing answers to questions that they did fully work through during the first pass, just because "on second thought, that other choice looks better." You might find this especially tempting if you were originally stuck between two answers. Try to resist this urge, though, because it's quite common for students to change correct answers to incorrect ones in the last few minutes, both because of stress and because the passage (if applicable) and question content are less fresh. This is a recipe for being tempted by an answer that is more speculative and less closely related to what the question is asking. It can be helpful to set personal rules regarding when you'll let yourself change an answer, and when you'll hold off. For example, you might only change your answer when you can decisively prove to yourself that your original choice was incorrect.

With practice, you'll become more adept at recognizing which questions will benefit from spending more time on them, and when changing your answer choice versus going with your gut tends to work in your favor. You can also detect patterns in the percentage of flagged questions you tend to answer incorrectly, versus the percentage of unflagged you answer incorrectly. Your Blueprint analytics page will help you spot these trends, and, if you're answering more unflagged questions incorrectly, then you may want to revisit the types of questions you identify as needing more time to review.

When you reach the **Section Review screen** or **Navigation Pane**, you'll see several options for reviewing questions. You can choose to review all questions, review incomplete questions only, or you can review flagged questions only.

First, check to make sure that there are no incomplete questions, as those should be your top priority. Then, work through your flagged questions, making note of approximately how many flagged questions there are to review, and how much time remains in that section. First, navigate to any questions you noted as top priority on your wet-erase board. If you still have time remaining after tackling those high priority questions, then you can begin to work through any other flagged questions until the section ends.

A final point to make here is that navigating through your flagged questions means dredging up the toughest, hardest problems in that section, which can negatively, and unfairly, influence your perception of how you did. Keep that in mind as you review, and, if you have the time, click through some of your unflagged questions to remind yourself that the number of questions you guessed on is likely quite small—and you took the time to feel confident about the many other questions that you didn't have to guess on.

6. Pacing Through Practice

Getting a feel for the right pacing on MCAT science sections takes practice. Your first full-length might be a bit of a wild card when it comes to timing, but by your second, third, and fourth full-lengths, you'll start to find your rhythm. You can "find your rhythm" more intentionally by carving out time to explicitly focus on **timed practice**. Just like developing any other skill, you can improve and refine your pacing strategies. However, in the earlier stages of your prep, you should be primarily focused on your content knowledge and reasoning-based performance.

As your content knowledge and reasoning skills improve, timed practice will not only help you maintain accuracy, but improve your efficiency, preparing you to do your best under the pressure of a ticking clock. Timed practice should always be some part of your MCAT prep, from your Diagnostic onwards, because , with practice, you will learn to work within the time limits and experience less anxiety due to the intense timing. In other words, the clock will become a background process running in the periphery, like how you stop noticing the sounds of rain outside after some time. It also won't be a complete new variable that you have to introduce late in your prep and learn to adjust to. You'll do most of your timed practice through full-length MCAT exams, although you should also use individual passages or section tests to really refine and improve your timing. Since individual science passages vary in length and number of associated questions, we recommend focusing on the average time spent across multiple, successive passages, rather than the time spent on an individual passage.

With timed practice, eventually you should be able to estimate, without looking at the timer, how much time you've spent on a given passage or series of questions and get a sense of whether your pacing is on target. Once you've been able to complete several trials with the appropriate pacing, then you can be confident that you'll get off to a strong start in each section.

If you're finding yourself behind your target pace, or even unable to get to the last few passages in a section, one way to jump-start this process is to take a few tests untimed with a stopwatch. You can use lap times to get an average time you spend on each passage to establish your baseline timing. Then you can work towards your pacing goal in incremental steps. If you're completing passages at a rate of 10 or 11 minutes per passage, for example, start by trying to shave 30 seconds or a minute off each passage, and then you can go from there. As you review practice passages, see if you can identify any timing issues specific to your situation so you can adopt strategies that will help. It can be helpful to get a sense of when time is being invested productively versus unproductively. Apparent issues with reading speed are often indicative of other issues, like re-reading paragraphs, or attention drifting elsewhere. You may also be misinterpreting parts of the passage, or reading the words without processing them in the context of the passage as a whole. The better you can identify what's affecting your timing most, the better you'll be able to implement a solution that'll be effective for you.

If you're on the other end of the spectrum and finishing with plenty of time to spare, then you're in a good position. But if you're missing questions, consider what the best use of that extra time might be. Fortunately you're in a position where you can afford to slow down, or spend a little more time on passages, and titrate your efforts to optimize your performance.

One of the major benefits of taking Blueprint's full-length MCAT exams is that you have a wealth of **analytics** available to you that you can use to troubleshoot your timing and performance. For example, you might notice that you're missing a lot of questions at the end of a section, or spending less time on questions at the end. This might suggest that you're running out of time, or running out of endurance and relying more on guessing. You might notice that you're spending too much time, or not enough time, on questions towards the beginning, suggesting that your pacing off the starting blocks needs fine-tuning. Maybe you're spending considerably more time on a small number of challenging questions, but still getting those questions wrong. This suggests that it could benefit you to spend that time elsewhere. Another possibility is that there are certain passages that tend to be real time sinks, so your practice should be focused on more efficient reading practices. Take advantage of all the data you have access to, and use it to your advantage!

Set goals for your timed practice for specific skills, such as performing calculations more efficiently, avoiding re-reading, or reducing the time spent focusing on details as opposed to the bigger picture. Setting specific goals is a lot more useful in practice than just shooting for a specific time goal on passages. For example, if you identify a specific timing issue that's affecting your performance, you can accomplish a lot more by setting a targeted goal, such as improving your highlighting strategy, than telling yourself to just buckle down and shave a minute or two off your time. Furthermore, focusing on incremental improvements — like cutting down 15 seconds on a passage, then 30 seconds, and so on — is more actionable and less stressful than restricting yourself to longer-term goals.

Ultimately, practice using real MCAT passages and content is the best kind of practice you can get during your MCAT prep. That said, you can always apply the same principles of efficiency to outside reading material. This may help you become more comfortable applying active reading methods to absorb and analyze totally new information. If you want these methods to work on your MCAT, the best advice we can give is to treat each practice test like a true simulation of your upcoming MCAT. Make each full-length practice test feel as real as possible. Go to bed and wake up at the times that you would on your exam date, and be okay with experiencing some of the adrenaline and test-taking jitters that you will on your actual MCAT. When that day comes, it'll feel like something you've already done a dozen times over.

7. Must-Knows

> Rough guidelines for timing in sciences: around four minutes for reading each passage, around four minutes for answering the associated questions.
  - To keep yourself on pace, check timer every two to three passages (~15 min).
  - Avoid superficial timing tricks (they hurt more than they help), like skipping seemingly "difficult" questions or passages.
  - If time runs low, speed-reading may be an option: read the first and last sentences of each paragraph, focusing on background and purpose, skim figures, then move on to questions.
> Some useful tips for efficiently getting through passages include:
  - Highlighting effectively.
  - Limiting yourself to strategic note-taking.
  - Minimizing re-reading (don't get caught up in irrelevant details. Decide at what point you will move on).
  - Avoid spending too much time on involved questions (flag them and move on).
> When doing practice materials:
  - Focus on pacing.
  - Become familiar with the clock.
  - Utilize analytics to identify points for improvement.
  - Set goals for your timed practice.

Applied Practice

The best MCAT practice is realistic, with detailed analytics to help you assess where things went wrong. For those reasons, we recommend completing practice questions in an online setting that simulates the real MCAT interface, and using the analytics provided to help you decide how to best move your studies forward.

CARS does not require knowledge of specific subject areas, but it does require development of strong test-taking skills. To ensure you are honing those skills as you work through this book, we suggest you go online after wrapping up each chapter and generate a Qbank Practice Set of 2-3 CARS passages to practice and review. While not every chapter of this book is directly applicable to CARS, regular CARS practice is key to test day success.

As a further supplement, given the importance of active learning for effective studying, we also suggest that you consult the Must-Knows at the end of each chapter of this Reasoning text as a basis for creating a study sheet. This is not a sheet to memorize in the more traditional sense of content memorization, but rather a quick reference of the most important strategies for you to refer to during and after practice in your early prep. Frequently revisiting the most important strategies for the MCAT - in both CARS and the Sciences - will help you continue to improve your performance.

This page left intentionally blank.

Math and Formulas

0. Introduction

Here's an MCAT paradox for you: the MCAT is definitely *not* a math test, but math is vital for MCAT success. What we mean by this is that the MCAT is interested in math for two main reasons. First, math is often the way that we express ideas about science, which is at the heart of the MCAT. Second, math serves as a way to evaluate your number sense and ability to reason about numerical quantities using techniques like rounding and estimation that are handy for clinicians in real-world settings. This, in turn, is why a calculator isn't available on the MCAT: the MCAT is simply not interested in math at that level of precision. As a result, when studying math for the MCAT, it's vital to focus on how it's tested. With that in mind, in this chapter, we'll take you on a journey from basic operations to more complicated concepts like logarithms and exponents, with constant reference to how these skills are tested within the framework of certain scientific concepts. We'll also pay special attention to common sources of errors and misconceptions.

1. Basic Operations and Algebra

At the core of most, if not all, quantitative MCAT questions are simple mathematical operations, from addition and subtraction to division and algebra. It might be tempting to skim any discussion of these topics, because they might seem laughably elementary compared to later, more complex mathematical concepts like logarithms and, of course, the extensive science material that is tested on the MCAT. However, since the name of the game on the MCAT is to get questions right, any common cause of mistakes deserves serious attention, and, in our experience, mistakes in even the simplest mathematical steps are more common than students think.

Possibly the most classic example of a "silly math mistake" is obtaining an answer with the wrong sign: negative instead of positive, for instance. The best way to avoid this is to be very careful when **subtracting a negative number**. Subtracting a negative number is identical to adding the absolute value of that number. For instance, 9–(-6) is the same as 9 + 6 (and equals 15). This probably isn't new to you, but especially when plugging values into an equation that involves subtraction, it's surprisingly easy to forget to write down one of the negative signs, or to simply see "9," "6," and "–" and think "3!" Likewise, care is needed when multiplying by negative numbers. In other words, if a minus sign is in the mix, it's worth slowing down to make sure that everything lines up.

Another common source of mistakes is **dividing by a number that is less than one**. Dividing any positive value by such a number will always result in a larger, or more positive, answer, while dividing any negative value by a number less than one will always yield a more negative answer. This can be a bit challenging to conceptualize. While $10 \div 5$ is quite obviously taking a group of 10 and dividing it into 5 smaller groups of 2, $10 \div 0.1$ is a bit more abstract.

Let's look at an example of how we can handle such situations by taking care to reason through our calculations step by step. For this example, we'll use the kinematics equation $v_f = v_i + at$. Suppose we're told that our initial velocity is 5 m/s and our object accelerates uniformly to 15 m/s over an interval of 0.5 seconds. What is the object's rate of acceleration? Well, let's start by plugging in the values we're provided This gives us 15 m/s = 5 m/s + 0.5a. With basic algebra, we can simplify this to 15 − 5 = 0.5a, or 10 = 0.5a. Now, all that's left is to divide 10 by 0.5, and we'll have our acceleration value. This is where we need to be careful! $10 \div 0.5$ is *not* 5, because whenever we divide a positive number by a value that is less than 1, we must obtain an answer that's larger, or more positive, than our original value. Five is less than 10, so 5 cannot be the right answer here. Instead, $10 \div 0.5 = 20$.

We can calculate $10 \div 0.5$ more intuitively, by asking ourselves "how many 0.5s fit into 10?" Another trick is to multiply both the top and bottom of our division expression by a value that transforms 0.5 into a value that is greater than 1. Specifically, multiplying both the top and bottom by 10 gives us 100/5, which is both exactly the same as our original expression and easier to solve. In some cases, it can also be helpful to switch over into fraction mode. In this example, $10 \div 0.5$ is the same as dividing 10 by 1/2, and if you're familiar with rules for multiplication and division using fractions, you should able to quickly see that you just need to multiply by the reciprocal of 1/2, or 2, to obtain the correct answer of 20.

Algebra errors are also quite common when manipulating equations. Most of these involve improper distribution when moving terms between the sides of an equation. As an example, take the kinematics equation $v_f^2 = v_i^2 + 2ad$. Imagine that the only information we have is that acceleration is equal to negative 0.5 m/s^2, and that we're trying to solve for displacement. First, we can plug in -0.5 for a, and multiply by 2 to give us $v_f^2 = v_i^2 - d$. Then, we subtract v_i^2 from both sides, yielding $v_f^2 - v_i^2 = -d$. Next up, we just need to divide both sides by -1 to get d isolated on the right side. But what is $(v_f^2 - v_i^2)/$-1? The most common mistake students make here is to only apply the negative sign to one of the terms on the left. In reality, since we're dividing the entire left side by -1, we need to apply a negative sign to both terms, yielding $-v_f^2 + v_i^2 = d$. This certainly isn't the only example of an algebra error—other potential pitfalls include situations where you're multiplying, dividing, or exponentiating algebraic terms in an equation—but it's an excellent example of the need to slow down and work through the operations systematically when manipulating equations.

The *math* in all of these examples isn't the hard part. The more difficult part is even getting to that point—that is, understanding the question stem, recognizing what equations to use, how to set up the problem, and moving variables around to isolate what we're solving for. Once we're at the point of substituting in numbers, and making sure that the signs line up, we've already done most of the conceptual heavy lifting, at which point the issue becomes making sure that the details are all correct.

This brings us to an important consideration that, on its surface, has nothing to do with arithmetic: how to reconcile what we've been discussing with the ever-present need to work quickly and efficiently on the MCAT. Time pressure is a very real aspect of this test, and for that reason we discuss it in much greater depth elsewhere. However, whenever you're doing a calculation question it's always worth taking an extra few seconds to work systematically and double-check your work, with a special focus on avoiding both the pitfalls that we've discussed here and any other mistakes that you find yourself making disproportionately often. If there's something particularly tricky about a certain question, it may even be worth flagging. After all, it's all about the points, and taking the time needed to do these questions the right way—that is, quickly, correctly, and not in a panic—is always a good investment.

2. Scientific Notation

Throughout the MCAT, you'll encounter a special method used by scientists (and others) to express numbers. This method is **scientific notation**, and its applications go far beyond MCAT passages and questions.

Scientific notation is distinct from standard notation, or, put simply, regular numbers. The numbers 6, 15, 0.0005, and 140,000 are all in standard notation. In fact, any number *can* be expressed in standard form, so you might wonder why we need a different notation format at all. Well, for numbers that are either very small or very large, standard notation gets pretty unwieldy. There are only so many times you can write "0.000002 meters" before you start to wonder if there's an easier way. What's more, it's all too easy to lose track of how many 0s there are if you have no better way of keeping track of them than trying to count how many times you said, or wrote, "0." Scientific notation makes values like this much more manageable. The secret is that it uses **exponents** to denote order of magnitude.

$$4.184 \times 10^3$$

$$\text{coefficient} \times \text{base}^{\text{exponent}}$$

Figure 1. Scientific notation

Let's use an example to investigate scientific notation in greater detail: 4.184×10^3 joules, or the number of joules in a Calorie. In this expression, some number—specifically 4.184—is multiplied by 10 to some exponent, which here is 3. We'll call the 4.184 part the coefficient, though you may have heard them called significand or mantissa. Values in scientific notation always have this structure: some coefficient multiplied by 10 to some exponent. In this case, 10^3 is equal to 1,000, so $4.184 \times 10^3 = 4.184 \times 1,000 = 4,184$.

Interestingly, we could actually write 4,184 in several other ways while still adhering to the constraints of scientific notation that we've defined so far. For example, we could write 41.84×10^2, or 418.4×10^1. These are all equal, but conventionally, we tend to use the notation in which the coefficient has a single digit before the decimal point, so the 4.184×10^3 version. This is called **normalized scientific notation**.

The coefficient can be positive or negative, so, for instance, if we've defined up as positive and down as negative, we might say that an object hurtling downward is traveling at a velocity of negative 300 meters per second, which is -3×10^2 in scientific notation. This is simple enough, but importantly, the *exponent* can also be positive or negative. For example, one piconewton (pN) is equal to 1×10^{-12} newtons. It's *essential* that you understand the difference between positive and negative exponents in scientific notation, so let's elaborate a little on this. When the base, 10, is raised to a positive exponent, the result is a value greater than 1, and 10 to the power of a *negative* number always equals a value less than 1, but greater than 0. The more negative the exponent, the smaller the value of the overall number. For example, $10^{-1} = 0.1$, $10^{-2} = 0.01$, $10^{-3} = 0.001$, and so on.

With practice, you'll quickly commit these values to memory, but converting between scientific and standard notation shouldn't rely on memory at all. Rather, you can use the relationship between the exponent in scientific notation and the position of the decimal point in standard notation to easily convert. Take our most recent example, 10^{-2}. This is equivalent to 1×10^{-2}, because one times any value just yields itself. First, write down our coefficient: 1, which is the same as 1.0. Then, since our exponent is -2, move the decimal point 2 places to the left. There's our 0.01! A simple way to check that you moved the decimal in the correct direction is to note that doing so made the value smaller, which corresponds perfectly to the fact that the exponent is negative. On the other hand, if we wanted to convert 3×10^4 to standard notation, we would write down our coefficient of 3.0, then move the decimal point 4 places to the right to yield the larger value of 30,000.

Where this becomes especially helpful is when dealing with units. Recall that the metric, or SI, system consists of a set of base units, like meters and seconds, each of which can be given a number of prefixes to indicate order of magnitude. Base units can be combined to yield derived units, such as newtons and joules, which can similarly be given prefixes to denote magnitude. For instance, we might read in a passage that a native (or folded) protein is unfolded in the lab by applying a 60 pN force. Here, our derived unit is newtons, and our prefix is "pico-", which stands for 10^{-12}, so we're dealing with a force of 60×10^{-12}, or 6×10^{-11}, newtons.

3. Operations and Scientific Notation

Like numbers in general, values in scientific notation can be subjected to mathematical operations. For our purposes, this really just means that they can be added or subtracted, and they can be multiplied or divided. The latter two operations—multiplication and division—are much more common on the MCAT than the former two, so let's start there. When **multiplying** a term in scientific notation by a value in standard notation—that is, a regular number—simply multiply the *coefficient* of the scientific-notation term by the standard-notation value. Take Avogadro's number, which is approximately 6.022×10^{23} items (typically atoms or molecules) per mole. To make our lives easier, let's round to 6×10^{23}, which is virtually always acceptable on the MCAT. Now, say that we have two moles of a certain compound. To find the number of molecules present, we just need to multiply 6×10^{23} by two. To do this, we just multiply 6 by 2, giving us an answer of 12×10^{23}, or more conventionally, 1.2×10^{24}. The same goes for dividing. If we had instead started with one mole and divided it equally into three containers, we'd divide 6 by 3, yielding an answer of 2×10^{23}. In the actual multiplication and division steps, the 10^{23} part doesn't even need to come into play.

If we have two numbers that are *both* in scientific notation, we need to multiply the coefficients and *add* the exponents together. This might seem counterintuitive. After all, the overall operation we're performing is multiplication, so it would seem natural to multiply the exponents too. To understand why we don't do this, let's look at an example involving force using the equation for power, or $P = Fv$. Say we're trying to calculate the power required to maintain a molecule at a constant velocity of 3×10^{-7} m/s when the frictional force opposing its motion is 2.5×10^{-12} N. To find power, we need to multiply these two terms, and if we follow the rules we outlined earlier, this means that we first multiply 3×2.5, giving us 7.5. Then, we *add* the exponents (-7 and -12) to yield a final value of 7.5×10^{-19} N·m/s, where N·m/s is equal J/s, or watts (W): exactly the units we would expect for power. This is a very small amount of power, but that corresponds reasonably well to what we'd expect, given that we're working with a tiny particle that's not moving fast. If we had multiplied the exponents, our result would be 7.5×10^{84}, which is MUCH too massive of a number to be correct here.

Given what we've covered so far, you might already be able to guess how **dividing** two terms in scientific notation works. We divide the coefficients, and we subtract the exponents. Unlike multiplying, however, with dividing it's important to be very clear about which term is the dividend, or number we're dividing, and which is the divisor, or the value we're dividing by. As an example, imagine that we're asked how many electrons correspond to a charge of -6.4×10^{-6} C, given that the charge of one electron is approximately -1.6×10^{-19} C. In short, then, we're dividing -6.4×10^{-6} by negative 1.6×10^{-19}. First, we can divide -6.4 by -1.6 to get 4. (This is easier than it looks, by the way. Either you can recognize that this is the same as $64 \div 16$, or you can work backwards and realize that 1.6×3.2, and $3.2 \times 2 = 6.4$, so 1.6 must go into 6.4 four times.) Second, we take -6 and subtract -19. This is the same as taking -6 + 19, giving us 13. Getting the order correct here is crucial! If we accidentally reverse these terms, we'll get an exponent with the wrong sign, specifically -13. Assuming we avoid that pitfall, we obtain the correct answer of 4×10^{13} electrons. If you're nervous about the potential for mistakes here, you can make a habit of doing a reality check after you finish any calculation involving division with scientific notation. In this case, 4×10^{13} seems reasonable enough, but if we had messed up and gotten 4×10^{-13}, an infinitesimally small fraction of one electron. Because that's not a physically meaningful idea, it can't be the right answer.

The nice thing about the problem we just did is that our dividend—the numerator, if we think in fraction terms—had a coefficient that was larger than that of our divisor. For most people, it's much easier to divide 6.4 by 1.6 than it would be to divide 0.64 by 1.6. But what if that's exactly what we were asked to do? Specifically, how would we go about dividing 0.64×10^{-5} by 1.6×10^{-19}? The key is to recognize that this is very similar to the problem we did immediately before (with the exception of dropping the negative signs, which we did for simplicity. If we manipulate the scientific notation of the numerator, we can change it to an equivalent value that *does* have a larger coefficient than our denominator. Just move the decimal point one position to the right and correspondingly decrease the exponent by one, and we get 6.4×10^{-6}, and can then divide by the denominator much more easily.

Last but not least, we have **addition** and **subtraction**. These work similarly to each other, but very differently from multiplication and division, so it's important to be careful. In particular, to add or subtract terms that are written in scientific notation, the base must have the same exponent. There's no adding or subtracting of exponents here! Instead, manipulate the terms until their exponents are the same, then add or subtract the coefficients. Say we have a velocity vector pointing upwards with a magnitude of 4×10^3 m/s and we want to add another vector, pointing the same direction, that has a magnitude of 8×10^5 meters per second. It's often easiest to convert the larger value to have the same exponent as the smaller one, rather than the other way around, because we can avoid dealing with coefficients that are less than 1. So here, we should convert 8×10^5 into 800×10^3, and from there, it's simple to add 4×10^3 to get our final answer: 804×10^3 m/s. If we wanted to subtract our second vector instead of adding it, we'd just take 4×10^3 and subtract 800×10^3, yielding -796×10^3 meters per second. The nice thing about addition and subtraction of terms in scientific notation is that it makes differences in magnitude crystal clear. Looking at 4×10^3 next to 8×10^5, these values might not have seemed too far apart, but looking at it next to 800×10^3 makes it obvious that the difference is greater than a hundredfold. In fact, the larger the difference in exponent, the more likely that we won't even need to take into account the smaller term, making our lives that much easier, and saving us crucial seconds.

4. Trigonometry

Trigonometry is a branch of math that deals with the angles and side lengths of triangles. Triangles might not seem to be all that MCAT-relevant, and trigonometry isn't tested in much depth on the exam. However, in the Chemical and Physical Foundations section, you can expect to regularly encounter questions that require a knowledge of basic trigonometric relationships, as well as knowing some common values.

We can begin with three core concepts in trigonometry: the trigonometric functions of **sine**, **cosine**, and **tangent**. As we talk through them, let's use a physics-related example. "A professional baseball pitcher throws a ball at an angle of 60° above the horizontal, with a total launch velocity of 20 m/s. What are the vertical and horizontal components of this velocity?" Before trying to solve, let's draw out our scenario. To do this, we should clarify what this first sentence even means. The horizontal is a straight line with no upward or downward slope, and this pitch was "above" the horizontal, so we need to draw another line sloping upward at an angle to our horizontal line. It's typically easiest to draw both lines stemming from the same point, although as long as your line slopes up and the angle between it and the horizontal is correct, you're good to go. As for what this angle should be, they gave it to us directly: 60°.

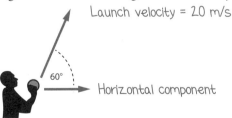

Figure 2. A ball thrown at a 60° angle to the horizontal

That takes care of the first part of this question, but we still need to determine where to put our 20 meters per second value, and what is meant by "vertical and horizontal components" of velocity. For the MCAT, these will always be **right triangles**, meaning triangles with one 90° angle. But in our pitcher example, we don't have a triangle - just two lines that form a 60° angle. To form a right triangle, just draw a perpendicular line connecting the two lines at the open end of the angle.

Right triangles have their own special terminology: the two shorter sides, which are the two that form the 90° angle, are called **legs**, while the longest side, the one opposite the 90-degree angle, is called the **hypotenuse**. The larger an angle, the longer the side opposite it will be. Here, the smallest angle is at the top, and it's opposite the shortest side: the horizontal leg. The largest angle is the 90° angle, and it's opposite the *longest* side: the hypotenuse. Since the hypotenuse represents the angle of the pitcher's throw, we can label it 20. The vertical and horizontal components of that velocity, then, must correspond to the lengths of the vertical and horizontal legs of the triangle.

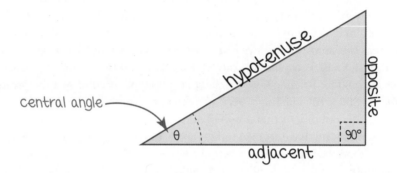

Figure 3. Sides of a right triangle

With our question stem fully drawn out, we can now return to our original goal: to understand the trig functions of sine, cosine, and tangent. Let's break them down one by one, starting with **sine**, which is defined as the ratio of the length of the side opposite the angle we care about to the length of the hypotenuse. Here, we care about the angle at which the pitcher threw the ball: 60°. The sine of 60° will be equal to the length of the opposite side over the length of the hypotenuse.

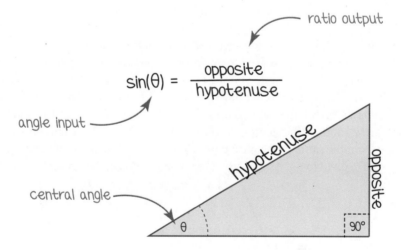

Figure 4. Definition of sine

Since the opposite side is the vertical leg, we must be on our way to getting the first half of our answer: the vertical component of the initial velocity. Plugging in values, $\sin(60°) = v_{initial\ vertical} \div 20$ m/s. Rearranging this equation gives us $v_{initial\ vertical} = 20$ m/s $\times \sin(60°)$. In fact, $\sin(60°)$ is about 0.866 (we'll talk more about this below), so for now, we can confidently say that $v_{initial\ vertical} = 20$ m/s $\times 0.866 \approx 17$ m/s.

How about the *horizontal* component of initial velocity? Here, we need to use the **cosine**, which represents the ratio of the side *adjacent* to the angle of interest to the hypotenuse, and is defined as the adjacent leg over the hypotenuse, relative to an angle. Therefore, the cosine of 60° equals our horizontal component of initial velocity, or $v_{initial\ horizontal}$, over 20 m/s, and rearranging gives us $v_{initial\ horizontal}$ equals $20 \times \cos(60°)$. Cosine of 60° is actually just 0.5, so $v_{initial\ horizontal}$ equals 20×0.5, or 10 meters per second.

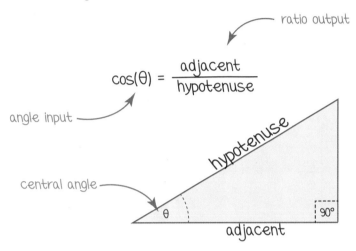

Figure 5. Definition of cosine

In addition to sine and cosine, there's also a third basic main trigonometric function: **tangent**, abbreviated "tan." This quantity represents the ratio of the opposite side to the adjacent side. In our projectile motion example, this would give us the vertical component of velocity over the horizontal component. Physically, that's not extremely useful, so tangent appears on the MCAT significantly less frequently than sine or cosine. However, it's still valuable to understand for the sake of completeness. If you find yourself forgetting any of these functions, you can use the common mnemonic "SOH CAH TOA," which stands for "sine is opposite over hypotenuse, cosine is adjacent over hypotenuse, and tangent is opposite over adjacent."

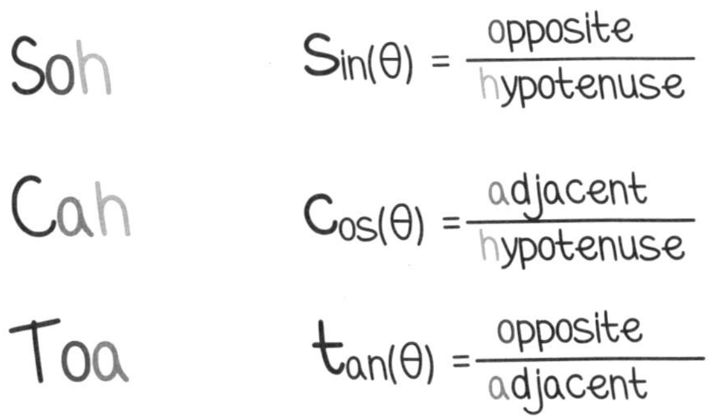

$$\text{Soh} \qquad \sin(\theta) = \frac{\text{opposite}}{\text{hypotenuse}}$$

$$\text{Cah} \qquad \cos(\theta) = \frac{\text{adjacent}}{\text{hypotenuse}}$$

$$\text{Toa} \qquad \tan(\theta) = \frac{\text{opposite}}{\text{adjacent}}$$

Figure 6. SOH CAH TOA: a mnemonic for trigonometric functions

The trigonometric relationships within two key types of triangles termed **special right triangles** are worth studying. These are the 45-45-90 and 30-60-90 triangles, where the numbers refer to the degrees of the triangles' three angles. Looking at the **30-60-90** triangle first, we can see that its smallest leg is opposite its 30° angle and has a length of x, which refers to some positive value. Its other leg, opposite the 60° angle, has a length of x times the square root of

3, and its hypotenuse has a length of 2x. Sine of 60°, then, has a value of (x × √3) divided by 2x, which simplifies to √3/2, or about 0.866. Then cosine of 60° equals x over 2x, which (unlike our previous value) we can actually calculate easily: 0.5. This triangle also tells us that the *sine* of 30° is 0.5, while the *cosine* of 30° is 0.866.

The **45-45-90** triangle has two identical non-right angles of 45°. These identical angles mean that its legs have identical side lengths, labeled x. Its hypotenuse then has a length of x × √2. Sine and cosine of 45 degrees therefore have the same value: 1/√2, which comes out to about 0.707.

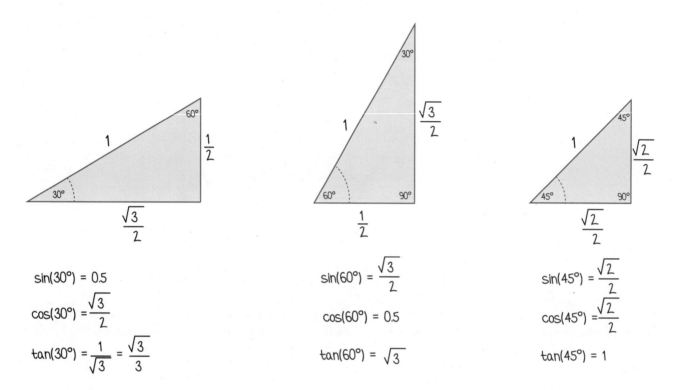

$$\sin(30°) = 0.5$$

$$\cos(30°) = \frac{\sqrt{3}}{2}$$

$$\tan(30°) = \frac{1}{\sqrt{3}} = \frac{\sqrt{3}}{3}$$

$$\sin(60°) = \frac{\sqrt{3}}{2}$$

$$\cos(60°) = 0.5$$

$$\tan(60°) = \sqrt{3}$$

$$\sin(45°) = \frac{\sqrt{2}}{2}$$

$$\cos(45°) = \frac{\sqrt{2}}{2}$$

$$\tan(45°) = 1$$

Figure 7. Special triangles

It's worthwhile to have at least a rough idea of these values memorized, since it's time-inefficient and subject to error to draw out the triangles every time. In addition to the values we've mentioned, it's worth knowing the sine and cosine of two more key angles: 0° and 90°. The sine of 0° is 0, while the sine of 90° is 1. Cosine values are simply reversed. The cosine of 0° is 1 and the cosine of 90° is 0. We highly encourage you to think critically about these values rather than just rely on rote memorization. In particular, throughout your prep, you'll occasionally encounter equations that include sine or cosine. Ask yourself questions like "would I expect this to have a small value if the angle is close to zero? Or what if the angle is exactly 0°? On the other hand, what if the angle is close to 90°?" By doing this, you'll gain a far more valuable understanding of what these equations actually mean, and you'll also have a better chance of being able to work out a sine or cosine value—especially those for 0° or 90° degrees.

Returning to our two special right triangles, you might be wondering where those variables and values—*x, 2x*, and so on—came from. The answer lies in the **Pythagorean theorem**, which relates the three sides of a right triangle according to the equation $A^2 + B^2 = C^2$ squared, where A and B are the legs and C is the hypotenuse. Looking at our 30-60-90 triangle and plugging in values gives us $x^2 + (x\sqrt{3})^2 = (2x)^2$. If we simplify, we get $x^2 + 3x^2 = 4x^2$, which is perfect. The 45-45-90 special right triangle similarly follows the Pythagorean theorem.

It's unlikely that the MCAT would ever ask you a question that directly focuses on the Pythagorean theorem as such, but it could come up in the context of problems where you have to estimate the magnitude of vectors. Generally, it's possible to solve such problems using graphical approaches to vector addition and subtraction that we discuss elsewhere, but having the Pythagorean theorem in your toolkit is a valuable backup. Plus, there are a few special cases where the Pythagorean theorem works out with whole numbers for all three sides of a triangle: namely, if the legs of a triangle have length units of 3 and 4, the hypotenuse will be 5 units long, and if the legs of a triangle are 5 and 12 units long, the hypotenuse will be 13 units long. These tidbits are by no means anywhere near as essential as having a good understanding of how the key trigonometric functions, especially sine and cosine, are defined, but they could come in handy.

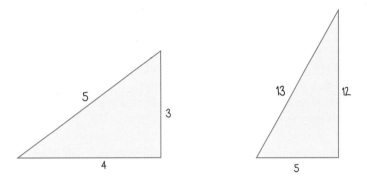

Figure 8. Special cases of the Pythagorean theorem

5. Fractions

You've probably dealt with fractions for most of your academic career, but using them in MCAT-style science questions can add a layer of difficulty that might throw you off. Fortunately, fractions appear on the MCAT in a limited number of contexts, the most common of which is in circuit-related equations. We'll talk in depth about how to solve those equations, but first, let's briefly discuss what fractions are and how to add and subtract them.

For our purposes, we'll use the term "**fraction**" to mean any term written as one value over another. These values might be numbers, variables, or a combination of the two, and the overall fraction might be less than, equal to, or greater than one, although you're most likely to see fractions that represent values less than one, like $\frac{1}{2}$ or $\frac{7}{10}$. The value on the top of the fraction, above the line, is called the numerator, and the value on the bottom is called the denominator. Often, fractions that contain only numbers can be easily converted into decimal form, since a fraction is simply its numerator divided by its denominator. For example, $\frac{1}{2}$ is equal to $1 \div 2$, or 0.5, and $\frac{7}{10}$ is equal to $7 \div 10$, or 0.7. In fact, in some cases you'll find that it's easier to convert fractions to decimals—or at least approximate decimal values—when working through a problem, but in other cases it makes sense to leave them in fraction form.

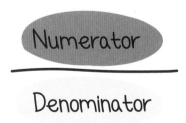

Figure 9. Numerator and denominator

The **denominator** is of particular note when dealing with fractions, because when adding or subtracting, the denominators of all fractions involved must be the same. As a simple example, let's say we're trying to add $\frac{1}{2}$ and $\frac{7}{10}$. To those unfamiliar with fractions, it's often tempting to try to add the numerators to get the numerator of the final answer and similarly to add the denominators to get the denominator of the final answer. This would give us an answer of $\frac{8}{12}$, which simplifies to $\frac{2}{3}$. If we didn't know this was the wrong approach before, we should be able to deduce that it is now that we have an answer, because $\frac{2}{3}$ (which can be rounded to 0.67) is actually *less* than $\frac{7}{10}$, which again, is 0.7. Our mistake was in adding unlike terms. $\frac{1}{2}$ tells us how many halves we have, and $\frac{7}{10}$ tells us how many tenths, so adding the two directly is an apples-and-oranges situation. Instead, we should manipulate one fraction to have the same denominator as the other, and *then* we can add directly. To do this, look at the denominators. Is one a factor of the other? In this case, two is a factor of ten, specifically 2×5 is 10. For that reason, we can multiply our $\frac{1}{2}$ term by $\frac{5}{5}$ to yield $\frac{5}{10}$.

Notice that, since we multiplied our denominator by 5 to get a new denominator of 10, we also had to multiply our numerator by 5. This is because we want to maintain the same value of our fraction while changing it to a different denominator. Multiplying by some value over that same value—be it $\frac{5}{5}$, or $\frac{17}{17}$, or $\frac{P}{P}$—is effectively multiplying by 1, which keeps our fraction the same numerically. So now, our addition problem is $\frac{5}{10} + \frac{7}{10}$. With our denominators the same, we can add our numerators to get an answer of $\frac{12}{10}$, or 1.2.

It's worth pausing briefly to discuss some pitfalls that can arise when doing math of this nature. First, notice that in the addition step we just performed, we only added the numerators, not the denominators. That is, we didn't end up with a final answer of $\frac{12}{20}$. The reasoning behind this is fairly intuitive; essentially, we had 5 of something (specifically, "10ths") and we added another 7 of that something, so we should end up with twelve of that same something, or twelve 10ths. But when time is ticking down in a section, it's easy to be hasty and add the denominators by accident. Similarly, it's common to make math mistakes in the denominator conversion step, where we multiplied both the numerator and the denominator of the fraction by 5. When rushed, it's really easy to forget the top part and only multiply the bottom by 5. As with math mistakes in general, it's worthwhile to spend a few extra seconds on each calculation-heavy problem to verify that you haven't made any errors.

In some cases, though, obtaining like denominators isn't quite this easy. That is, in the above example, since 2 is a factor of 10, we were easily able to convert our $\frac{1}{2}$ term into $\frac{5}{10}$. But what if one denominator isn't a factor of the other? As an example, take $\frac{1}{3} + \frac{1}{8}$. Three isn't a factor of eight, or vice versa, so what do we do? Situations like this just involve one extra step: specifically, identifying a larger value that is a multiple of both denominators, then manipulating both fractions to have that value as the denominator. An easy way to do this is simply to multiply the denominators together, which here yields 24. We can convert $\frac{1}{3}$ into 24ths by multiplying by $\frac{8}{8}$, and we can convert $\frac{1}{8}$ into 24ths by multiplying by $\frac{3}{3}$. This translates our addition problem into $\frac{8}{24}$ plus $\frac{3}{24}$, making it easy to see our final answer: $\frac{11}{24}$. And there we have it: adding fractions is simple! Subtracting fractions works exactly the same way, particularly in that the denominators of all fractions involved must be the same.

Let's put what we've discussed into practice in the context of **circuits.** Within the scope of MCAT physics are two fraction-heavy circuit equations: one for finding the equivalent resistance of a system with resistors in parallel, and one for finding the equivalent capacitance of a system with capacitors in series. Respectively, these equations are $\frac{1}{R_{total}} = \frac{1}{R_1} + \frac{1}{R_2} + \dots$, continued for all parallel resistor elements, and $\frac{1}{C_{total}} = \frac{1}{C_1} + \frac{1}{C_2} + \dots$, continued for all series capacitor elements. The process of solving these two equations is identical, so let's work through an example of the first one, and you can use the same steps to solve the second if it arises.

Let's say that we have a circuit with three resistors: two 6 Ω resistors and a 12 Ω resistor. One of the 6 Ω resistors is on its own branch of the circuit. The remaining two resistors are in series with each other on a second, parallel branch. What is the total equivalent resistance of the circuit?

Our first step here should be to combine series resistors where possible, since resistors in series add linearly. Here, that means we can combine the 6 Ω and 12 Ω resistors that are on the same branch to form one equivalent 18 Ω resistor. But we're stuck here, because we now have one 6 Ω resistor in *parallel* with our 18 Ω combined resistor, and we have to use our fraction equation: $\frac{1}{R_{total}} = \frac{1}{6} + \frac{1}{18}$. One potential pitfall right off the bat: do *not* equate this to

R_{total} = 6 + 18! We're often so accustomed to the algebraic mantra of "doing the same thing to both sides" that we might think this practice extends to, say, taking the reciprocal of all the terms on both sides, but this is not mathematically correct when multiple added or subtracted terms are present on either side of the equation. Instead, we should solve the right side of our equation, then solve for R_{total}. To add $\frac{1}{6} + \frac{1}{18}$ we just need to manipulate these terms to have the same denominator. 6 is a factor of 18, so we can multiply $\frac{1}{6}$ by $\frac{3}{3}$ to yield $\frac{3}{18}$. Next, we add our fractions: $\frac{3}{18} + \frac{1}{18} = \frac{4}{18} = \frac{2}{9}$. And finally, we also need to remind ourselves that $\frac{2}{9}$ is *not* R_{total}! It's $\frac{1}{R_{total}}$, so now that we have a single term on each side of the equation $\frac{1}{R_{total}} = \frac{2}{9}$, we can take the reciprocal of both terms to give us $R_{total} = \frac{9}{2}$. This has a decimal value of 4.5. So 4.5 Ω is our answer!

Let's wrap up with a brief mention of multiplying and dividing fractions. Unlike addition and subtraction, these operations do not require the denominators of the fractions involved to be the same. Instead, for multiplication, just multiply the numerators to obtain the numerator of the product, and multiply the denominators to obtain the denominator of the product. For instance, multiplying $\frac{2}{3}$ by $\frac{7}{8}$ gives us a product of $\frac{14}{24}$, which simplifies to $\frac{7}{12}$. In previous math classes, you may have learned techniques to simplify fractions even before multiplying, through a technique termed cross-cancellation. That is, if the numerator of one fraction and the denominator of the other have a common factor, we can divide both by that factor and effectively cancel it out, and since we're doing the same thing to both numerator and denominator, the value of the multiplication product does not change. Here, both 2 (in the numerator of one fraction) and 8 (in the denominator of the other) have a common factor of 2, so we can divide both by 2 and transform our expression into $\frac{1}{3} \times \frac{7}{4}$. The product, of course, is the same: $\frac{7}{12}$.

Finally, we have dividing fractions. The key to remember is that dividing by a fraction is the same as multiplying by that fraction's reciprocal. That is, if we're dividing $\frac{1}{10}$ by $\frac{1}{2}$, this is the same as multiplying $\frac{1}{10}$ by $\frac{1}{2}$'s reciprocal, which is 2 (or, to keep it as a full fraction, $\frac{2}{1}$). $\frac{1}{10} \times \frac{2}{1}$ is simple: $\frac{2}{10}$, or $\frac{1}{5}$! Understanding this concept can be useful because, as we've mentioned before, dividing by values that are less than 1 can be a minefield of potential errors for some students. If you're asked to divide 28 by 0.25, and you find it easier to think in fractional terms, just convert 0.25 to $\frac{1}{4}$ and divide 28 by $\frac{1}{4}$. We can easily see that this is equivalent to *multiplying* 28 × 4, giving us 112. Even if this isn't the primary method you use to solve a given problem, it can serve as a great way to check your work and ensure that you haven't fallen victim to a common error.

6. Exponents and Roots

In MCAT-relevant math formulas, you'll notice plenty of linear relationships, where an increase or decrease in one variable results in a directly proportional increase or decrease in the other. However, you'll also frequently encounter **exponential relationships**, where one variable might be proportional to the other variable squared, cubed, or raised to some other power. Exponents and roots are particularly common in general chemistry in the context of equilibrium, solubility, and acid-base chemistry, although they can be found in equations ranging from physics to biology.

Exponentiation is a mathematical operation in which one term is raised to the power of another. The term that is raised to some power—in other words, the term at the bottom—is called the base, and the power is called the exponent. Examples of exponentiation include 2^2, 14^3, v^2, $Ae^{-\frac{Ea}{RT}}$, and countless more—including, in fact, all values written in scientific notation. Raising a value to some exponent is tantamount to multiplying it by itself, that exponent number of times. 2^2, then, is 2 × 2, and 14^3 is 14 × 14 × 14. This might seem pretty simple, and in fact, it is; the most common sources of MCAT errors involving exponentiation result not from a lack of understanding of how it works, but rather from careless errors, such as forgetting to square the velocity term when plugging it into an equation like $KE = \frac{1}{2}mv^2$.

This is where units can be particularly helpful; if you forget to square a term, you'll correspondingly fail to square its units, and this will result in a units mismatch that you can use as a heads-up that you made a mistake. In this example, energy has units of joules (J), which are equivalent to $\frac{kg \cdot m^2}{s}$; if we had simply plugged in velocity as meters per second without squaring it, we would get units of $\frac{kg \cdot m}{s}$ on the right. This presence of different units on the left and right sides tells us loud and clear that we need to go back and rework the problem.

Things can get a little trickier when dealing with base values less than one. For example, what's 0.4^2? If you're thinking 1.6, you've fallen victim to a mistake that has ensnared countless students over the years. In particular, raising a positive value that's less than 1 to a positive exponent should always result in a smaller value. In more informal terms, since we multiplied 0.4 by itself (0.4), we need to get an answer smaller than 0.4, since 0.4×1 would equal 0.4, and we multiplied by a value *less* than 1. The true answer is 0.16. If this concept tends to trip you up, it can help to convert any decimal value into scientific notation before squaring it. In this case, 0.4 is equal to 4×10^{-1}. To square a number in scientific notation, you must square the coefficient (here, 4) and *multiply* the exponent by 2, the exponent to which you're raising it. This gives us an answer of 16×10^{-2}, which we can convert back into decimal form to get 0.16. In some cases, it can also be helpful to convert to fractions when exponentiating base values that are less than one. In this case, we could convert 0.4 to $\frac{4}{10}$, and apply familiar rules of multiplying fractions to determine that $\frac{4}{10} \times \frac{4}{10} = \frac{16}{100}$, or 0.16.

Let's solidify what we've covered so far using an example. A circuit has an equivalent resistance of 8 Ω and a current of 0.06 A. How much power is generated by the circuit? To solve, we can use the power equation $P = I^2 \times R$; all we need to do is plug in our given values. This gives us $P = (0.06 \text{ A})^2 \times 8 \text{ Ω}$. Rather than risk making a mistake squaring the decimal, we can convert 0.06 A into 6×10^{-2} A and square that value to give us 36×10^{-4}, or 3.6×10^{-3}, A^2. Finally, multiplying that value by 8 Ω gives us a final answer of about 30×10^{-3}, or 3×10^{-2}, watts (W). As a gut check, this is equal to 0.03 watts, which is a small value, but not unexpectedly so given that our current was also very small.

We've been dealing quite a bit already with **negative exponents**, which can be significantly harder to grasp than positive ones. Like many other confusing concepts in math, this is largely because they're difficult to picture mentally. It's easy enough, after all, to imagine 4^2 as 4 multiplied by itself, or 4 times 4. It's much harder to imagine 4^{-2}. In fact, this value is equal to $\frac{1}{4^2}$. Fortunately, for the MCAT, though, the vast majority of the time you'll see negative exponents will be in scientific notation, meaning that you'll be dealing exclusively with 10 as the base— 10^{-2}, 10^{-6}, and so on. The key to remember here is that the *more negative* the exponent, the *smaller* the overall value. 10^{-6}, then, is smaller than 10^{-2}.

Even simpler than negative exponents are negative bases, because they follow the same rules of multiplication that you should already be very familiar with. However, they're worth mentioning as cases where mistakes in sign can occur if you're not careful. For instance, say that you need to square -2 (-2^2). This is the same as multiplying -2 by itself, and two negatives multiplied together make a positive; the answer, then, is 4, but it's easy to slip up and write down -4 if you're not keeping a watchful eye. If we instead were asked to cube -2 (-2^3), our answer would be -8, because an odd number of negative values multiplied together yields a negative answer.

With exponents out of the way, let's move on to a closely related concept: **roots**. You've most commonly seen roots written as a radical sign over some value. Most often, you'll see only the radical sign and the value underneath it. This is a square root, with the "2" for the root implied. Occasionally, you may also see a small number, termed the "index," written above the left side of the radical. This indicates that we're dealing with a root that isn't a square root, for instance a cube root if the index is 3.

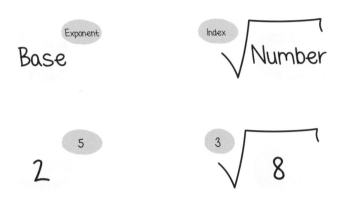

Figure 10. Notation for powers and roots

On the MCAT, the overwhelming majority of roots that you'll deal with are **square roots**, so let's focus on those. Taking a square root of a number is the same as asking yourself "what value squared would equal this number?" For instance, taking $\sqrt{64}$ is asking yourself what value squared equals 64, and the answer should come easily from memory: 8. Numbers like 64—and 4 and 16 and 36 and 100—are "perfect squares," meaning that they have whole-number square roots. We've typically memorized these perfect squares from a young age, at least up to 121 or so, but taking the square root of a non-perfect square might seem more intimidating. Keep in mind that, on the MCAT, rounding and estimation are so widely acceptable that even square-rooting non-perfect squares becomes a simple exercise. For instance, say that one step of a problem requires you to take $\sqrt{50}$. 50 is only slightly greater than 49, which is 7^2. Thus, rounding our answer to 7 is absolutely fine. Or maybe we're attempting to take $\sqrt{90}$. This lies pretty much midway between the perfect squares 81 and 100, so it's fine to say our answer lies somewhere between 9 and 10.

If you think back to our discussion of exponentiation, you'll recall that things got a little trickier when we started to talk about base values that are less than 1. The same is true of roots, for essentially the same reason. Take a situation in which $p^2 = 0.64$, where we're asked to solve for p. In other words, we're looking for $\sqrt{0.64}$. It's very tempting to think that 0.08 must be our answer, because $8^2 = 64$. But in fact, 0.08—as a value less than 1—must yield a number *smaller* than itself when it's squared, meaning that 0.08 cannot possibly be the square root of the much larger value 0.64. Instead, our answer is 0.8. Again, if this is confusing or if you find yourself repeatedly getting problems wrong due to slip-ups with this concept, it may be very helpful to convert to scientific notation. Here, we could convert 0.64 to 64 $\times 10^{-2}$. To take the square root of a value in scientific notation, just square-root the coefficient (here, 64) and cut the exponent in half. Our answer, then, is 8×10^{-1}, which is equivalent to 0.8.

7. Exponents and Roots in Solubility

Let's apply the knowledge presented above about exponents and roots in the setting of a solubility-related example. What is the concentration of carbonate in a saturated solution of $PbCO_3$ at standard temperature, given that the K_{sp} of $PbCO_3$ under standard conditions is approximately 1.5×10^{-13}? First, let's write out our dissociation equation: $PbCO_3 \leftrightarrow Pb^{2+} + CO_3^{2-}$. Next, we use this to find our K_{sp} equation: $K_{sp} = [Pb^{2+}] \times [CO_3^{2-}]$. We know that for every "x" amount of $PbCO_3$ that dissociates, we get "x" amount of Pb^{2+} ions and "x" amount of CO_3^{2-} ions. We can therefore plug x into the K_{sp} equation for both terms, yielding 1.5×10^{-13} equals x squared. Our final step is to take the square root of our scientific-notation term. Here is where we run into trouble: we know that square-rooting such a term involves taking the square root of the coefficient and halving the exponent. But this coefficient is an ugly term to square-root, and the exponent is odd, which, when halved, will lead to a decimal in our product's exponent. This is where being able to manipulate scientific notation really comes in handy. If we identify that 1.5 is pretty close to 1.6, and that 1.6 looks like 16—a term that is *very* easy to square-root—we can transform our value into 15×10^{-14}, which is close enough to 16×10^{-14}. Now the coefficient is easy to square root *and* the exponent is even! Taking the square root of this term gives us a final answer of about 4×10^{-7}. Our last step is to refresh our memory regarding what this value is, and in fact, it's "x," which we earlier said was equal to the concentration of CO_3^{2-}. We have our answer!

You now have all of the tools you need to approach exponent- and root-related MCAT problems. But some questions—solubility ones in particular—do get a bit more complicated, so let's work through a couple more examples. First, we'll tackle a problem in which our solid dissociates into more than two ions, which, as we'll see, can add a layer of complexity: "The molar solubility of calcium hydroxide is approximately 1.12×10^{-2}. Find the K_{sp} of this compound."

Calcium hydroxide has a formula of $Ca(OH)_2$. This means that its dissociation equation is: $Ca(OH)_2 \leftrightarrow Ca^{2+} + 2\ OH^-$. Its K_{sp} equation, then, is $K_{sp} = [Ca^{2+}] \times [OH^-]^2$. That's all well and good, but how can we translate between K_{sp} and molar solubility? Well, molar solubility refers to the number of moles of solute, here $Ca(OH)_2$, that are dissolved in a saturated one-liter solution. So we're looking for the amount of $Ca(OH)_2$ that dissolves. Let's call that amount "x," meaning that "x" stands for our molar solubility. Now, we need to figure out what, in terms of x, we need to plug into our K_{sp} equation. For every "x" amount of $Ca(OH)_2$ that dissolves, we get "x" amount of Ca^{2+} ions, but we get $2x$ amount of OH^- ions. So we should plug in x for $[Ca^{2+}]$ in the K_{sp} equation, and plug in $2x$ for $[OH^-]$.

We can simplify the right side of the equation and thereby equate K_{sp} to some term that includes x. But this is where we need to be careful! On the right side, we see a "$2x$" term in parentheses, and that term is squared. It's tempting to simplify this to "$2x^2$" but since the *entire* term—not just x—was present in the parentheses, we need to square the entire term. $(2x)^2$ is $4x^2$, so our entire right side simplifies to $4x^3$. Now, we have our simplified equation: $K_{sp} = 4x^3$.

What were we asked to do again? Well, we were given the molar solubility, which we called x, and we were asked to find the K_{sp}. We can now plug our 1.12×10^{-2} molar solubility value in for x and solve. First, we need to raise 1.12×10^{-2} to the 3rd power. This involves cubing *both* the coefficient and the exponent. We absolutely don't need to cube 1.12 in any sort of exact manner, so let's say it's somewhere in the neighborhood of 1.4. Then, to find $(10^{-2})^3$, we just multiply the exponents, giving us 10^{-6}. Finally, multiply by 4 to yield our final answer: about 5.6×10^{-6}, which is extremely close to the known K_{sp} of calcium hydroxide, 5.5×10^{-6}.

Another useful example of exponents and roots is the common ion effect. Consider silver chloride, AgCl, which has a K_{sp} of 1.77×10^{-10} under standard conditions. Let's first consider what this value implies for dissolving AgCl in pure water. We can write the given solubility product as $K_{sp} = 1.77 \times 10^{-10} = [Ag^+] \times [Cl^-]$. Then, we can substitute x for the concentration of Ag^+ and Cl^- ions, giving us $1.77 \times 10^{-10} = x^2$. Square-rooting both sides yields a value for x that is about 1.3×10^{-5} molar.

To be clear, what we have just found is that 1.3×10^{-5} molar is the maximum concentration of AgCl that we can have suspended in solution before some will start to precipitate out. Now, let's imagine that we dissolve AgCl in a solution of 0.5 molar NaCl. In this case, the $[Cl^-]$ term will automatically be 0.5 M. Since this amount dwarfs the amount of Cl^- that we would reasonably expect from the dissolution of AgCl, we can neglect the amount of chloride ion that comes from AgCl to simplify our calculations. We get $1.77 \times 10^{-10} = x \times 0.5$, and dividing both sides by 0.5 yields $3.54 \times 10^{-10} = x$.

This shows that *dramatically* less AgCl—close to 50,000 times less—will dissolve now that we have flooded the reaction environment with Cl^-. This is the common ion effect in action—and a fantastic example of how the rules of exponentiation can be applied to a realistic general chemistry example, allowing us to efficiently derive the correct answer by systematically and carefully applying these rules to scientific notation.

8. Logarithms

A **logarithm**, or "log" for short, is the inverse of an exponent. Put simply, this means that the logarithm of a number denotes the exponent to which another value (termed the *base*) must be raised to equal the original number. Let's illustrate this with an example: $\log_{10} 1000 = 3$.

Here, we're taking the base-10 logarithm of 1000, and we find that it equals 3. This must mean that 3 is the exponent to which we must raise 10 to get a final product of 1000—in other words, $10^3 = 1000$. We know from our understanding of exponents that this is correct. In fact, one common method to remember that this is the case is to draw out the logarithmic equation, then have the base move to the other side of the equation and "bump up" the logarithm. In our example above, 10 would move to the other side and "bump up" 3 to yield 10^3. A noteworthy point here is that a base of 10 is extremely common, in math in general and on the MCAT, to the point that sometimes, the "10" is not explicitly written. If you see a logarithmic expression where no base is included, then you can safely assume that you're dealing with a base-10 logarithm.

Given that exponents are involved in a number of MCAT formulas and relationships, it's not surprising that logarithms should be closely involved in some, too. Namely, an understanding of logs is crucial to mastery of two MCAT topics: acid-base chemistry and decibels. Logarithms are also found in a handful of other MCAT-relevant equations, but before diving into those applications, let's outline a few simple rules that you should be familiar with, called the "log rules."

First, the logarithm of 1, regardless of the base, is always equal to 0. This is because any number raised to a power of 0 will always yield an answer of 1. Second, log of some value (we'll call it x) to that same base, x, must always equal 1. This should be similarly intuitive if we use our "bump up" trick; of course $x^1 = x$ and so $\log_x(x) = 1$! Less common, but still worth being familiar with, are rules for combining and splitting up logarithms. To illustrate these rules, we'll imagine we have two values: N and M, where N and M could refer simply to numbers, variables, or even more complex terms. Our first rule is $\log(N \times M) = \log(N) + \log(M)$. This means that, for example, $\log(6x)$ is the same as $\log(6) + \log(x)$. A similar rule is that $\log(N \div M) = \log(N) - \log(M)$. A final, somewhat different rule is that the negative log of any term is equal to log of 1 over that term.

OPERATION	EXPRESSION
Multiplication split into addition	$\log(N \times M) = \log(N) + \log(M)$
Division split into subtraction	$\log(N \div M) = \log(N) - \log(M)$
Logarithmic identity	$\log_x(x) = 1$
Negative log	$-\log(N) = \log(1/N)$

Figure 11. Laws of logarithms

We can use these rules to derive an equation that is a key component of acid-base chemistry: the **Henderson-Hasselbalch equation**. This equation states that for a buffer solution, pH equals pKa plus the logarithm of the concentration of conjugate base (which we can term A⁻) over the concentration of original acid (which we can term HA). Let's try to derive this equation, starting from the simple dissociation reaction of the generic weak acid HA (which makes sense because a buffer should always consist of a weak acid and its conjugate). While you would never be asked to perform this derivation directly on the MCAT, doing it now can both reinforce the log rules we discussed earlier AND emphasize that the equations covered on the MCAT truly aren't random, but rather are derived from basic, core concepts and describe fundamental rules.

We start with our generic weak acid, HA. HA dissociates in water into H^+ (or more specifically, H_3O^+, but we'll stick with H^+) and A^-. We can therefore write our K_a equation as $K_a = \frac{[H^+][A^-]}{[HA]}$, all at equilibrium. The Henderson-Hasselbalch equation is used to calculate pH, so let's get H^+ by itself on one side of the equation. At this point, we have $[H^+] = \frac{[HA]K_a}{[A^-]}$. Next, we can take the negative log of both sides. On the left, this gives us $-\log([H^+])$, which is pH. On the right, we have $-\log\frac{[HA]K_a}{[A^-]}$. Using our log rules, we can split up this term into $-\log(K_a) + -\log\frac{[HA]}{[A^-]}$ which we can simplify further to just $pK_a - \log\frac{[HA]}{[A^-]}$. Finally, using our final log rule, we can translate this to $pK_a + \log\frac{[A^-]}{[HA]}$, and we have our Henderson-Hasselbalch equation: $pH = pK_a + \log\frac{[A^-]}{[HA]}$. Again, you'll never need to work through this derivation step-by-step for any MCAT question or passage, but it's is a valuable cognitive exercise. Hopefully it makes the slew of acid-base equations and relationships seem just a little bit more connected.

With log rules under our belt, let's move on to talk about how logs actually appear in MCAT problems. Let's start with a simple example: finding the pH of a strong acid. What's the pH of a 0.01 M solution of hydroiodic acid? Well, we know that HI is strong, so it fully dissociates—meaning that our solution also has an H^+, or more technically has an H_3O^+, with a concentration of 0.01 molar. Since pH is the negative log of H_3O^+ concentration, we can say that $pH = -\log(0.01)$. To make things really easy, all we need to do is convert into scientific notation. 0.01 is equivalent to 1×10^{-2}, so we're taking the negative log of 1×10^{-2}. One logarithm trick that we haven't mentioned yet, but that's extremely helpful, is that the logarithm of 1×10 raised to any power is equal to that power. Here, that means that the log of $1 \times 10^{-2} = -2$. We're taking the *negative* log, not just the log, so our answer is simply $-\log(1 \times 10^{-2}) = 2$. The pH of our 0.01 M HI solution is 2.

What if we instead had been trying to find the pH of a 0.05 M HI solution? Here, we're asked to take the negative log of 0.05, which is 5×10^{-2}. Since our coefficient isn't 1 here, we can't simply take the negative value of the exponent. Instead, we can approach this in one of multiple ways. First is the "common-sense estimation" method. 5×10^{-2} falls between 1×10^{-2} and 1×10^{-1}. The pH of this solution, then, should fall somewhere between 2 and 1—probably close to the middle, at 1.5—and that's virtually always enough to get the right answer on MCAT questions. However, you might have trouble keeping your negative exponents straight here. It's common to mistakenly think that 5×10^{-2} falls between 10^{-2} and 10^{-3}, for instance. If this gives you a lot of trouble, you can use a different trick that isn't subject to this concern. Simply take the coefficient and move the decimal place one position to the left. Here, that gives us 0.5. Next, take the positive value of the exponent and subtract that adjusted coefficient value. In this case, this means we take 2 and subtract 0.5. Our answer is 1.5, and this method, like the previous one, will easily get us close enough to select an answer.

Things get a little more complicated when dealing with the pH of a weak acid. This is because, as you should recall, weak acids don't dissociate completely in water, meaning that the equilibrium H_3O^+ concentration for such a species is different from the original concentration of the acid itself. Say we have a 0.1 M solution of benzoic acid at standard temperature. Given that the K_a of benzoic acid is 6.5×10^{-5}, what is the pH of the solution? To solve, we first need to determine the concentration of each species at equilibrium. This is something we've done before in the context of solubility, but acid-base chemistry can be a little bit tougher to keep track of, given that the concentration of the reactant (the acid molecule) is involved in the K_a equation, unlike the concentration of the solid reactant in the K_{sp} equation. To keep track of all of our concentrations, let's use a device called an ICE table, where ICE stands for "*i*nitial concentration," "*c*hange in concentration," and "*e*quilibrium concentration."

As always, our best first bet is to write out our dissociation equation. Benzoic acid, or $HC_7H_5O_2$, dissociates into H_3O^+ and its own conjugate base, $C_7H_5O_2^-$, yielding the equation $HC_7H_5O_2 \leftrightarrow H_3O^+ + C_7H_5O_2^-$. Next, we fill in our I, or "initial," row. Initial concentration of benzoic acid is 0.1 Molar, and initial concentrations of our product ions are zero. For our C, or "change," row, we can say that some amount (termed "x") of benzoic acid dissociates, and that same amount of each product ion is formed. Finally, we simply add the I and C values in each column to obtain that column's E, or equilibrium, value: $0.1-x$ for benzoic acid, and x for our two ion products. Now that we have equilibrium concentrations for all species, even though they're in terms of x, we can plug them into the equilibrium expression for the dissociation of benzoic acid.

SPECIES	INITIAL	CHANGE	EQUILIBRIUM
$HC_7H_5O_2$	0.1	-x	0.1 - x
$C_7H_5O_2^-$	0	+x	x
H^+	0	+x	x

Figure 12. ICE table for the dissociation of benzoic acid in water

Doing so yields an equation of $K_a = 6.5 \times 10^{-5} = \frac{x^2}{0.1\,M\,-\,x}$. Since benzoic acid is a weak acid, x is likely to be small—much smaller than 0.1 molar—so we can drop the "-x" term from the denominator, since it'll have a negligible effect on our final answer. Then, multiply 6.5×10^{-5} by 0.1 to get 6.5×10^{-6}. Finally, we square-root both sides to yield an answer of about 2.5×10^{-3}.

At this point, we know that x is equal to 2.5×10^{-3}. Meanwhile, x represents our H_3O^+ concentration, so the -log(x) will give us our pH. Therefore, our final step is to take -log(2.5×10^{-3}). Using our estimation technique, we can see that 2.5×10^{-3} falls somewhere between 1×10^{-3} and 1×10^{-2}, so our answer should fall somewhere between 3 and 2—probably closer to 3, since 2.5 isn't that much greater than 1. Or using our alternative trick, we'd get 3−0.25, for an answer of about 2.75.

Finally, it's worth mentioning the other main MCAT-relevant area that involves logarithms: calculating the intensity of sound in decibels. The decibel scale is a logarithmic scale that expresses the intensity of a sound as a ratio to that of the smallest intensity detectable by humans, which is 1×10^{-12} W/m^2. The decibel equation is $dB = 10\log\frac{I}{I_0}$, where I is the intensity of the sound being measured and I_0 is the reference intensity. This is typically 1×10^{-12} value unless another sound is specified as a point of comparison. The decibel scale follows the rules of logarithms that you've already learned, so nothing about it should come as a surprise, but the fact that it's multiplied by 10 does sometimes throw students off.

Let's try a practice problem just to ensure it makes sense. How many times more intense is a 75 dB sound than a 35 dB sound? Well, here, the decibel difference between the sounds is 40 dB. This means that we can plug in and get $40\,dB = 10\log\frac{I}{I_0}$. We're solving for $\frac{I}{I_0}$ here, assuming that I is our 75 dB sound and I_0 is our point of comparison, which is our 35 dB sound. So let's divide both sides by 10, giving us $4\,dB = 10\log\frac{I}{I_0}$. Finally, since our base is 10 here, we can translate this equation into $10^4 = \frac{I}{I_0}$, and we have our answer: our sound is 10^4 as intense as the reference sound.

9. Units

As a reminder, **units** are important because they help us keep track of what we're using a number to quantify. The cool thing about units, from a mathematical point of view, is that we can treat them as algebraic variables that we can manipulate and solve for. So, just like how $(x / y) \times y = x$, miles per hour × hours = miles. This fact might already be familiar to you from previous coursework, but it has a few implications.

First, doing algebra with units is a way to check your work, and to verify that you're using the correct form of an equation. That is, when taking the MCAT, you'll likely have to pull at least a few equations from memory to use when answering a question, and it's very normal to second-guess whether you're putting the right variables in the right places, especially if the equation isn't particularly intuitive.

For example, let's consider the equations for standing waves in a closed pipe. There are two relevant equations: one for wavelength, and one for frequency. Let's look at the one for frequency, which is $f = n\frac{v}{4L}$, where n is an odd number corresponding to the harmonic, v is the velocity of the wave, and L is the length of the tube. There are multiple ways in which this equation could pose difficulties, but let's focus on just one. What if you're having trouble remembering which variables go in which equation, and whether they go in the numerator or denominator? Here's where units can come to the rescue, because whatever expression we use to calculate frequency must work out to the units we use for frequency, which is hertz (Hz), or $\frac{1}{seconds}$.

So, let's analyze our equation, $f = n\frac{v}{4L}$. Frequency has units of Hz, or $\frac{1}{seconds}$, velocity has units of $\frac{distance}{time}$, or $\frac{meters}{seconds}$, and L has units of distance, which we can represent as meters. Both n and 4 are unitless constants that we can ignore for these purposes, so we just need to figure out the units $\frac{v}{L}$. Doing some quick algebra, we can take the expression of $\frac{m}{s}$, m, and rewrite it to $\frac{m}{s} \times \frac{1}{m}$. Then, the meters term cancels out and we're left with $\frac{1}{s}$, which is just what we need for frequency. This kind of units check can be very useful to make sure that we wrote the equation out correctly. If, instead, we had put L in the numerator and v in the denominator, we'd wind up with units of seconds, which doesn't match up with the units of frequency.

But what if we were dealing with *different* units of distance? For instance, what if we were given information about the length of the pipe in feet and needed to calculate wavelength, but all the answer choices were in meters? Or, even more plausibly, what if there was a mismatch in scale, like if the question gave us information in meters, but all the answers were in millimeters? From the point of view of unit checking, as a way to make sure we're putting the right variables in the right place of the equation, all we have to do is make sure the same *type* of units end up in the same place on either side of the equation, without worrying so much about what those units are. That is, in this case, as long as we see some unit for distance in the same place on both sides of the equation, we know that we've set up the problem correctly. However, when the time comes to match our units to the correct answer choices, we need to make sure that the *specific* units line up.

This is where **unit conversion** comes in. To convert between units, we can utilize the concept of dimensional analysis. If we're given an equivalence relationship between two units, like 1 foot = 0.3 meters, we can write that as a fraction in the form of $\frac{1\,ft}{0.3\,m}$ or, alternatively, as $\frac{0.3\,m}{1\,ft}$. Because 1 foot and 0.3 meters are equal, those fractions both equal 1, meaning that we can multiply any other value by that fraction without changing its magnitude. While doing so, we're simultaneously doing algebra with the units, which results in them being changed.

Let's look at this more concretely: what if we had a value of 10 feet that we needed to change into meters? We could take 10 feet, and then multiply it by $\frac{0.3\,m}{1\,ft}$. As we do so, the units of feet cancel out, so that we're left with 10×0.3 m = 3 m, and we've successfully converted from feet to meters. Let's explore one common source of error in these conversions. We mentioned that we could also write this fraction as $\frac{1\,ft}{0.3\,m}$. So why did we use $\frac{0.3\,m}{1\,ft}$ instead? The idea here is that we pick whichever way makes the units work out. Let's see what would happen if we made the incorrect choice of multiplying $\frac{10\,ft \times 1\,ft}{0.3\,m}$. If we work through the math, that will give us a value of 33.3 feet-squared divided by meters. This isn't wrong *mathematically*, but it's wrong for our physics problem-solving purposes because it doesn't accomplish our goal, which was converting to meters.

Students often wonder whether they need to know conversions like 1 foot = 0.3 meters, or 1 kilometer = 1,000 meters. The answer to this is simple: yes and no. You do *not* need to memorize long lists of random conversions, especially conversions between metric or SI units, and traditional (also known as imperial) units like pounds and feet. If you do encounter a strange or unusual unit on the MCAT, the test will give you the information you need to work with it. That said, it is generally a good idea to be familiar with some common conversions, like knowing that a meter is slightly more than three feet, that a kilometer is slightly less than two-thirds of a mile, that a kilogram is about 2.2 pounds, and being able to convert between degrees Fahrenheit and Celsius. Being able to do these common conversions can help you better grasp physical or experimental setups described using those units.

However, you *do* have to be very comfortable going back and forth between different orders of magnitude using SI units and their associated prefixes. This means being able to quickly calculate conversions like 30 milligrams = 0.03 grams. A thorough familiarity with scientific notation pays off in this regard. Although certain conversions, like milligrams to grams, may become second nature as you practice, it's *always* an option to convert everything to scientific notation and work through the conversion step by step. For example, we could say that 30 milligrams = 30×10^{-3} grams, or 3×10^{-2} grams. From here, we can easily see that this is equal to 0.03 grams.

Relatedly, a common question is "what units do we have to know for the MCAT?" The short answer is that since it's a good idea to study units as part of learning each equation, you should know the units that correspond to each equation that is covered in MCAT prep. However, there are some important nuances when we dig deeper. For one, we can certainly prioritize the base SI units, including meters, kilograms, seconds, amperes, kelvin, and moles, as well as especially common derived units, such as hertz for frequency, newtons for force, pascals for pressure, joules for energy, watts for power, coulombs for charge, volts for electric potential, and teslas for the strength of magnetic fields.

Upon further reflection, however, it may not be entirely obvious what it means to "know" a unit. Let's consider joules, which we encounter all the time in bioenergetics and areas of physics relating to energy. On one hand, "knowing" what a joule is could be as simple as associating it with energy. And that really is the *bare* minimum that you should know. On the other end of the spectrum, you could imagine being able to rattle off the fact that a joule is defined in SI base units as a kilogram meter squared over seconds squared, and could also be defined in terms of SI derived units as $C \times V$, or $W \times s$, or $Pa \times m^3$, or newtons times meters. However, here's the issue: while there's not really such a thing as knowing too much about units, that way of approaching it also kind of misses the point. You *could* get a question that just directly asks about alternative ways that a joule could be defined— it's not impossible—but the better approach is to try to understand how these definitions of joules fit into different contexts where energy pops up in physics.

As an example of what this cognitive process looks like, we should first understand that work is defined in terms of energy, so any time we encounter work in an equation, we'll be dealing with joules. Work is often first introduced through the example of applying a certain force over a certain distance. The units of force are newtons, and those of distance are meters, so energy, or joules, can be defined as newton-meters. Moving on, power is defined as work divided by time. We could therefore rewrite this equation to define work as power multiplied by time. Since power has units of watts, this gives us the definition of joules as watts times seconds. The definition of joules as pascals times meters cubed is a bit more involved. Pressure is defined most basically as force per unit area, or newtons divided by meters squared. Multiplying both the numerator and denominator by distance, we get newton-meters divided by meters cubed. Since, as we just saw, newton-meters are equivalent to joules, we find that a pascal is equal to a joule divided by meters cubed. This is insightful in its own right, because it tells us that pressure is a way that fluids can store energy, plus we can rearrange it to define a joule as a pascal times meters cubed. Finally, the definition of joules as coulombs times volts is grounded in the idea that it takes work to move a charge, expressed in coulombs, against an electric potential gradient, expressed in volts.

The takeaway point is that units are both an important tool for mathematical hygiene, which can help you avoid making preventable mistakes, and an excellent lens through which to assess your mastery of physics concepts as you study, allowing you to identify concepts that you may need to review further.

10. Choosing Equations

At the end of the day, getting a high MCAT score means correctly answering questions. Doing so is where all the various skills that you hone through MCAT prep must be integrated. This is particularly true for answering quantitative questions, which can require *both* that your overall question analysis skills be on point *and* that you execute flawlessly in terms of math. With that in mind, let's conclude our study of math and formulas by tying all the threads together.

As for any question, the first step when answering a quantitative question is to understand what it's asking. We present a step-by-step approach to answering science questions in considerable depth elsewhere, so there's no need to reiterate every cognitive step, but identifying which equation to use is an absolutely crucial part of the process. It can be tempting to rush through this part, for a couple reasons. First, we tend to make automatic associations with certain scientific key words and specific equations, like how "frequency" might automatically make you think of the equation $v = \lambda f$. Second, time pressure is *always* in the back of our minds, but taking some extra seconds to double-check this choice can avoid wasted effort.

Remember that **equations are tools**, and we need to pick the right tool for the job. This means that the equation or equations should contain variables related to the information presented in the question stem *and* yield a calculated result that corresponds to the answer choices. So, to return to our example of frequency, although v equals lambda f is an important equation dealing with frequency, if a question is asking about the energy of an electromagnetic wave as it relates to its frequency, $E = hf$ might be a better choice. Or if we're dealing with the frequency of standing waves in an open or closed pipe, we might need one of those equations, such as $f = \frac{nv}{2L}$ for an open pipe.

Another possibility is that the passage could us a *new* equation related to frequency, perhaps in the setting of an experiment. Not to worry. The beautiful thing about passages is that no matter how involved or intimidating they seem, they *must* be accessible on the basis of core MCAT content knowledge. Of course, "accessible" doesn't mean "easy"—the information you need might be buried in a blizzard of confusing terminology and acronyms—but the information *will* be there. This means that the key to handling novel equations is to leverage passage information to understand the point of the equation, and how it fits into the broader ideas discussed in the passage. Work through each variable in the equation one-by-one, making sure that you account for every variable. Even if you've never seen a certain symbol before, again, it must be defined somewhere.

Once you've identified what each variable refers to, then it's time to translate the equation into words. Virtually any new equation can be boiled down to a statement that some variable of interest—let's call it X for convenience—has a direct or inverse relationship with one or more other variables, which we can call Y and Z. As a brief refresher, a **direct relationship** between X and Y means that if X goes up, so does Y, and vice versa, while an **inverse relationship** between X and Z means that if X goes up, Z goes down, and vice versa. Therefore, it's usually possible to rephrase a new equation in simple terms as something like "more X means more Y," or "more X means less Z," which will set you up to apply that equation appropriately.

Once you've got your equation set up, it may be time to start calculating, unless, that is, the question only necessitates proportional reasoning. Keep an eye out for that possibility, because if that's the case, you can generally substitute in simple algebraic values, like $2x$ or $3x$, to perform the calculation. You may even be able to reason through the problem using simple inequalities, like v_2 is greater than v_1 when comparing two velocities. It's also possible that they could give you a set of answer choices with values pre-substituted in, in which case your task is to identify which values correspond to which variables, and based on that, the correct way to set up the equation. Using your wet-erase board to write out the equation may help you to systematize your thinking if faced with such a problem.

Another caveat is that the solution may wind up requiring more than one equation. For example, a question asking about the energy delivered by EM radiation of a certain wavelength would require you to combine the two equations $E = hf$, which links energy to frequency, and $c = \lambda f$, which links frequency to wavelength for EM radiation. Therefore, you have two options: either calculate frequency first and then use that numerical value to calculate wavelength, or combine the two equations into a single one, $E = \frac{hc}{m}$. In fact, the latter approach is common enough that the combined equation is often given as one to memorize separately, but it's still an excellent example of the basic dilemma: do you prefer doing two sets of calculations, but with simpler setups, or a single calculation that's somewhat more complex? Either approach is OK. Practice both ways, and figure out which works better for you.

To summarize, it's remarkably common for the source of mistakes on quantitative MCAT questions to occur in the problem-solving steps that take place before you ever write down a number. Sometimes it can be easy to feel like the core of quantitative questions is the math itself, which can make you rush through the preceding steps. In reality, though, both stages of problem-solving matter, and investing some extra care into selecting an appropriate equation can pay off.

11. Calculations in Practice

When faced with a quantitative question, once you've set up your equations and actually started writing down numbers, it's time to do some math. The key to doing math on the MCAT without a calculator—in addition to knowing the basic mechanics cold—is skilled estimation and rounding. Let's work with the equation $E = \frac{hc}{m}$, which can be obtained by combining $E = hf$ and $c = \lambda f$, to calculate the energy of a single photon of 580 nm wavelength light.

First, we need to assemble our variables. Planck's constant, or h, is 6.62×10^{-34} meters squared times kilograms over seconds. There's no need to memorize this, though, because you'll be given this value if it comes up. Then, the speed of light in a vacuum, c, is 3×10^8 m/s. This constant, in contrast, *is* worth knowing. Next, we have our wavelength of 580 nanometers. This equals 580×10^{-9} meters, but we'll probably have an easier time working with this value if we convert it to normalized scientific notation, or 5.8×10^{-7} meters. Now we've got a fraction with two terms in the numerator and one in the denominator. Let's handle the numerator first, and then divide by the denominator. As we do so, we have two tasks: to estimate efficiently, and to work skillfully with scientific notation.

$$E = \frac{(6.62 \times 10^{-34})(3 \times 10^{-8})}{5.8 \times 10^{-7}}$$

$$E = \frac{(6.62 \times 10^{-34} \frac{\text{kgm}^2}{\text{s}})(3 \times 10^{-8} \frac{\text{m}}{\text{s}})}{5.8 \times 10^{-7} \text{m}}$$

Figure 13. Composite equation for calculating the energy of a photon.

Once the time comes to do nitty-gritty calculations, it may be helpful to toss out the units and just operate with numbers. This keeps things cleaner and reduces the number of items that you have to keep track of while you're doing the math. However, if you have any doubt about how you've set up the equation, it's always possible to do a quick units check to make sure it lines up. Then substitute in the numbers. Now, as we mentioned, estimation is vital, but it's not necessarily obvious how precise we need to be. With that in mind, let's first work through this example using relatively careful estimation, and then we'll explore what would happen if we used very rough estimation strategies instead.

Our numerator is 6.62×10^{-34} multiplied by 3×10^8. Let's first handle the coefficient, or the thing that comes before the "× 10" in scientific notation. We can definitely get rid of the "2" in 6.62. To make life easier, we might handle the 6 in the tenths digit by recognizing that 6.6 is a little bit more than halfway between 6 and 7. Therefore, instead of multiplying 6.6 × 3, we can recognize that 6 × 3 is 18, and 7 × 3 is 21, and we need something closer to 21 than to 18—so how about 20? That's a nice round number, so let's use it. And, by the way, it turns out that 6.6 × 3 is 19.8, which we would just round up to 20 in the next step anyway. Now, let's turn to the exponents, which we need to add together, since we're multiplying in scientific notation. By doing so, we get −34 + 8 = −26.

We now have 20×10^{-26} in the numerator, and we need to divide this by 5.8×10^{-7}. On one hand, we *could* take 20×10^{-26} and convert it into normalized scientific notation as 2.0×10^{-25}, but if we anticipate the division task that awaits us, it might be easier to estimate a value for 20 divided by 5.8 than for 2.0 divided by 5.8, so we can just leave the numerator as is right now. Let's adopt the same estimation strategy that we used above: 5.8 can be rounded up to 6, and now we have to estimate 20 divided by 6. Since 18 divided by 6 is 3, we need something slightly higher than 3, but not by too much, since 6 × 4 would be 24. Let's guess 3.25. If we want to be extra careful here, we can note that rounding 5.8 up to 6 in a division problem means that our estimate would be lower than the real value. If this isn't completely intuitive, the rationale here is that higher numbers in the denominator give lower absolute values when you carry out the division operation. We could account for this source of error by adding another one-tenth or so to the final value. This would give us 3.35, which is pretty close to the actual value of 20 divided by 5.8, which is 3.45.

Recalling that even 20 was an estimation that we used instead of 19.8, we might wonder about the error induced by that term. It turns out that 19.8/5.8 is 3.41, so we're very much in the ballpark. Returning to the orders of magnitude, when dividing in scientific notation, we subtract the denominator from the numerator, so we get (-26)–(-7), or (-26)+7, or -19. Our final estimated answer, then, is 3.35×10^{-19}, which is very similar to the answer of 3.42×10^{-19} that we would have gotten if we had used everything out to the hundredths digits starting with 6.62 for Planck's constant.

What if we were really in a rush, and just rounded 6.62 up to 7 and 5.8 up to 6? Well, then the coefficient in our numerator would be 7×3, or 21, which we'd have to divide by 6. We might be able to recognize that $21 \div 6 = 3.5$, because 21 is exactly halfway between 18, or 6×3, and 24, or 6×4. That's remarkably close to the completely precise answer of 3.42. Even if we don't recognize $21 \div 6$ as being equal to precisely 3.5, hopefully we can at least recognize that it's 3 point something, which may be all we need to answer the question.

Depending on how the answer choices are set up, an estimate of "about 3×10^{-19}" might be fine, because the answer choices could be something like:

(A) 3.[something] $\times 10^{-19}$ J—which is correct.

(B) 3.[something] $\times 10^{-33}$ J—which is what you would have gotten if you had made a mistake in handling the powers of 10 in the final division step, either by adding them or by getting tripped up with the math involved in subtracting a negative number.

(C) 3.[something] $\times 10^{-21}$ J—which you would get by writing 580 nm as 5.8×10^{-9} m, which would actually be 5.8 nm, instead of converting properly to write it as 5.8×10^{-7} m.

(D) 8.[something] $\times 10^{-19}$ J—which reflects a random mistake with the coefficient calculations, like inadvertently using 8×10^8 m/s for the speed of light instead of 3×10^8, as 3 and 8 look similar.

As this example implies, incorrect answers often reflect **predictable mistakes**. In addition to the possibilities we just discussed, incorrect answers may use the wrong units, be obtained from correct calculations made using the wrong equation, reflect having plugged in the wrong values, and so on. So, just because you calculate something that matches up with an answer choice doesn't automatically mean that you're correct. But perhaps even more importantly, it can be helpful to briefly skim over the answer choices before you get too deep in calculations. First, before you switch over to numbers-only mode, it's good to double-check that your equations will result in something that yields the same units as the answer choices. If the answer choices don't all have the same units, then that's a sign that you need to pay especially careful attention to the units involved. Second, a quick overview of the answer choices can give you a sense of the level of precision needed. Occasionally, you may even be so lucky as to get answer choices where the coefficient differs, but the order of magnitude is always the same, or vice versa, which is a signal that you can disregard whatever aspect of the scientific notation calculations that you don't actually need. Regardless, the key is to work systematically and to tailor your calculations to the requirements of the question.

12. Math and Formulas in a Practice Passage

As always, the proof is in the pudding, which while you're studying for the MCAT means realistic practice. Therefore, let's work through a sample passage that's heavy on equations as a way of synthesizing everything that we've covered:

> The circulatory system can be modeled as a series of anatomically complicated pipes linked to a pump. making the physical properties of fluids and their flow highly relevant for physicians. A fluid undergoing laminar flow as it flows through a tube of length L and radius r experiences a pressure drop (ΔP) from one end of the tube to the other, as expressed through Poiseuille's law (Equation 1), in which μ is the viscosity of the fluid and Q is its flow rate.

Equation 1
$$\Delta P = \frac{8nLQ}{r\,r^4}$$

> The flow of a fluid is equal to its velocity multiplied by the cross-sectional area through which it passes. Combining this information with Poiseuille's law indicates that there is a relationship between the velocity of fluid flowing through a cylindrical tube and the length of that tube, as shown in Equation 2.

Equation 2
$$v^{-1} = \frac{8n}{\Delta P r^2}$$

> To empirically verify this relationship, students conducted an experiment in which they attached plastic tubing with a radius of 2.00 ± 0.05 mm to a hole at the bottom of a water tank that was filled with water to a height of 0.43 ± 0.01 m above the center of the tube, and positioned such that the tubing lay flat on the ground. Water was allowed to flow into the beaker for 30 ± 0.2 s and the volume of water collected in the beaker was measured. The pressure difference across the tube was kept constant by maintaining the water level at 0.43 ± 0.01 m. The experimental setup is shown in Figure 1.

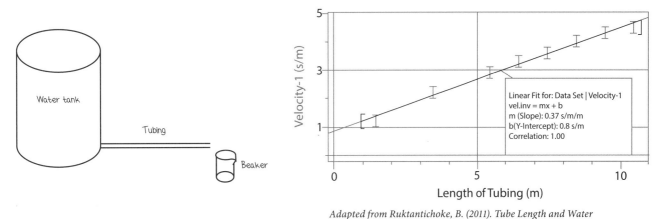

Adapted from Ruktantichoke, B. (2011). Tube Length and Water Flow. ISB Journal of Physics (June) under CC-BY 4.0

Figure 1. Experimental setup   **Figure 2.** Experimental results

The results of this experiment were graphed, as shown below in Figure 2.

The first paragraph introduces **Poiseuille's law,** which many students are not very comfortable with. The good news, though, is that the passage gives us Poiseuille's law in Equation 1, and spells out what the variables refer to in paragraph one.

The second paragraph reminds us that the rate of flow of a fluid is equal to its velocity multiplied by the cross-sectional area that it's traveling through. This relationship is used to derive Equation 2, which the passage describes as articulating a relationship between the velocity of fluid flowing through a cylindrical tube and that tube's length. Let's take a closer look at Equation 2.

The first thing to notice about this equation is that it's formulated in terms of *inverse* velocity, as denoted by the v^{-1} term, which is equal to $1/v$. Inverse velocity has a direct relationship with viscosity and length and an inverse relationship with the pressure drop and radius. Since the passage implies that we should focus on the relationship between velocity and length of the tube, we can translate this into more accessible language by noting that velocity has an *inverse* relationship with length. The fact that this is an inverse relationship is extremely important, and the way that the passage presents this as v^{-1} instead of $1/v$ may even be a hint that misinterpreting this relationship as direct might be a trap set by passage writers.

Moving into paragraph three, we get some information about an experiment that students conducted to verify this relationship. This wording is a dead giveaway that we'll be dealing with a Lab Manual passage, and indeed, the rest of the paragraph fills us in about the details of their setup, as illustrated in Figure 1. Don't agonize about the details, as long as you can visualize what they're doing.

Then we get the results in Figure 2. As always, when analyzing a figure, we should take a careful look at the axes to understand what's being measured. The x-axis, corresponding to the independent variable, shows length in meters. The scale implies that the students were using some pretty long tubing setups, on the scale of up to 10 meters, which is kind of weird, but who knows—maybe they had an enormous physics lab and a surplus of tubing. Glancing upward to look at what's plotted, it seems like the students conducted eight experiments with different lengths of tubing and then fitted a line to that experimental data. Looking at the y-axis, the first thing we might notice is that it's labeled "Velocity"—but here again, we have to be more careful, and notice that it's actually *inverse* velocity, or v^{-1}, which is why we see units of s/m instead of m/s. Now, let's look at the linear plot again. We see a linear increase, so this reflects a *direct* relationship between tubing length and inverse velocity, or an *inverse* relationship between tubing length and velocity. This corresponds to what Equation 2 predicts, so everything's in order—although we might also notice that Figure 2 is a *second* place where reading too quickly might make it easy to overlook that these equations deal with *inverse* velocity. This observation should confirm our intuition that we should be on the lookout for this issue when problem-solving. Speaking of which, it's time to move onto the questions, which we'll present one-by-one.

> 1. Based on Figure 2, what velocity would be predicted for water exiting the water tank through a 3-cm-long tube?
>
> A. 0.5 m/s
>
> B. 0.8 m/s
>
> C. 1.25 m/s
>
> D. 2 m/s

Question 1 asks us to predict the velocity of water exiting a 3-centimeter tube based on Figure 2. The fact that the question specifically references Figure 2 indicates that we should answer the question based on that figure, *not* by attempting to calculate it from scratch using a formula. As such, it initially seems like we just need to go to the figure and read a number off of the chart. And that's true, but we have to keep in mind that it's unlikely, albeit not impossible, for the MCAT to just ask you to literally read a simple graph with no other complications. Therefore, we need to be careful for potential traps. The first such trap has to do with units. The question stem asks for a 3 *centimeter* long tube, but the x-axis gives us units of meters. 3 cm is just 3/100ths of a meter, so in essence, this question is asking us what value we would extrapolate for the *y*-intercept. OK, so that looks like it'll be about 0.8. But now we need to ask—0.8 *what*? Now, hopefully we noticed when we were reading the passage that the y-axis here is inverse velocity, in units of seconds per meter, but even if not, now we have a second chance. Therefore, the right answer will be 1/0.8, which we can quickly estimate as being a little bit greater than 1, so choice C, 1.25 meters per second, fits the bill perfectly. Note that we didn't have to be too precise about either that estimation step *or* reading the y-intercept as 0.8. It would have been perfectly fine to say, "the y-intercept is a little bit less than 1, so 1 over the y-intercept will be a little bit more than 1." This question reinforces a valuable lesson: we can often be quick and imprecise with the actual calculations, but we *must* be very careful and deliberate about how we set up the problem.

Turning to the incorrect answer choices, choice A can be obtained by incorrectly reading up from $x = 3$ meters instead of $x = 0.03$ meters, but correctly calculating the reciprocal of the obtained y value of 2. Choice B, 0.8 m/s, corresponds to what would happen if you correctly recognized that 3 centimeters is equivalent to 0.03 meters, making it essentially the y-intercept, but used this value directly instead of taking the reciprocal. Finally, choice D, 2 meters per second, is the worst of both worlds, in that it is obtained by incorrectly using the x-axis value of 3 meters instead of 0.03 meters *and* failing to recognize the need to take the reciprocal of the inverse velocity values on the y-axis. Note, though, that choice D might be most tempting if you were in a rush, and just wanted to choose a value corresponding to something on the graph based on eyeballing the axes.

2. If the tubing were modified by narrowing its middle section slightly as shown below, the water moving through the narrower section would:

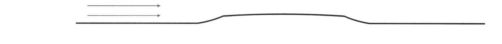

A. move more slowly than the water moving through the wider section of the tubing.

B. exert more pressure on the walls of the tubing.

C. move more slowly than the water exiting the tubing.

D. exert less pressure on the walls of the tubing.

Question 2 might not initially seem quantitative, as neither the question nor the answer choices contain any numbers, but appearances can be deceiving. The question asks about the relationship between the width of the middle section of tubing and two other variables: velocity and pressure. And, of course, relationships among variables are expressed using equations. We can tackle the velocity part of the question by using the continuity equation for fluids, or $A_1v_1 = A_2v_2$. This principle states that within a closed system, the flow rate of a fluid remains constant. As a consequence, if a pipe gets wider, the fluid moving through it will slow down, and vice versa. Therefore, narrowing the tubing, as the question stem describes, will make the fluid go faster. This alone lets us eliminate answer choices A and C.

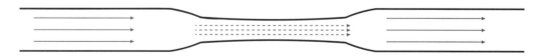

Figure 14. Visualization of continuity equation. Length of each vector represents flow velocity.

Now, to bring pressure into the picture, we'll need **Bernoulli's law**. We can handle this the long way or the short way. The long way is to write out Bernouilli's law: $\rho gh_1 + \frac{1}{2}\rho v_1^2 + P_1 = \rho gh_2 + \frac{1}{2}\rho v_2^2 + P_2$. The tubing is described as flat, so we can discard the term for gravitational potential energy. Then we can do some algebra and write an expression for P_2, which is what answer choices B and D deal with: $P_2 = \frac{1}{2}\rho v_1^2 - \frac{1}{2}\rho v_2^2 + P_1$. Our v_2 is greater than v_1, so $\frac{1}{2}\rho v_1^2 - \frac{1}{2}\rho v_2^2$ will be a negative number, which we can call $-K$, and we can rewrite the equation to read $P_2 = P_1 - K$, which tells us that P_2 will be smaller than P_1, so we can choose choice D.

Or, if that gives you a headache, we can do it the short way. Conceptually, Bernoulli's law is basically conservation of energy for fluids, which can contain energy in the form of gravitational potential energy, kinetic energy, and pressure. We don't care about gravitational potential energy, so we're left with kinetic energy and pressure. If velocity goes up, so does kinetic energy, so for energy to be conserved, pressure must go down. This points us to choice D. In fact, the relationships between radius, velocity, and pressure are tested often enough with fluids that we do recommend becoming familiar with them, to the point that questions on these relationships become automatic. Nonetheless, this question illustrates the point that it really pays off to understand the relationships encoded by equations, rather than just memorizing them so that you can plug and chug.

    3. According to Equation 2, which of the following variables does NOT show an inverse relationship with the velocity of a fluid moving through a tube?

    I. Radius of the pipe
    II. Viscosity of the fluid
    III. Length of the tube

    A. I only

    B. II only

    C. II and III only

    D. I, II, and III

Question 3 explicitly asks you to evaluate Equation 2 qualitatively. This is both a Roman numeral question and a *not* question, so it's especially important to translate the question stem into a clear sense of what we're looking for, and then proceed systematically. If a variable shows an inverse relationship with velocity, we'll need to eliminate it, and if a variable has a direct relationship—or, conceivably, no relationship at all—with velocity, we must choose a Roman numeral answer that includes it. All three of these variables are in Equation 2: viscosity and length are in the numerator, and radius is in the denominator, so it might be tempting to say that viscosity and length show a direct relationship and radius has an inverse relationship—but hold up! As we've discussed, this equation is written in terms of *inverse* velocity. Therefore, viscosity and length have a *direct* relationship with *inverse* velocity, meaning that they have an inverse relationship with plain old velocity. The same relationship tells us that the radius must have a direct relationship with velocity. Based on this reasoning, the correct answer is A, or Roman numeral I only. Even if you get lost within this thicket of double- and triple-negatives, it should be possible to eliminate B by recognizing that viscosity and length co-occur in the numerator of Equation 2, so it would make no sense for the answer to include one and not the other, and to eliminate D by realizing that the structure of the equation means that it would make no sense to pick all three variables.

    4. If a 6-meter tube used with the students' experimental setup were twisted downward at the end so that the water exited the tubing at 1m below the bottom of the water tank, what would be the measured velocity of the water?

CHAPTER 11: MATH AND FORMULAS

A. 0.33 m/s

B. 3 m/s

C. 4.5 m/s

D. 5.4 m/s

Finally, with Question 4, we have what seems like more of a traditional physics question. The first step is to visualize the setup described in the question. We're thinking about fluids, and we're given information about gravitational potential energy and velocity. Therefore, Bernoulli's law seems like a good fit. We can discard the pressure term of the equation because there's no mention of either container being pressurized, so we can assume that the pressure on both sides of the setup will just be atmospheric pressure, or close enough as to make no real difference.

Let's set up the y-axis so that the point where the tubing exits from the water tank is $y_1 = 1$ m and the point where it exits the tubing is 0 m ($y_2 = 0$ m). This allows us to get rid of the $\rho g h_2$ term, and if we factor out density, we get the much simpler equation of $\frac{1}{2}v_1^2 + gy_1 = \frac{1}{2}v_2^2$. Let's multiply through by two, and take the square root, which will give us an equation stating that $v_2 = \sqrt{v_1^2 + 2gy_1}$. So what's v_1? Well, based on the question stem, a reasonable starting point would be the exiting velocity observed with a 6-meter tube laid flat. Turning to Figure 2, we can estimate the inverse velocity as 3 seconds/meter, meaning that the actual velocity would be ⅓ meters/second. We can use 10 m/s² g, and y is of course 1 meter, so we get the final velocity as the square root of one-third squared, or one-ninth, plus 20. This is basically equivalent to the square root of 20. Well, $\sqrt{25} = 5$, and $\sqrt{16} = 4$, so we can estimate our answer as about 4.5 m/s, or choice C. Let's look at the incorrect answer choices. Choice A is just the velocity of water exiting a 6-meter flat tube according to Figure 2, and choice B is the inverse velocity read directly from the y-axis. As such, both of these answer choices reflect a misunderstanding of the problem setup. Choice D, 5.4 meters per second, would be obtained if you used 3 meters per second for v_1 instead of ⅓ meters per second in the final calculation, which is the same conceptual mistake as in choice B, just later on in the process.

An interesting point about this question is that since we cancelled out the pressure and density terms, we could also have solved this problem using the kinematics equation $v_2^2 = v_1^2 + 2ad$, or for that matter, simple conservation of kinetic and potential energy. Bernoulli's law might have been overkill, but at the same time, it might be better to use a more powerful equation than is really necessary, and then have to cancel out some terms, than to waste time spinning our wheels about what to do.

This passage was definitely tricky. However, the passage itself, as well as its accompanying questions, illustrated some important points about how to reason using math and formulas on the MCAT, which we can summarize as follows: read carefully, reason about the relationships encoded by equations, and take care to understand what each question is asking for. Rapid calculation skills are helpful, but they're a secondary concern.

As a final point to mull over in your head, those key points for applying math and formulas on the MCAT overlap are highly reminiscent of the skills needed to succeed on the MCAT more broadly, including the CARS section. That is, all these seemingly-separate skills are actually working towards a similar goal. Food for thought.

215

13. Must-Knows

> Basic operations and algebra: familiar, but there are some pitfalls.
  - Double-check work when subtracting a negative number, e.g., $9 - (-6) = 9 + 6 = 15$.
  - Remember that dividing by a number less than 1 yields a larger number, e.g. $10/0.5 = 20$.
  - Algebra errors can crop up, so be careful to work systematically despite need for efficiency.
> Scientific notation: coefficient $\times$ 10 to some power, e.g. $4.184 \times 10^3 = 4,184$.
  - Multiplying scientific notation term by a standard term (regular number) = coefficient $\times$ the regular number. The same logic holds for division.
  - Multiplying two scientific notation terms: multiply coefficients, add exponents of 10.
  - Dividing two scientific notation terms: divide coefficient, subtract exponents of 10.
  - To add/subtract scientific notation terms, they must be converted into terms with the same exponents.
> Trigonometry: used on MCAT primarily to resolve vectors into x- and y-components.
  - Key underlying insight: Pythagorean theorem for right triangles: $A^2 + B^2 = C^2$, where A and B are the legs and C is the hypotenuse.
  - "SOH CAH TOA": sine = opposite/hypotenuse, cosine = adjacent/hypotenuse, tangent = opposite/adjacent.
  - Key values of sine: $\sin(0°) = 0$, $\sin(30°) = \frac{1}{2}$, $\sin(45°) = \frac{\sqrt{2}}{2}$, $\sin(60°) = \frac{\sqrt{3}}{2}$, $\sin(90°)$.
  - Key values of cosine: $\cos(0°) = 1$, $\cos(30°) = \frac{\sqrt{3}}{2}$, $\cos(45°) = \frac{\sqrt{2}}{2}$, $\cos(60°) = \frac{1}{2}$, $\cos(90°) = 0$.
  - Special cases of the Pythagorean theorem: sides of 3, 4, 5 and 5, 12, 13.
> Fractions: may be familiar, but worth reviewing a few sources of common errors:
  - To multiply fractions, multiply numerators and denominators.
  - To divide fractions, invert the fraction that is the divisor and then multiply.
  - To add/subtract fractions, convert denominators to be the same, then add numerators.
> Exponents: when multiplying/dividing expressions with exponents (like in scientific notation), add/subtract the exponents. When exponentiating expressions with exponents, multiply the exponents.
  - Negative exponents do not yield negative numbers, instead $2^{-2} = 1/2^2$, so negative exponents of positive numbers yield numbers between 0 and 1.
> Logarithms = inverse of exponents, so $\log_{10}(1000) = 3$ because $10^3 = 1000$.
  - Log rules: $\log(N \times M) = \log(N) + \log(M)$, $\log(N \div M) = \log(N) - \log(M)$, $\log_x(x) = 1$, $\log(1) = 0$.
> Units: being able to convert using fractions is essential (dimensional analysis), checking units can help make sense of equations and solidify science knowledge.
> Choosing equations is like picking the right tool for the job: study equations and approach questions with that in mind.

Applied Practice

The best MCAT practice is realistic, with detailed analytics to help you assess where things went wrong. For those reasons, we recommend completing practice questions in an online setting that simulates the real MCAT interface, and using the analytics provided to help you decide how to best move your studies forward.

CARS does not require knowledge of specific subject areas, but it does require development of strong test-taking skills. To ensure you are honing those skills as you work through this book, we suggest you go online after wrapping up each chapter and generate a Qbank Practice Set of 2-3 CARS passages to practice and review. While not every chapter of this book is directly applicable to CARS, regular CARS practice is key to test day success.

As a further supplement, given the importance of active learning for effective studying, we also suggest that you consult the Must-Knows at the end of each chapter of this Reasoning text as a basis for creating a study sheet. This is not a sheet to memorize in the more traditional sense of content memorization, but rather a quick reference of the most important strategies for you to refer to during and after practice in your early prep. Frequently revisiting the most important strategies for the MCAT - in both CARS and the Sciences - will help you continue to improve your performance.

This page left intentionally blank.

Analyzing Figures

0. Introduction

Peer-reviewed scientific articles are at the heart of how scientists convey information about new discoveries, and they often display important information presented in the figures. This is why analyzing and interpreting figures, taken directly from primary research articles, is a major part of the MCAT. Although this can be a hurdle in studying for the test, the ability to effectively interpret scientific figures really *will* pay off down the road in your career in medicine.

In this chapter, we'll alternate between discussing specific techniques for analyzing figures (in Sections 1, 3, and 5) and putting them into practice through breaking down sample passages (in Sections 2, 4, and 6).

1. Analyzing Figures: Foundational Techniques

For our purposes, **figures** are kind of a double-edged sword. The good news is that the figure, along with whatever wording may introduce it in the passage, *has* to contain all the information that you need, although you may also need to apply some content knowledge in order to understand what the figure communicates. The bad news is that the information we need from the figure might not be presented in the most obvious way. Our task as efficient passage-readers and figure-interpreters is to learn systematic ways of understanding what the figure or table is telling us. This is especially important for figures that present experimental findings.

The first question we need to ask when presented with experimental results is: what are the independent and dependent variables? As a brief reminder, **independent variables** are the parameters that are manipulated in an experiment, and **dependent variables** are the outcomes that are measured. Another way of framing this is that you need to figure out what the researchers are measuring, in response to changes in one or more parameters. In an experiment, researchers directly manipulate the independent variable, like in a study where several groups might receive different doses of a drug. When the independent variable cannot be randomly assigned, like age or gender, researchers use pre-existing variability in the independent variable to analyze some set of outcomes. This is known as a quasi-experiment. Whether a graph displays results from an experiment or quasi-experiment, the independent variables are almost always shown on the x-axis, and dependent variables on the y-axis.

For tables, there's not really a fixed guideline about which variables are presented where. It often depends on how many variables of each type exist, as well as the table's layout, so you have to cross-reference the table with the experimental procedure to understand which values correspond to certain experimental conditions, and which are the measured outcomes. At the end of the day, studying figure and table axes isn't a substitute for analyzing the experimental design from the passage to determine the independent and dependent variables. If you know what the researchers changed and what they measured before you even get to the figure, you'll be in good shape. However, taking time to analyze the axes can help you check whether you've fully understood the experimental setup, and potentially alert you to any misunderstandings that might have crept in. Therefore, it's still good practice.

In an ideal world, figures would always be labeled with clear descriptions of the relevant variables. But that's not always the case. After all, scientists love abbreviations, so your figure might have some unfamiliar-looking terms on the axes. However, the passage *must* explain to you somewhere what any nonstandard acronyms or abbreviations mean. First, look at the figure itself to see if the information you need is buried there, and then look at the figure caption. It's often the case that the caption will contain key information needed to decipher a figure. If that doesn't work, then turn to the passage. Look in particular at the paragraphs before and after a figure, which are likely to introduce the figure in some way, either directly or indirectly, by providing context for the experiment. This is one place where careful highlighting pays off. If you've highlighted new terms and acronyms in the passage, you'll rapidly be able to locate what you're looking for. If highlighting isn't your style, fortunately acronyms tend to stand out in a field of text when you're scanning the passage.

Often, though, technical terms like "the CD38 glycoprotein" or "the Annexin 5 protein" are used as proxy markers for some biological process, like T-cell activation or apoptosis. These molecules give us a convenient way to measure and quantify these processes in the lab.

That said, recognizing the different molecules and terms that make up a graph is half the battle. You also must identify the independent and dependent variables to understand the graph. Even if you don't usually stop to spell out your thinking, like explicitly saying in your head "the independent variable is X, and the dependent variable is Y," understanding this is a prerequisite for making any sense out of the figure whatsoever. Therefore, it's worth taking a second to make sure that you take the time to get this step right.

Here's a routine workflow that we suggest for analyzing a figure. First, read the caption. Some captions are more informative than others, but they all provide at least a sense of what the figure is trying to communicate in the context of the passage as a whole. With that in mind, your second step should be to read the axes of a figure, or the column and row legends of a table. Compare these to what you know about the experimental setup: what is it that the researchers are changing (the independent variables), and what outcomes are they measuring (the dependent variables)? This is how you determine what the figure is *actually* telling you. Your third step is to note the units. Understanding the units can be especially important for questions that ask you to apply the information contained in the figure, and taking a moment to do a quick unit check can also help you verify whether you've properly understood the axis labels. Plus, making incorrect assumptions about the units in a figure is an *incredibly* common source of errors. Fnally, you're ready to jump into the figure or table itself and make it tell a story.

"Make it tell a story" might sound a little strange to you, but we mean this very seriously. Even if scientists don't call journal club "story time," an expert-level ability to read the scientific literature involves developing the skill of converting an intimidating-looking or abstruse figure into a summary of what it's telling the reader. Doing so allows us to take a complicated-looking figure, and make a one- or two-sentence summary about what's significant or meaningful about it. This ability to make a figure tell a story is the key to answering questions about experimental design or statistical reasoning based on a figure.

This is a skill that you build with practice. With that in mind, we recommend making it part of your routine when reviewing practice materials to take time to thoroughly analyze entire passages and all their figures, especially unclear or difficult figures. Without the stress of the clock, how would you summarize the figures? How do they fit into what the passage presents in the text? Most crucially, what in the figure actually gives you the information you need? The more you carefully analyze figures in passages in a stress-free setting, the more you'll build up your mental muscles to interpret figures quickly and effectively under test-like conditions.

There are also some tips that can help you tell a story based on a figure. Once you've understood the axes of a figure a helpful technique is to try to understand the default behavior of the system being investigated; what does the baseline look like before we start poking and prodding it with chemicals and other interventions? If any experimental conditions are labeled as controls, those are a great place to start. You can then explore how changing various parameters yields changes in the dependent variable, and relate that to the information in the passage to build a picture of why these parameters matter. Even if there's not a control group, it may still be possible to identify something that approximates a baseline, normal, or default condition, and then go from there. If more than one independent variable is changed (for example, it may be that multiple substrates are removed from a culture medium, or multiple genes are silenced) then focus on one at a time, comparing its effects on the outcome measured to the control condition.

If you're feeling stuck, another approach is to work backwards, by first identifying any extreme values and seeing what conditions induce those extreme results, and contrasting them with conditions that yield more moderate outcomes. Fortunately, on the MCAT, typically the results presented will be fairly clear-cut: there won't be much of a gray area in determining which effects were meaningful or different from the control. Additionally, be on the lookout for any trends you can observe, like positive or negative correlations, and linear or nonlinear relationships between variables. We also need to synthesize that information and figure out what it means. For this, information from elsewhere in the passage can provide useful context.

Now, we're not entirely done with the topic of figure analysis. There are definitely more nuances and pitfalls to consider, as we'll explore later in this chapter. Nonetheless, the techniques we've presented here are really at the heart of figure analysis and interpretation for the MCAT, and even just developing this set of core techniques will help you avoid many incorrect answers designed to trap students who rush through figures, don't pay attention to units, or make hasty assumptions about what figures mean. Our next step will be to look at a practice passage and see how we can deploy these techniques to our advantage.

2. Practice Passage 1

Let's take a more concrete look at how to put the foundational techniques of figure analysis into practice, using the following passage:

Tetrodotoxin (TTX) is a potent sodium channel blocker that functions as a neurotoxin. It is present in several species of marine life, most notably pufferfish, and several incidents of TTX poisoning occur each year due to improper food preparation. However, three voltage-gated sodium channel isoforms in mammals are TTX-resistant: $Na_v1.5$, which is expressed in cardiac tissue, and $Na_v1.8$ and $Na_v1.9$, which are expressed in nociceptors.

In light of findings that some receptors may co-localize to lipid rafts, which potentially regulate the trafficking, clustering, and electrophysiological properties of ion channels, a study was conducted to determine whether $Na_v1.8$ is located in lipid rafts in dorsal root ganglion (DRG) neurons in a rat model.

Fluorescent immunohistochemistry was used to visualize Na$_v$1.8 channels at various locations along the axon of DRG neurons, as shown in Figure 1.

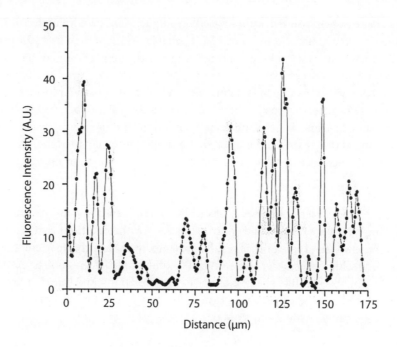

Figure 1. Clustering of Na$_v$1.8 along the axons of DRG neurons

Next, the co-localization of Na$_v$1.8 with flotillin-1 (a protein marker of lipid rafts), GM1 (a lipid marker of lipid rafts), and transferrin receptor (a marker of non-raft areas) was investigated by extracting membrane samples containing lipid rafts, centrifuging the samples on an iodixanol density gradient, and performing western blotting and dot-blot analysis of the resulting nine fractions.

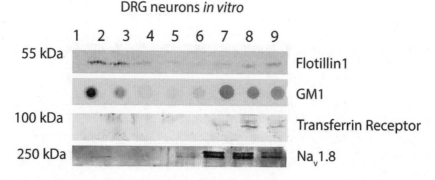

Figure 2. Co-localization of Na$_v$1.8 with lipid rafts in vitro

To investigate the impact of lipid raft destabilization on signal transmission via Na$_v$1.8, a fluorescent Ca^{2+} indicator, Fluo4, was used to measure the speed of signal transmission in response to mechanostimulation along the axons of four groups of DRG neurons: a control group (CTR), a cholesterol-treated group (CHOL), a group that received 7-ketocholesterol (7KC) treatment, and a group that was treated with methyl-β-cyclodextrin (MβCD). 7KC is a cholesterol analogue that has negative effects on lipid raft stability, and MβCD depletes cholesterol from the cell membrane.

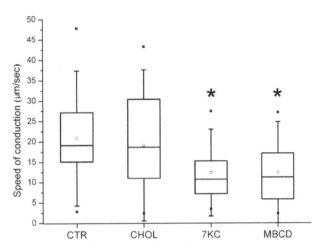

Figure 3. Speed of propagation of Fluo4-tagged signals in response to mechanostimulation. *: p<0.05 vs. CTR.

The first paragraph is largely background information. The information that TTX is a sodium channel blocker could serve as a pretext for a question to ask about the effects of this kind of neurotoxin, or about ion channels in general, but beyond that, our main takeaways are that TTX exists, that some voltage-gated sodium channels are resistant to it, and that these channels are referred to using the abbreviation Na_v followed by a number between one and two.

Things get a bit more interesting in the second paragraph. We're told that lipid rafts may play a role in the function of ion channels, and that researchers were interested in determining whether $Na_v1.8$ is co-located with lipid rafts in a rat model. Now we've got a research question to investigate! A quick skim of the passage indicates that it contains three figures, so hopefully they'll all work together to answer that question. Finally, the last sentence of the second paragraph tells us that $Na_v1.8$ channels were visualized using fluorescent immunohistochemistry at various points along the axon. Familiarity with immunohistochemistry can't hurt, but we're also told what the point of this experiment was, so we can interpret the figure even if we're not immunohistochemistry wizards.

Now, let's look at the figure itself, and work systematically. That means not getting distracted by all the peaks in the graph until we've laid the groundwork for understanding what the graph means. The figure caption builds slightly on the description in the previous paragraph by specifying that this figure illustrates the clustering of $Na_v1.8$ along the axon. Now let's take a look at the axes. On the x-axis, we see distance, and on the y-axis, we see fluorescence intensity. What's going on here is that distance along the axon body is the independent variable, and the researchers are trying to figure out how this fluorescence intensity changes as a function of location along the axon.

We now have a non-obvious question: what does fluorescence intensity mean? We're not given many details about the fluorescent immunohistochemistry procedure, but we should be able to infer that immunohistochemistry is a way to selectively identify compounds or biological structures of interest using antibodies, and one way to visualize the compounds of interest is by conjugating the antibodies with a fluorescent marker. Therefore, fluorescence signals indicate the presence of $Na_v1.8$ channels. Even if we're fuzzy on the details, the figure caption and description at the end of paragraph two help provide context by explaining that this procedure was done to localize these $Na_v1.8$ channels. Therefore, the dependent variable should tell us something about the location of $Na_v1.8$ channels. We can make a reasonable inference that the intensity of the fluorescence signals corresponds to the presence of these channels.

Next, let's look at the units. Distance is measured in micrometers. Pretty straightforward, but worth making a note of so that we can use the appropriate conversions if a question asks us to do some calculations involving distance. Fluorescence intensity is measured in AU, which stands for absorbance units. Again, even if you're shaky on that, context indicates that AU must be some measure of intensity. So, how does this information help us answer the question that the researchers are trying to answer? Like we said, fluorescence intensity must be an indicator of whether $Na_v1.8$ channels are present. We can assume that greater intensity corresponds to a greater density of these receptors, although we should steer clear of oversimplifications like the idea that a y-axis value of 20 means that there are 20 of these channels in a given place.

Now we can meaningfully interpret this graph. The fluorescence intensity jumps up and down, seemingly at random, as we move down the x-axis. We can conclude based on this that the $Na_v1.8$ channels aren't distributed smoothly or continuously along the axon. Instead, as the figure caption suggests, they appear to be clustered in various locations. This figure doesn't tell us anything about *which* locations these channels cluster in, or why, although based on the context provided in paragraph two, we might be wondering if this clustering has anything to do with lipid rafts. Centering our interpretation on the experimental hypothesis, and the questions posed by the researchers, is sure to make our analysis more effective, and help us connect the dots between multiple, related figures, as we'll see next.

And indeed, the next paragraph returns to this theme of lipid raft localization. Paragraph three is actually a single sentence, but it's a long and dense one, so let's break it down. We're told that the researchers were interested in investigating whether $Na_v1.8$ channels are co-localized with two markers of lipid rafts—one of proteins and one of lipids—or with a marker of non-lipid-raft areas. It sounds like this sub-experiment will give us a more direct answer about whether the clustering we observed in Figure 1 occurred because $Na_v1.8$ channels are embedded within lipid rafts. We're also given some details about *how* this sub-experiment was done, but we don't really have to agonize over the details. Basically, we're going to get nine sub-samples, and blotting was used to identify the molecules of interest.

Moving to the figure itself, the caption doesn't really add much to what we already figured out based on the passage text. But it's still always worth checking, as sometimes the figure caption can be informative. Now, let's look at the figure itself. Though presented as a figure, it has a tabular organization of rows and columns. The columns are labeled 1 to 9, which may seem puzzling, but the previous paragraph indicates that these correspond to the nine fractions that were obtained by density-gradient centrifugation. That's literally all we know about these nine samples, so if we need to know anything else about them, we should be able to derive that information from the figure or from any of the remaining passage text. The right-hand side of this figure tells us that these rows correspond to flotillin-1, GM1, transferrin receptor, and $Na_v1.8$, moving from top to bottom, and the left-hand side gives us some kind of protein ladder indicating the relative size of these components in kilodaltons. The independent variable here is the density-based fraction—that is, locations 1 to 9—and the dependent variable is whether a given protein is visualized using blotting.

Let's make this figure tell a story. Paragraph three tells us that the point of this sub-experiment is to investigate co-localization. That's confirmed by the figure caption, so let's look for co-localization. Remember, we're not all that interested in flotillin-1, GM1, or the transferrin receptor in isolation. What we're interested in is flotillin-1 and GM1 as markers of lipid rafts, and transferrin as a marker of non-raft areas. First off, let's define the fractions containing lipid rafts, and the fractions containing non-raft areas. The lipid raft markers flotillin-1 and GM1 are enriched in fractions 2, 3, and 4, and flotillin-1 is also enriched in fractions 8 and 9, whereas the transferrin receptor appears in fractions 8 and 9. Thus, we can conclude that fractions 2, 3, and 4 are a clearly lipid raft portion, and fractions 8 and 9 likely contain non-raft portions of the membrane, or perhaps a mixture of lipid raft and non-lipid-raft structures.

Here, we can see that $Na_v1.8$ tends to show up in fractions 2 and 3, the same density fractions as lipid raft markers flotillin1 and GM1. Thus, Figure 2 provides support for the idea that $Na_v1.8$ channels are located within lipid rafts.

Next, let's move to paragraph four, which should set us up for Figure 3. We're again told that the purpose of this next sub-experiment is that the researchers want to see whether disrupting lipid rafts will affect the degree to which $Na_v1.8$ channels can transmit signals. We see that there are four experimental conditions. The control group should show us the baseline behavior. The effects of the cholesterol treatment might not be obvious, but we know that lipid rafts are rich in cholesterol molecules, so it would be reasonable to infer that this treatment will promote the stability of lipid rafts, or enrich the membrane in lipid rafts. We're then told that 7KC has negative effects on lipid raft stability, and that MβCD depletes cholesterol from the cell membrane. Again, since lipid rafts are rich in cholesterol, we might guess that MβCD treatment isn't great for lipid raft stability. Essentially we have a baseline condition, a pro-lipid raft condition, and two anti-raft conditions.

Let's look at the figure. The figure caption re-emphasizes that the graph illustrates the propagation speed of signals, as visualized through Fluo4 tagging. We're also told that the asterisk indicates statistically significant differences versus the control group. Therefore, we rely on those indicators to determine which of these effects are meaningful, rather than leaving it up to our own impressions. Now let's move to the axes. The x-axis contains four labels, one for each of the experimental groups that we already discussed. However, if you skimmed over the descriptions of 7KC and MβCD while reading paragraph four, this should be your signal that yes, you really do have to understand what's going on with these groups. The y-axis is pretty straightforward: conduction speed, with units of micrometers per second. So, the experimental groups are our independent variable, and conduction velocity is our dependent variable.

What story does Figure 3 tell us? The 7KC and MβCD groups show decreased conduction speed compared to the control group and the cholesterol-treated group. Integrating this with what we figured out and discussed earlier about the impacts of 7KC and MβCD, we can conclude that destabilizing lipid rafts interferes with the ability of $Na_v1.8$ channels to transmit signals promptly. That's kind of like a double negative: if we *interfere* with lipid raft stability, and that *inhibits* signal propagation, that must mean that lipid rafts are essential or at least important to $Na_v1.8$ signal propagation. In any case, these findings suggest both that $Na_v1.8$ channels are co-located with lipid rafts and that lipid rafts make some contribution to the optimal function of $Na_v1.8$ channels. Circling back to the question that researchers asked at the beginning of the passage: are these TTX-resistant channels embedded in lipid rafts? The answer seems to be "yes," and it also seems that lipid rafts contribute to their proper function.

Before we pat ourselves on the back, congratulate ourselves on a well-analyzed passage, and move on, there's one important general point to make. Did you notice how working through the initial steps of figure analysis was slow and systematic, but then once we did the preparatory work of reading the figure caption and axes, identifying the independent and dependent variables, and noting the units, the puzzle pieces just fell into place? The figures in MCAT passages aren't tricky puzzles that were put there to torture you. Instead, their goal is to transmit information, in a condensed and concise way. One mistake students often make is to rush into a figure and try to pick out the major trends first, and only then retroactively trying to figure out what the various experimental conditions are, and how the figure fits into the bigger questions posed by the researchers. Putting in the upfront investment of time and energy into systematically working through what the figure is trying to say is the key that unlocks the treasure box of information contained in the figure. If you're going to do all the work of interpreting a figure, you might as well start with the basics and build up from there in a logical progression. Doing this consistently will both help you avoid test-taking panic and help you interpret figures accurately every time.

Doing all of this *while* maintaining appropriate pacing may seem challenging. However, as you practice, the basics will become more automatic. Although the variety of possible scientific figures may seem near-infinite, the reality is that there's a finite number of ways that figures can be set up, and the scientific process has an inherent logic to it. So it will get easier, and quicker, with careful practice. In the meantime, if you're pressed for time and encounter an extremely bewildering figure, it can be OK to take a pass on interpreting it, and then come back to it if a question asks about it. However, be sure at least to read and make note of the figure caption. That way, even if you don't have the time to work through the details of what a figure is showing, at least you know what it's about in general terms, so you can efficiently return to it if needed. Regardless, though, don't forget that figure analysis isn't magic—it's a skill, and like any other skill, practice makes perfect!

3. Figure Types

A major distinction exists between tables and graphs, which affects how you'll approach them. Since **tables** often present numerical data, you have to be more active to visualize the relationships between different variables. You might even find yourself imagining what a line graph or a bar graph would look like based on the table. Another tricky aspect is that there's not a single consistent convention for which variables are arranged in columns and which are arranged in rows. As a result, you can't take shortcuts with tables. You have to take the time to figure out what the labels for each column and row mean in the context of the passage, and assign independent and dependent variables as appropriate. This means looking for definitions of any abbreviations or technical terms, noticing the units, and understanding how those variables fit into the questions the researchers are investigating.

With graphs, you'll most often encounter line graphs and bar graphs, although pie charts are also possible. One thing worth noticing here is that there's a link between the kind of graph used and whether a variable is continuous or categorical. A **continuous variable** is a variable that you can measure on a spectrum. For example, height is a continuous variable. Some people are 70 inches tall, some are 69 inches tall, some are 71 inches tall. A **categorical variable** has discrete categories or groups that data can fall into. Examples of this include blood type, or states in the U.S., or dog breed. To take height, we could transform height into a categorical variable by deciding that people with a height over 72 inches are "tall," those with a height under 60 inches are "short," and those in between are, well, in between.

Line graphs are used for continuous variables, as the shape of the line makes it easier to visualize how the dependent variable, on the y-axis, changes as you increase or decrease the value of the independent variable shown on the x-axis. In contrast, **bar graphs** and **pie charts** are usually used to illustrate categorical variables. The principal difference between bar graphs and pie charts is that bar graphs show absolute values of some dependent variable, while pie charts are specialized for showing the distribution of categories in terms of percentage of the whole. If you're reading a passage that describes multiple distinct experimental groups, expect a bar graph. If you're reading about how researchers were trying to figure out how a certain outcome variable changes in response to variation in a continuous parameter, like time, expect a line graph. If researchers administered a survey to determine the percentage of respondents that fit certain criteria, then you might see a pie chart.

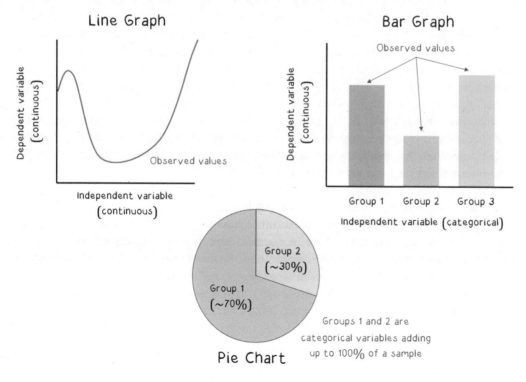

Figure 1. Line graphs, bar graphs, and pie charts

However, graphs don't always fit our expectations of a single variable on the x-axis, a single variable on the y-axis, and a linear scaling of units. More **complicated graphs** can be a source of confusion, so it's worth taking time to focus on some common ways that line graphs can be made more complex. One way is to have **multiple lines or curves** shown, or **clustered bar columns**. More often than not, these correspond to different experimental groups, or different independent variables, so be sure to pay attention to the visual cues, like dotted versus solid lines, or shaded versus unshaded bars, that are used to indicate various groups. Furthermore, focus on just one independent variable at a time. If a clustered bar graph shows the effects of both morning beverage and sleep debt on MCAT score, first just evaluate the effect of morning beverage, and then evaluate the effect of sleep debt. When you answer a question based on this graph type, be sure to double-check that you're answering based on the correct line or curve.

Another way that scientists compress more information into a line graph is to layer **multiple axes**. In particular, you might see a situation where there are two y-axes, one on the left and one on the right. These charts are used to compare two sets of trends, or similar outcome measures that have different scales, or relative versus absolute values of a parameter. The key for these graphs is to use the correct y-axis when answering a question. Often, such charts will have multiple lines or curves, in which case some form of coding, usually based on color or shape, will be used to indicate which y-axis corresponds to which data set. This type of chart organization is not common on the MCAT, but it can occur. If you do encounter one, you're almost guaranteed to run into a question where the trap answers involve making the wrong choice about which y-axis to use. The take-away point is to be careful when analyzing a graph like this, and to double-check your work. As always, all the information that you need will be on the graph, but it might just be a little bit more difficult to disentangle.

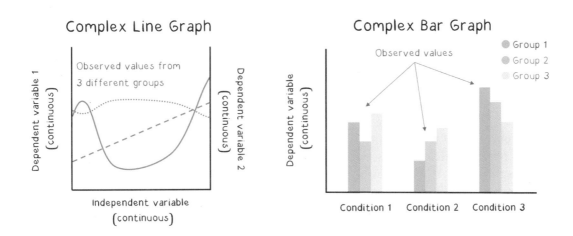

Figure 2. Complex line and bar graphs

Another complication can occur when the axes are based on **logarithmic scales**. Log-log plots, where both the x- and y-axes are log-transformed, and semi-log plots, where just one axis is log-transformed, are useful ways of visualizing nonlinear relationships. Recall that a linear equation has the form $y = mx + b$. In other words, in a linear relationship, y is proportional to x, the slope of the line is indicated by m, and the y-intercept is shown by b. In a nonlinear, power-law relationship, y is proportional to x to some other power. Let's say that $y = mx^k$. If k = 2, and we graphed this directly, we'd get a familiar parabolic curve. Anyway, though, let's see what happens if we take the logarithm of both sides of this equation: $\log(y) = \log(mx^k)$. We can simplify the expression on the right to $\log(m) + k\cdot\log(x)$, so $\log(y) = \log(m) + k\cdot\log(x)$. This is now an equation for a linear graph on logarithmic axes! So if we plot it along logarithmic axes, we'll get this nice-looking line, and its slope will be k, or the exponent that x was raised to.

Log-log graphs like this are often used to visualize power law relationships because they make it easier to visualize and extrapolate the relationship.

Let's switch this up a bit, and consider a relationship where y is proportional to 10^x, or even let's say x multiplied by some constant. Such an equation could be something random-looking like $y = 2.7 \times 10^{0.25x}$. We can use a more general form of these equations: $y = k \times 10^{mx}$. If we take the logarithm of each side, we basically get rid of the 10, so using the logarithm rules, we get $\log(y) = \log(k) + mx$, or $\log(y) = mx + \log(k)$. Again, we can use this to form a nice-looking linear graph using one logarithmic and one non-logarithmic axis, where the slope winds up being equal to the value used to multiply x in the original exponential relationship. Note here, though, that there's only a log on one side of the equation. This is a **semi-log**, or a log-lin plot.

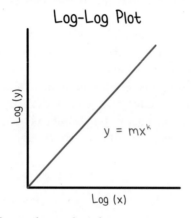 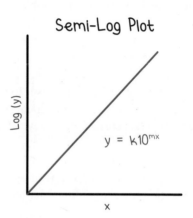

Figure 3. Log-log and semi-log plots

Now, if this discussion is inducing math anxiety in you, don't panic! To summarize:

> A linear-looking graph on a log-log plot is actually a power-law relationship, like $y = x^2$.
> A linear-looking graph on a semi-log plot is an exponential relationship, like $y = 10^x$.

More broadly, logarithms are a way to visually smooth out huge quantitative variations in magnitude. With something that ranges from values of 1, or 10^0, to 10^{12} (that is, *trillion*fold variation) we can use logarithms to view that range on a scale of 1 to 12. Therefore, if you see an axis labeled as the log of something, understand that the log-transformation masks huge variation in the values, and that you therefore need to be careful to take that into account if you do math using those numbers. The most common mistake that students make with log plots on the MCAT is simply failing to notice that an axis is log-transformed! That's a relatively straightforward pitfall to avoid, and you don't need expertise on how log plots are *derived* in order to be able to apply simple processes of exponentiation and logarithmic transformation to convert to and from log values if needed.

You should also be on the lookout for specialized types of graphs that are studied in relation to specific content areas. Some examples include Michaelis-Menten and Lineweaver-Burk graphs for enzymes, or hemoglobin-oxygen binding curves. On one hand, the general principles of analyzing graphs certainly still apply here, and it can't hurt to identify independent and dependent variables, pay attention to units, and so on. On the other hand, these are specific enough topics that you should also study them in the context of the corresponding content areas.

Last but not least, chemical structures, equations, and reaction diagrams are an important subset of figures that often cause confusion. In our experience, an important aspect of these figures is recognizing that they usually contain WAY more information than you actually need. This is a double-edged sword. On one hand, a consequence is that you shouldn't be intimidated by a frightening-looking organic reaction diagram, the kind of thing that nightmares are made of in o-chem classes, because many of the details are likely to be irrelevant. On the other hand, though, it's important to cultivate the skill of trying to pick out the subset of information that *is* relevant. For chemical structures, that might include noticing important functional groups. For chemical equations, that could mean paying attention to things like any accompanying ΔG values or important products. For organic reaction diagrams, that means comparing reactants to products to figure out what's changed, as well as noticing any important-looking reagents or side processes.

Most importantly, derive the information you need to make sense of the passage. If the passage spends a lot of time talking about a complicated series of steps in some reaction scheme, it can be helpful to corroborate that with a visual depiction of the reaction mechanism if provided. For chemistry-related figures, it's especially helpful to link the diagram with the text in the passage itself, because the passage will likely contain clues about what parts of the diagram matter. In other words, the passage helps you make an informed choice about what to focus on, as you don't have infinite time or mental energy. This applies to all figures. They're not independent of the passage, and you should try to avoid rushing in a way that causes you to *only* look at a figure or table in the absence of context. As always, remember that the passage *has* to give you all the information that you need to decipher a figure or table, in combination with standard background content knowledge. Therefore, try not to let a confusing-looking figure or table rattle you and induce you to pick an answer choice based on shaky reasoning. Instead, stay cool, stay systematic, and consult the figure legend, figure caption, *and* the passage text as needed in order to demystify the figure.

4. Practice Passage 2

Let's put some of the figure analysis skills into practice by working through a passage that requires skillful analysis of multiple figure types. As passage context is always helpful for getting the most out of figures, we'll analyze both the passage text and the figures, but with a special focus on figure interpretation.

The aldol condensation reaction is widely used in industry as a tool for forming C–C bonds. In these reactions, C–C bond formation proceeds via condensation between a molecule containing a carbonyl group and another molecule containing an activated methylene group. Aldol condensations involve reactions forming β-hydroxy aldehydes (β-aldol) or β-hydroxy ketones (β-ketol), either by self-condensation or mixed condensation of aldehydes and ketones. Then, via the dehydration of the intermediate β-aldol or β-ketol, α,β-unsaturated aldehydes or α,β-unsaturated ketones are formed.

However, a concern in applying aldol condensation reactions for industrial purposes is that side reactions are common, potentially yielding multiple outputs in addition to the desired product. Furthermore, it is easier to hydrogenate α,β-unsaturated carbonyls into saturated carbonyls than into unsaturated alcohols, as thermodynamics favor the hydrogenation of C=C bonds over C=O bonds. Figure 1 shows possible pathways for reactions involving methyl ethyl ketone (MEK), under basic and acidic conditions and with metal catalysts.

Figure 1. Reaction pathways for methyl ethyl ketone (MEK). MVK: methyl vinyl ketone

Researchers developed a novel 15% Cu–ZrO$_2$ catalyst with the goal of synthesizing 5-methyl-3-heptanone from MEK and tested it at various temperatures. The results are shown in Figure 2.

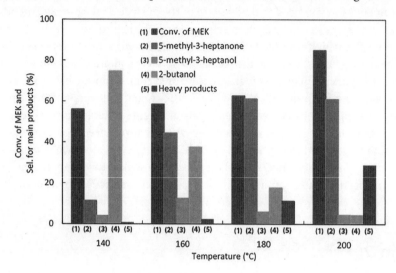

Figure 2. Conversion of MEK at various temperatures using 15% Cu–ZrO$_2$ catalyst and an H$_2$/MEK molar ratio of 2. Heavy products: those with 12+ carbon chains

A follow-up experiment investigated how varying the H$_2$/MEK molar ratio at a constant temperature (180°C) would affect the distribution of products, as shown below in Figure 3.

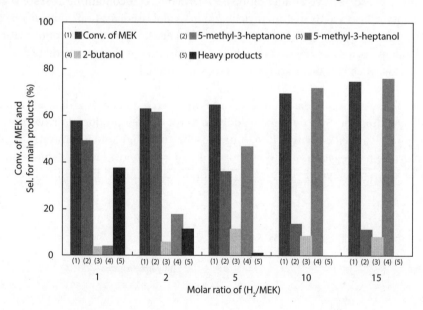

Figure 3. Conversion of MEK using a 15% Cu–ZrO$_2$ catalyst at 180°C with various H$_2$/MEK molar ratios. Heavy products: those with 12+ carbon chains

The Cu–ZrO$_2$ catalyst was also compared to similar catalysts with other metals, and it was found that at 180°C and an H$_2$/MEK molar ratio of 2, Ni–ZrO$_2$ showed similar efficacy and selectivity for 5-methyl-3-heptanone, despite showing a lower H$_2$ uptake rate.

The first paragraph of this passage is on the long side, but it's fairly informational. Though the passage on the aldol reaction may be the stuff of nightmares, we should stay calm and see whether the passage provides information that can help refresh our memory. It does remind us that the aldol reaction first results in a condensed molecule containing both a carbonyl group and a hydroxyl group on the β carbon, which is located two carbons away from the carbonyl carbon. Then, a dehydration step removes that hydroxyl group, yielding an α,β-unsaturated aldehyde or ketone. If these terms don't immediately click, see if any of these structures are illustrated in Figure 1. Indeed they are.

Moving onto the second paragraph, we learn that side reactions are a concern in industrial applications, and that unsaturated alcohols are apparently difficult to form, because it's easier to hydrogenate, or reduce, the C=C bond than the C=O bond. It's worth making note of this, especially because the term "thermodynamic" is used, which may be a link to important testable content. Then we get an introduction to Figure 1, stating that Figure 1 shows us various things that can happen to methyl ethyl ketone, or MEK.

This figure seems like a doozy, as it contains eight chemical structures and six reaction arrows. Where should we start here? Remember that understanding the context of the passage is the best way to approach complicated chemical diagrams, because the passage tells us what's important. The previous paragraph mentioned that side products are a concern with aldol reactions, so let's approach the figure through that lens. The paragraph and the figure caption both tell us that this figure is all about what happens to MEK, so let's find MEK up in the top left and go from there. Well, there are three things that can happen to MEK. One of them is labeled "aldol reaction," so that's obviously the aldol reaction, which also has the bonus of giving us a quick refresher of what this reaction looks like. The other options seem to involve adding or losing H_2, and result in four-carbon molecules: either 2-butanol or MVK. The figure caption tells us that MVK is methyl vinyl ketone. The paths that yield four-carbon molecules seem like dead ends. So these are presumably side reactions that MEK can undergo instead of the aldol reaction.

Let's pick up the thread of the aldol reaction, then. We get a product labeled "β-hydroxy ketone," like what was discussed in the first paragraph. Depending on our comfort with organic chemistry, this is a great time to remind ourselves of what that means structurally. We see the ketone structure with the carbonyl carbon on the right, and then on the β-carbon—two carbons down the chain—we see a hydroxyl group. We now follow the downward arrow, and see that a dehydration reaction takes place under acidic conditions. That is, we lose the –OH group and form a double bond between the β carbon and the carbon that is in between the beta carbon and the carbonyl carbon— the α carbon. This is an α,β-unsaturated ketone: ketone because we have a carbonyl carbon flanked by other carbons, and α,β-unsaturated because we have a double bond between the α carbon and the β carbon, so this bond is *less* saturated with hydrogens than before. Now, as we move from left to right along the bottom of the figure, we see what happens if we hydrogenate this product in the presence of a metal catalyst. The first round of reduction gets rid of the carbon-carbon double bond, yielding 5-methyl-3-heptanone. The second step reduces the carbonyl carbon, yielding 5-methyl-3-heptanol. The fact that we first reduce the C=C bond corresponds to what paragraph two told us about the relative ease of forming saturated aldehydes or ketones compared to unsaturated alcohols.

Paragraph three is short. The passage tells us about a novel catalyst that the researchers wanted to test what happened at various temperatures, with the goal of obtaining 5-methyl-3-heptanone. This brings us to Figure 2, which is pretty busy. The figure caption reminds us that this is about the conversion of MEK at various temperatures. Now let's review the axes. The x-axis is labeled temperature in units of degrees Celsius. There are four different temperature groups in this bar graph, each of which contains five bars, labeled 1 through 5. This is a clustered bar graph! We might immediately see that groups 1 through 5 are defined in the figure legend, above the bars, but let's pause and look at the y-axis. Here we see that the y-axis is labeled "conversion of MEK and selection for main products," with units in percentages. Look at the figure legends to figure out what groups 1 through 5 are. Group 1 is the conversion of MEK (so this is presumably the percentage of MEK that gets turned into something else) and the other groups are various possible products.

As we have figured out the basics of the graph, let's try to make it tell a story. There are 20 different bars, which is a lot to visually make sense of. Let's tease apart the two variables—temperature and products formed—and evaluate the effect of temperature on each product individually. Let's pick each of the groups, 1 through 5, one at a time, and mentally sketch curves of what happens as we increase the temperature. If we start with (1), conversion of MEK, we can see that it increases as temperature increases, first gradually, and then sharply at 200°C. So the hotter it gets, the more MEK reacts. What about (2), 5-methyl-3-heptanone? This is probably worth investigating, because paragraph three did tell us that this is what the researchers wanted to synthesize, and Figure 1 shows us that it corresponds to the aldol reaction. Likewise, we can observe that the yield of 5-methyl-4-heptanone increases sharply between 140°C and 180°C, and then levels off around 60%. Group (3) looks like a pretty minor product throughout, and the passage doesn't really talk about 5-methyl heptanol anyway, so let's not invest any more mental energy there. Group (4), 2-butanol, starts off high, and then plunges as we increase the temperature. Finally, heavy products (which the figure caption tells us are 12+ carbon compounds) increase in number as temperature increases, but they still remain a minor product. So, summarizing, the main point here is that temperature makes a major difference in terms of whether MEK undergoes the aldol reaction, which we see more often at higher temperatures, or whether MEK just gets turned into 2-butanol instead, which predominates at lower temperatures.

Paragraph four introduces a figure. We're told that now the researchers tried varying the H_2/MEK molar ratio to see what would happen. Let's pause for a second to make sure we understand what this means. A higher H_2/MEK molar ratio means a relatively hydrogen-rich environment, and vice versa. So this is an investigation of whether making more hydrogen available affects the choice of reaction pathway.

So now we see Figure 3, which is also pretty busy. But lucky for us, it has the same basic setup as Figure 2. The x-axis is different, because we're investigating different H_2/MEK molar ratios, but otherwise, the organization of the figure is the same. So the legwork we did with the previous figure will pay off here too, and we can jump right into trying to tell a story, using our same strategy of disentangling the two variables by examining the effect of temperature on groups (1) through (5) in order. Group (1) is the overall conversion of MEK, which seems to increase fairly steadily as hydrogen availability increases. Group (2), 5-methyl-3-heptanone, is the product of the aldol reaction. The yield of (2) jumps up as we move from a molar ratio of 1 to 2, and then crashes as we increase the molar ratio further. This seems to suggest that MEK likes to undergo the aldol reaction in lower-hydrogen environments, but not in higher-hydrogen environments. As in Figure 2, group (3) looks like it's just some minor side reactions, so let's skip it, but if a question asks about 5-methyl-3-heptanol, we know where to go. For group (4), though, 2-butanol, we see the opposite pattern—at low hydrogen molar ratios, barely any MEK gets converted to 2-butanol, but at higher ratios, 2-butanol comprises the vast majority of products from MEK. Apparently 2-butanol *loves* hydrogen. Now, finally, let's take a look at these heavy products. They only occur with relatively low hydrogen/MEK ratios, and drop off to basically nothing by the time we hit a molar ratio of 5. So, looking at this from the point of view of the passage as a whole, which is concerned with pathways competing with the aldol reaction, it appears that the aldol reaction is favored in environments with some hydrogen, and that as we increase the amount of hydrogen, the butanol-producing side reaction becomes predominant.

Finally, the last paragraph contains a little bit more information about how a similar-looking catalyst, Ni–ZrO$_2$, showed similar results. This is a random factoid, but we make a quick note of it in case a question brings up zirconium or the choice of a different catalyst.

Now, let's take stock of what we've done here. We've made our way through a dense-looking passage with some very busy figures, but we managed to distill a coherent story out of it. Namely, chemists want to figure out ways to favor the aldol reaction, instead of side reactions. At least with this experimental setup, the aldol reaction was favored by high temperatures and relatively low availability of hydrogen, while the side reaction producing butanol was favored by lower temperatures and a hydrogen-rich environment. Having done this, we now have a coherent picture in our minds we can use to start answering questions, and a good jumping-off point for thinking about deeper questions, like what these findings might imply about the mechanisms and thermodynamics of these reactions.

As always, we should emphasize that we didn't reach these conclusions by magic. Instead, we carefully read the figures and invested the effort in understanding how each figure was designed, and, most crucially, how each figure was related to the context established by the passage. In other words, the passage text basically told us what was important, and what we needed to focus on, and then we found the important details in the figures. This is a pattern you'll see again and again in MCAT materials, so keep this example passage in mind as you move forward, as an illustration of how systematic, text-rooted analyses can help make sense of even very dense-looking figures!

5. Statistical Significance and Figure Analysis

Statistical significance is a major aspect of how experimental findings are presented on the MCAT in figures and tables. Fortunately, though, there's a simple rule that will allow you to succeed in the vast majority of cases:

> If a figure or table on the MCAT presents statistical significance, only statistically significant differences, which are indicated by a p-value less than 0.05, should be interpreted as "real" for the purposes of answering passage-based questions.

There. That's it. That rule *will* take care of the vast majority of circumstances that you run into on the MCAT. But we want to equip you with the expertise needed to handle anything you might run into.

The first part of that rule reads "***If a figure or table presents statistical significance...***" This implies two things: first, that we have to be able to recognize how statistical significance is presented, and second, that some figures do present this information and others don't. As a starting point, we should familiarize ourselves with some common ways of indicating statistical significance. One of the most frequent ways of indicating statistical significance you'll encounter is an asterisk (*), multiple asterisks (** or ***), (†) a dagger, or the double-dagger (‡). These marks can show up in tables, and figures, where they frequently occur together with a bar or some other indication of which pieces of data are being compared. Different symbols indicate different levels of statistical significance. For example, a single asterisk might indicate p-values less than 0.05, two asterisks might mean that p is less than 0.01, three asterisks might mean that p is less than 0.001, and so on. While these are common strategies, the passage writers *have to* indicate statistical significance somehow, and they have to describe what the symbols mean.

Now, what about that idea that some figures present this information and others don't? To fully answer this, we need to take a somewhat deeper dive into what ***p*-values** mean. Some familiar tests used to calculate p-values include the chi-square test and the t-test, although others also exist. The most appropriate test is chosen based on the characteristics of the data. That said, the details really don't matter for our purposes. We can just assume that the researchers knew what they were doing. This, by the way, is a dangerous assumption in life, but it's OK for the MCAT.

In any case, though, a p-value refers to the probability that we observed the result we did, by chance, when in fact the null hypothesis is true, generally meaning that there's no real difference between the means. A p-value of 0.05, therefore, indicates that this probability would only be 5%, and that's commonly considered the threshold for statistical significance.

It is worth clarifying the definition of a **null hypothesis**. Sometimes people say that the null hypothesis is what we're trying to disprove. That can be helpful to some extent, but it also can be misleading. Here's another way of thinking about it. If we're doing an experiment, we want our results to be interesting, or to at least have the possibility interesting. "Interesting" only makes sense relative to some baseline or default assumption, and we can think of that default expectation as the null hypothesis.

The null hypothesis has to be defined in context. So, for example, say we're conducting an experiment on whether people prefer cookies or cupcakes, and find that of our sample of 1000 respondents, 990 prefer cupcakes. From the point of view that cookies and cupcakes are comparably tasty, that would be a highly surprising finding. However, from the point of view that cupcakes are obviously far superior to cookies, our discovery wouldn't be too surprising. We can translate these points of views into null hypotheses if we articulate our expectations more precisely. The point of view that cookies and cupcakes are comparably tasty might translate into a null hypothesis that the distribution of preferences for one over the other would be largely random. The latter point of view, that cupcakes are superior to cookies, might translate into a null hypothesis that the vast majority of people would prefer cupcakes. So, which null hypothesis is right? Well, both and neither. It's kind of a meaningless question. That said, in actual practice, it's far more common for null hypotheses to state that no difference is expected to exist between the groups being investigated, so calibrate your expectations accordingly.

A further fun fact about statistical practice in the real world is that researchers often don't state the null hypothesis explicitly. So you should be prepared to make appropriate inferences. For example, a statement like "$p<0.05$ versus control" could be spelled out as saying that "there is a less than 5% chance of observing these findings by chance based on the null hypothesis that there is no underlying difference between the control group and experimental group."

Of course, low-probability events *can* certainly occur. After all, *someone* wins the lottery every now and again, right? So a finding of $p<0.05$ doesn't exclude the possibility that an observed difference *was* due solely to chance. With that in mind, you might ask "What's so special about a p-value of 0.05?" Believe it or not, the answer is basically "why not?" In all seriousness, that threshold was just proposed as one of many possibilities, and it kind of took on a life of its own. As it happens, some fields, like experimental physics, where measurements are very precise, prefer lower p-values. Anyway, although it's good to be aware that such differences could still be due to chance, for our purposes, we can use 0.05 as a rule of thumb.

Now that we've established that a statistically significant difference is one that is highly unlikely to have occurred by chance given a certain null hypothesis—usually indicating no difference—let's talk about **misconceptions about statistical significance**. First off, statistical significance implies *nothing* about whether a finding is meaningful for anyone. One of the main reasons for this is **effect size**. Especially given a very large sample size, it's entirely possible for researchers to find a very real—and therefore statistically significant—but very small difference. A vivid example of this occurred when researchers announced with high certainty that processed red meat (e.g. bacon) is a carcinogen. Innumerable news articles rushed to point out that while that might be true, the amount it raises any one person's likelihood of developing colorectal cancer is quite small, so it doesn't necessarily make sense to make lifestyle changes based on this finding. In other words, scientists better not try to separate Americans from their bacon. That's the difference between statistical significance and effect size in a nutshell.

To tackle another misconception, statistical significance is also not the same thing as the standard deviation. The **standard deviation** of a dataset is a measure of the degree to which the data points are dispersed, and its cousin, the standard error of the mean, normalizes for the size of the population being sampled. On one hand, if there's an even distribution of values in the population, or what is technically called a "normal distribution," the finding that a measured value is one or two standard deviations above the mean does in some sense indicate that it's a relatively less probable observation. But on the other hand, we have to be careful, for a few reasons. First, a single standard deviation on each side of the mean contains only 68% of the population. We have to get up to *two* standard deviations to reach the threshold of 95% that we've used before for statistical significance. Second, measures of dispersal, like the standard deviation and standard error of the mean, don't explicitly refer to a null hypothesis, which—as we've discussed—is a key part of what statistical significance means. Third, we don't always know whether the values of some parameter are distributed evenly in the population. If, for instance, we have a situation where there's a bunch of very low values and a bunch of very high values, but nothing in between, the standard deviation isn't really helpful. Researchers have come up with many different ways of handling these issues, which go beyond our scope, but we're building up to a very practical point.

At the beginning of this discussion, we mentioned that not all figures show information about statistical significance. Instead, many figures use error bars to show standard deviations or standard errors of the mean, as a way of indicating the dispersal or clustering of the data. There's a very common misconception that non-overlapping error bars mean that a difference is statistically significant, and that overlapping error bars mean that a difference is not statistically significant. However, *this is not true.* Even if all the assumptions we need to stipulate hold true, like there being a normal distribution and so on, a ± 1 standard deviation range will still capture 68% of the population, which is not at all like the threshold of p being less than 0.05 that we use for statistical significance. That said, for the purposes of the MCAT, if a figure doesn't contain any indicator of statistical significance, we can use that rule of thumb about overlapping or non-overlapping standard deviations or error bars, in which non-overlapping results can be considered to reflect a "real" (at least for our purposes) difference. However, we need to be much more cautious about differences with overlapping standard deviations or error bars.

What if a figure presents you with just the data points, without any additional information like error bars or statistical significance? This can certainly happen, especially for experiments with very small sample sizes or for experimental results in lab-manual-type passages. Basically, in such situations, you need to use your judgment to identify trends in the data. However, the MCAT will structure any related questions to avoid situations where a difference might seem significant to one student, but not to another. They'll only ask you to make deductions within the bounds of what's generally considered reasonable, and there will always be a clear and objective explanation for why the correct answer choice is correct.

As a final note, don't forget that statistical significance, by itself, doesn't allow you to reach a conclusion one way or another about whether a **cause-and-effect** relationship exists between two variables. This can be the case because, as we discussed, random things *do* happen, so statistical significance doesn't rule out the possibility of an observed relationship just being an unlikely coincidence. It can also be because establishing a cause-and-effect relationship requires specific choices in terms of experimental design. In particular, statistical significance can be calculated for observed correlations. Never forget, though, that correlation does not equal causation! That is, just because two events cluster together, that doesn't mean that one causes the other. This is true even if the claims of correlation are bolstered with statistical significance.

So, let's end this discussion with the same rule of thumb that we presented at the beginning:

> If a figure or table on the MCAT presents statistical significance, only statistically significant differences, which are indicated by a p-value less than 0.05, should be interpreted as "real" for the purposes of answering passage-based questions.

That really *is* an excellent rule of thumb, but hopefully by now you have a better sense of some of the underlying issues and of some ways of approaching figures that might not fit your initial expectations.

6. Practice Passage 3

Let's put the points we discussed about statistical significance into practice by working through a passage with lots of figures and indicators of statistical significance. As always, we'll focus on both the text of the passages and the figures, because the text generally provides important clues for understanding the context of figures and how they relate to the questions that scientists are exploring.

> Lung squamous cell carcinoma (LSCC) is a subtype of lung cancer characterized by a poor therapeutic response, a high relapse rate, and poor prognosis. Forkhead box transcription factor A2 (FOXA2) regulates the expression of genes critical to lung morphogenesis, and may function as a suppressor of tumor metastasis in human lung cancers. Loss of FOXA2 expression is common in lung cancer cell lines, and squamous cell carcinomas are negative for FOXA2 staining.

Curcumin, a compound derived from the turmeric plant, has been suggested to show anti-cancer activity by inhibiting cell proliferation and metastasis, inducing apoptosis, and enhancing chemotherapeutic efficiency. An experiment investigated the effects of curcumin on cell proliferation and FOXA2 expression in the NCI-H292 line of human LSCC cells. First, cell proliferation was assessed in response to various doses of curcumin and incubation periods through optical density (OD) measurements using a cell counting kit, and apoptosis was quantified directly and through relative caspase-3/7 activity, as shown in Figure 1.

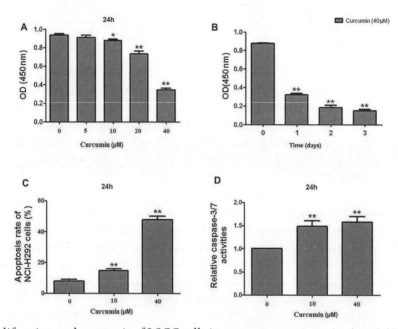

Figure 1. Proliferation and apoptosis of LSCC cells in response to curcumin. $*p < 0.05$, $**p < 0.01$

Next, an analysis was conducted of the effects of curcumin on FOXA2 expression over the course of 48 hours. FOXA2 expression was analyzed both by quantitative reverse-transcription PCR and by relative quantification of FOXA2 protein levels in comparison to β-actin as a control (Figure 2).

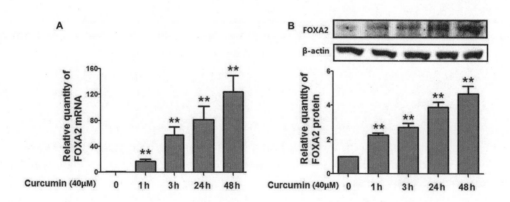

Figure 2. FOXA2 mRNA and protein expression after curcumin administration. $**p < 0.01$

To clarify whether curcumin-mediated changes in FOXA2 expression influenced proliferation and apoptosis, a knockdown experiment was conducted using control or FOXA2-specific small interfering RNA (siRNA).

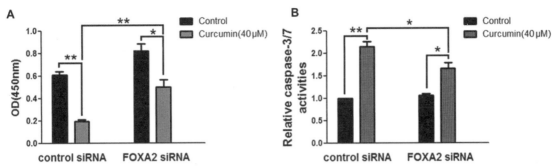

Figure 3. FOXA2 mediation of curcumin-induced effects on proliferation and apoptosis. *$p< 0.05$, **$p< 0.01$

Further investigation additionally revealed that curcumin downregulated signaling via STAT3, an upstream regulator of FOXA2. Furthermore, curcumin was found to upregulate SOCS1 and SOCS3, which are inhibitors of STAT3.

Adapted from Tang, L., Liu, J., Zhu, L., Chen, Q., Meng, Z., Sun, L., ... & Wang, X. (2018). Curcumin Inhibits Growth of Human NCI-H292 Lung Squamous Cell Carcinoma Cells by Increasing FOXA2 Expression. Frontiers in pharmacology, 9, 60 under CC-BY.

The first paragraph gives us some general information about LSCC, but more importantly for our purposes, introduces a transcription factor called FOXA2. We're told that FOXA2 helps prevent metastasis, and is often lost in cancer cells. This is mostly background information, but it should help calibrate our expectation for the idea that FOXA2 expression is basically "good"—at least in the context of cancer—and loss of FOXA2 is a sign of bad news.

The second paragraph pivots to curcumin, which apparently has shown various anti-cancer properties, and we're told that researchers investigated the effects of curcumin on cell proliferation and FOXA2 expression. Before we even see the results, we can integrate this information with what we were told in the first paragraph to anticipate that curcumin might be expected to reduce cell proliferation—which is part of how malignant cancers exert harmful effects—and either increase FOXA2 expression or promote stably high levels of FOXA2 expression. Next, we're given some information about what's in Figure 1, which we're told will contain information about proliferation and apoptosis.

Now let's take a closer look at Figure 1. The figure caption re-emphasizes that it shows information about the proliferation and apoptosis of LSCC cells. This figure contains four different graphs, so we need to know which is which. A great way of figuring this out is to look at the y-axes. One of them is labeled "apoptosis," which is clear. Two others are labeled OD at 450 nm, and the fourth shows relative caspase 3 and 7 activity. So, we need to figure out how these graphs correspond to the big-picture topics of proliferation and apoptosis. To do so, we can check the figure legend and caption, but that doesn't help, so we have to return to the previous paragraph. We're told that OD measurements were made to track proliferation, and that caspase 3/7 activity was a measure of apoptosis. So the top two graphs show cancer cells' proliferation in response to curcumin, and the bottom two graphs show two different measures of apoptosis. Cool! Now we've got somewhere to start.

Figure 1A shows that for a 24-hour incubation period, increasing doses of curcumin result in decreased cell proliferation, with statistical significance kicking in at 10 micromolar and even stronger statistical significance at higher doses. The figure doesn't specify what exactly these *p*-values are comparing, but based on context, we can infer that it's relative to 0 micromolar curcumin. Figure 1B then shows that for a constant—and high—dose of curcumin, we get decreased proliferation with longer exposure, again with statistical significance kicking in at around 1 day. Looking at the bottom two figures, we also see that curcumin causes increased apoptosis, starting at doses of 10 micromolar. Note that in Figure 1C, even though the apoptosis rate jumps up sharply when we go from 10 to 40 micromolar concentrations of curcumin, the indicator of statistical significance is the same as we see for 10 micromolar. So the effect size may be larger, but it's not necessarily more significant compared to the no-curcumin group, and we aren't given a p-value comparing the effects of 10 versus 40 micromolar curcumin, so we need to be cautious about concluding that more curcumin is necessarily better. Graphs like these that show the relationship between treatment dosage and outcome are called dose-response curves, and when the effect size appears to be trending in the up or down direction with increasing dose, generally this can be considered a dose-dependent relationship for the purposes of the MCAT.

In any case, though, Figure 1 seems to confirm the possibility that curcumin might exert anti-cancer effects. But we haven't heard anything about FOXA2 yet. Not surprisingly, that's where paragraph three comes in. This paragraph introduces a new sub-experiment analyzing FOXA2 mRNA and protein expression. We can briefly note the methods—PCR and some form of blotting—but the key point is that now we're measuring FOXA2.

So let's jump to Figure 2. We have two graphs. Let's look at the y-axes. Figure 2A contains information on mRNA expression, and Figure 2B presents data on protein expression, complete with actual pictures of blots to help show things more clearly. The x-axes show time points, and the figure legend indicates that we're dealing with a dose of 40 micromolar curcumin. Looking at the trends, we see a clear tendency for curcumin to increase FOXA2 expression, even starting at 1 hour. Again, although the changes become statistically significant starting at 1 hour, and the magnitude of the changes increases over time, we only get information about statistical significance versus the 0-hour condition. Therefore, we'd have to be careful, for instance, about concluding whether 24 hours of administration would be "enough" for some purpose or whether an additional 24 hours, pushing us to 48 hours in total, would help.

So, at this point, we have two useful pieces of information: curcumin favorably impacts proliferation and apoptosis in tumor cells, and it increases FOXA2 levels. But are these two observations causally linked? Paragraph four briefly introduces a new experiment that was conducted to clarify this point through a knockdown model involving anti-FOXA2 siRNA. As a refresher, siRNAs function by "silencing" other RNA expression pathways, so a cell treated with FOXA2 siRNA is essentially equivalent to a cell that no longer meaningfully expresses FOXA2 proteins. Turning to Figure 3, we see that the point of this figure is to present the degree to which FOXA2 mediates the effects of curcumin on proliferation and apoptosis. This lines up with what the paragraph tells us. However, the figure itself is very dense, so let's take a closer look.

As always, the first thing we should do with a figure is look at the axes to see more specifically what it's measuring. In this case, for both Figures 3A and 3B, the x-axes involve comparisons between a control group, marked in black, and a curcumin group, marked in gray, in a control siRNA group and a FOXA2 siRNA group. The y-axis for Figure 3A is marked OD (450 nm), which should remind us of what we saw in Figure 1—this is a proxy measure of proliferation. Likewise, as in Figure 1, caspase 3/7 expression is a marker of apoptosis. Looking first at Figure 3A, we can see that in both siRNA groups, curcumin reduced proliferation compared to control. This isn't surprising, since we saw the same thing in Figure 1. The question is whether curcumin had the same effect in both groups. This is where the various asterisks come in. Two out of the three sets of asterisks—on the left and right of Figure 3A—are placed above short lines that connect the two bars in each siRNA group. That means that these values for significance—$p<0.01$ on the left and $p<0.05$ on the right—are for the changes within each siRNA group that occurred in response to curcumin administration. The asterisks in the middle and on top are placed above lines that connect the two curcumin groups. This means that a very significant difference—$p<0.01$—exists between the two curcumin groups. The proliferation was higher in the curcumin group in the FOXA2 siRNA group than in the curcumin group in the control siRNA group. In other words, knocking down FOXA2 made curcumin *less* effective at inhibiting proliferation in these cells. This, in turn, implies that FOXA2 must play a role in mediating the anti-proliferative effects of curcumin.

Turning to Figure 3B, luckily, we don't have to start from scratch. The architecture of the figure is the same, it's just looking at apoptosis instead of proliferation. And indeed, we see a similar pattern. As in Figure 1, curcumin promotes apoptosis, but that top asterisk, associated with the line connecting the two curcumin groups, shows that it did so less effectively in the group where *FOXA2* was knocked down. This provides another piece of evidence suggesting that FOXA2 mediates the anti-cancer effects of curcumin. Of course, we should note that the effects of curcumin still do persist in the *FOXA2* siRNA groups—they're just weaker—so we shouldn't conclude that the effects of curcumin are *entirely* due to FOXA2.

Finally, as if that wasn't enough, paragraph five gives us some brief information about how curcumin might exert its effects on FOXA2: namely, curcumin upregulates SOCS1 and SOCS3, which are inhibitors of STAT3, which is itself a regulator of FOXA2. We're not given any other notable information about SOCS1, SOCS3, or STAT3, so we can just make note of this in case a question asks about it. In fact, this pathway might be something we'd want to jot down on our wet-erase board to keep these relationships straight.

To summarize, although we had to work through a lot of figures—and this *is* about as complicated in this regard as you'll ever see on the MCAT—we've ended up with a pretty coherent story. That is, curcumin increases the expression of FOXA2, an anti-metastasis transcription factor, which contributes to its ability to reduce proliferation and promote apoptosis. With this summary in mind, you'll be well-positioned to answer any questions that require interpreting data, extrapolating it, or assessing new possibilities in light of experimental findings.

Once more, note how we used the basic fundamentals of figure analysis that we discussed earlier in the chapter. That is, we read the figure captions and the axes, figured out what was being measured in response to which conditions, linked the figures back to the text of the passage to help understand how the experiments fit together, and then found a way to make the figures tell a story. The only real difference here is that we used more specific expertise about statistical significance to help us understand the conclusions more precisely. So remember, for all that this was a dense passage, the ultimate message here is encouraging: even the densest of passages and busiest of figures can be tackled through a systematic approach yoked to a solid understanding of what statistical significance does and doesn't tell us.

7. Must-Knows

> Figures *must* contain all the necessary information, but extracting that information can take some effort.
> Always identify independent variables (manipulated in an experiment, almost always on x-axis) and dependent variables (outcomes measured, almost always on y-axis).
> Figure captions and discussion in passage also provide valuable context.
> Suggested workflow:
  – Read the figure caption to understand what the figure conveys in the overall context of the passage.
  – Read the axes of a figure or the column/row labels of a table.
  – Make a note of the units.
  – Make the figure tell the story.
> Some tips for figure analysis:
  – Try to understand the default behavior in the system being presented and then analyze what happens when conditions are changed.
  – Work backwards from looking at extreme values and trying to understand what makes them extreme.
> Types of figures/diagrams:
  – Tables: specialize in quantitative or yes/no data. May be useful to envision a graph.
  – Line graphs: used for continuous variables (those that form a continuum, like height).
  – Bar graphs: useful for categorical independent variables (those that reflect categories/groups) and continuous dependent variables.
  – Pie charts: specialize in showing percentages.
  – Complex graphs: might have multiple lines/curves (for multiple experimental groups), multiple y-axes (for multiple dependent variables), or clustered bar graphs. Moral of the story is to be careful.
> Scale of axes can vary:
  – Log-log plots: both x- and y-axes are log-transformed. Linear plot corresponds to a power-law relationship (like $y=x^2$).
  – Semi-log (log-lin) plots: only one axis is log-transformed. Linear plot corresponds to an exponential relationship (like $y = 10^x$).
  – Point of log transformation is to visually smooth out huge variations in magnitude.
> Statistical significance: basic guideline is that if figure or table on the MCAT presents statistical significance, only statistically significant differences, which are indicated by a p-value less than 0.05, should be interpreted as "real" for the purposes of answering passage-based questions.
> Some caveats on statistical significance:
  – Look out for how significance is presented, e.g. an asterisk (*), multiple asterisks (** or ***), a dagger (†), or a double-dagger (‡).
  – p-values: the probability that we observed the result we did, or an even more extreme result, by chance when in fact the null hypothesis is true.
  – Usually, the null hypothesis is that no significant difference exists between groups, but not always, so keep an eye out to understand what researchers are trying to figure out.
  – Statistical significance is not the same as effect size (magnitude of the effect). An effect can be significant, or real, but very small.
  – Standard deviation is a measure of dispersal in a data set—not the same thing as statistical significance, although it can provide useful clues about magnitude of differences.
  – Statistical significance does not automatically indicate a cause-and-effect relationship.

Applied Practice

The best MCAT practice is realistic, with detailed analytics to help you assess where things went wrong. For those reasons, we recommend completing practice questions in an online setting that simulates the real MCAT interface, and using the analytics provided to help you decide how to best move your studies forward.

CARS does not require knowledge of specific subject areas, but it does require development of strong test-taking skills. To ensure you are honing those skills as you work through this book, we suggest you go online after wrapping up each chapter and generate a Qbank Practice Set of 2-3 CARS passages to practice and review. While not every chapter of this book is directly applicable to CARS, regular CARS practice is key to test day success.

As a further supplement, given the importance of active learning for effective studying, we also suggest that you consult the Must-Knows at the end of each chapter of this Reasoning text as a basis for creating a study sheet. This is not a sheet to memorize in the more traditional sense of content memorization, but rather a quick reference of the most important strategies for you to refer to during and after practice in your early prep. Frequently revisiting the most important strategies for the MCAT - in both CARS and the Sciences - will help you continue to improve your performance.

This page left intentionally blank.

Experimental Design

0. Introduction

We cover the nuts and bolts of experimental design in Chapter 1 of the Psychology and Sociology textbook since the subject tends to be most directly tested in that section of the MCAT. However, primary research passages are extremely common on the MCAT, so a strong understanding of experimental design pays off throughout the exam. What this means is that in addition to learning the terminology related to research design, it's also important to get the hang of how experimental design is presented in passages throughout the MCAT, even if the questions never ask about it specifically. Understanding the design of an experiment will help you understand its results, which in turn establishes a framework for answering passage-based questions.

1. Experimental Design in a Practice Passage

Physicians and scientists must be able to interpret research findings in a well-informed, critical way, so it's no surprise that the MCAT emphasizes this skill. For this reason, let's take the terms and concepts concerning experimental design (which, again, are further outlined in Chapter 1 of the Psychology and Sociology textbook) and combine them with the general critical reading skills we've covered in earlier chapters by analyzing this Psych/Soc passage:

Strong social support networks have long been linked to more positive measures of health, including lower rates of depression, metabolic disorders, and cardiovascular disease. In fact, social isolation is considered a risk factor for increased mortality. The health implications of functional social networks have generated considerable interest among the medical community in their potential to prevent and mitigate risk factors for chronic illness.

In recent decades, social networking sites (SNS) have begun to alter the ways in which individuals interact with their social networks. To investigate the effect of SNS on the management of hypertension, researchers conducted a single-blind randomized controlled trial in which 30 hypertensive patients were randomized to the intervention, consisting of access to an SNS for patients with hypertension, or to the control group, who received access to an informational website. Systolic blood pressure measurements were recorded at rest over the course of the experiment (Figure 1).

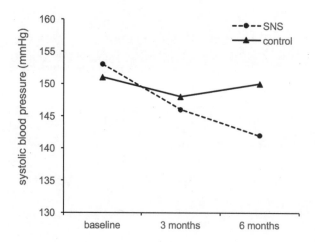

Figure 1. Systolic blood pressure in SNS and control participants

Self-esteem levels were also monitored over the course of the experiment to better elucidate the mechanisms behind the intervention response (Figure 2).

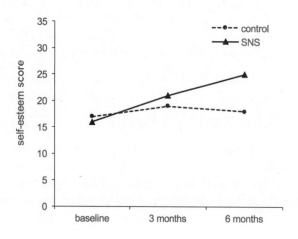

Figure 2. Self-esteem levels in SNS and control participants

To investigate the response to the intervention by participant age, blood pressure measurements were compared among intervention participants categorized into three age groups (Figure 3).

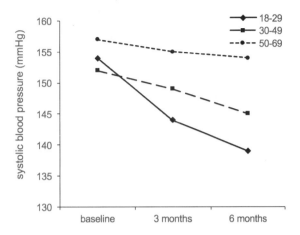

Figure 3. Systolic blood pressure among SNS participants with high and low self-esteem

This passage begins by presenting some background information in its introduction, like all primary research passages do. Such information, including the fact that social isolation is considered to be a risk factor for increased mortality sets up the hypothesis, or the entire basis for the experiment. By understanding the scientific context in which the experiment was developed, you gain insight into its significance, the purpose of its methods, and the questions it's designed to answer, which will help you make sense of the results. This passage in particular looks at the strength of social support networks and their mitigating effect on chronic health conditions.

In the next paragraph, the focus of the passage narrows to present the researchers' specific interest in the effects of social networking sites on hypertension. Although the passage does not specifically spell out a hypothesis using explicit wording like "the hypothesis of this study was _____," we can infer a likely hypothesis from context. Since we're told that having a robust social network has positive effects on health, the most likely hypothesis is that social networking sites have a positive effect on hypertension, namely a reduction in blood pressure. By the way, here's an insider tip: on the MCAT, and in most published papers, the results nearly always corroborate the experimental hypothesis. That's not necessarily a great thing for science, as it leads to a phenomenon called publication bias in which only significant or interesting results are published, but it's helpful for us because reflecting back on the hypothesis can help you interpret experimental results.

If we were the researchers investigating this question, and we wanted to prove once and for all whether social networking has an effect on hypertension, what kind of study design should we implement? Our study would more directly address this question if we can demonstrate causality, not just an association between the two. The gold standard for determining causation is an **experiment**. Experiments require manipulation of some independent variable in order to observe changes in the dependent variable or measured outcome. The researchers do precisely that! To study the effect of social networking sites on hypertension, they simply ask participants to use a social networking site and then measure how their blood pressure changes.

However, to help consolidate our knowledge of experimental design, let's also briefly discuss other possible ways of investigating this question. Sometimes it's not possible or ethical to manipulate the independent variable. For instance, what if we wanted to study the effects of something, like concussions, on blood pressure? We can't reasonably enroll people in a study, whack them upside the head to the point of inflicting serious damage, and then measure their blood pressure. Instead, we'd have to use an **observational study design**, meaning we observe the effect of something (disease, treatment, etc.) without affecting who is exposed or not exposed. The major weakness with this study design is that we can't determine causation. After all, if blood pressure increases after a concussion, it's hard to conclude whether that occurred due to the concussion itself, or due to some underlying factor that predisposed the individual to both a concussion and hypertension, or perhaps long-standing hypertension predisposed the individual to a concussion. Interestingly, though, for the study described in the passage, it's hard to see how an observational design would even work. The author mentions a social networking service specifically for people with hypertension, and there are probably not many people in the population as a whole who just happen to join such a network without any additional prodding.

For the study presented in this passage, it should be both possible and ethical to ask participants to join a social networking site and then measure the effects on blood pressure. That is, unless a subset of recruited participants opt out of the study because they happen to believe participating in social media is immoral and a scourge on humanity. This non-random sampling of the population would introduce a form of selection bias into the study known as **sampling bias**, in which the study population doesn't perfectly represent the intended population as a whole. That doesn't mean we toss this entire study out, but it does mean we have to factor in each source of bias when we interpret the study's conclusions.

Sampling bias is an important concern. For instance, women are nearly 3 times more likely to die after a heart attack and their symptoms are more likely to be characterized as "atypical," which reflects the fact that early heart disease studies were conducted in all male patients. Similarly, until very recently, car manufacturers only tested car safety using crash dummies modeled after the male physique. It's not a coincidence that women in car accidents are 47% more likely to be seriously injured and 17% more likely to die than men are. Selecting a representative sample on the basis of gender, age, and as many other criteria as possible has real consequences.

The larger the **sample size**, the more likely it is to be representative of the entire population, and the greater the study's statistical **power** will be. With a sample of just 10 people, it's quite possible that well over 50% of the participants could identify as men. With a sample size of 100 or 1000, we're much more likely to capture a gender distribution that's proportional to that in the target population. A sample size of 30 isn't all that large, so we should keep that in mind if we're asked about potential study design flaws.

While we're selecting as representative a sample as possible, let's consider any other flaws we need to watch out for. What would be the problem with just taking 30 people with hypertension off the street, creating social networking accounts for all of them, and measuring their blood pressure in a few months? Imagine that average systolic blood pressure decreases by 10 points over the course of the study. This design may sound appealing, but it actually has serious problems.

The most obvious flaw is that there are no **controls**. How can we conclude that blood pressure didn't decrease due to the placebo effect and participants' frequent interactions with clinical research coordinators? Or maybe blood pressure naturally tends to decrease during times of the year that are less stressful, like summertime or right after the holidays? To control for this, the experimental design should include control groups. Specifically, we're going to want an equal number of hypertensive patients who do not receive the intervention (which is access to a social networking site) but who receive some kind of analogous control condition instead, like access to an informational website. This controls for the effect of increased online access to information about their condition while allowing researchers to isolate the effect of interactions with social networks. For another example, let's say we were testing a novel treatment for a medical condition. In this case, the control group would receive the standard treatment for that condition, as denying the standard form of medical care would be unethical. These are examples of **negative controls**, which, as a reminder, are conditions expected to produce a negative response. **Positive controls**, on the other hand, are expected to produce a positive result and are often included in assays to confirm that the assay is working.

Furthermore, it's not a good idea to let participants choose whether they want to belong to the intervention or control group, as self-selection will introduce another source of sampling bias into the study. For this reason, the gold standard for experimental design is random assignment of participants to each study condition, or **randomization**.

This type of study design constitutes what's known as a randomized controlled trial, in which participants are randomized to the intervention and the control.

Another step that can be taken to minimize bias is to blind study participants to the procedures each participant undergoes. This is described as a single-blind study design. Here's a question: since double-blinding provides even more validity to the study, why do you think the participants and researchers weren't both blinded? And which group do you think was not blind to the procedures? Well, it's one thing to give participants a sugar pill and convince them that they're taking a miracle drug, but it's quite another to hide the study procedures from participants logging into a social networking site. Sometimes it's just not possible to conceal the study procedures from the participants, in which case a single-blind study design, where only the researchers are blinded to these procedures, is the way to go.

So, let's return to our passage here. It may seem like we've gone on quite a digression, but this was a digression with a purpose. When scientists or anyone with extensive background in analyzing research first skim through an abstract, they might not pause and explicitly think through all of this stuff we've discussed about blinding, controls, experimental versus cross-sectional design, and so on. But it all will be in the back of their minds, and building that skill is the point of this exercise. That is, a sentence like "researchers conducted a single-blind randomized controlled trial in which 30 patients were randomized to the intervention, or to the control group" conveys a surprisingly large amount of information both about what the researchers did and didn't do. Linking this information with an understanding of the hypothesis under investigation and its broader content sets the stage for analyzing the results.

2. Interpreting Experimental Results in a Passage

The effort we put into understanding this experiment's design will help us make sense of its results, starting with Figure 1, replicated below:

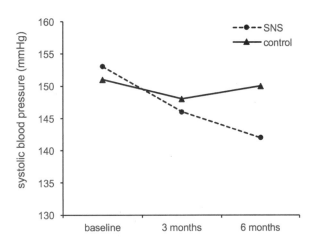

Figure 1. Systolic blood pressure in SNS and control participants

The axes on this figure correspond to the independent and dependent variables of the study, namely the duration of access to a social networking site or a control website on the x-axis and systolic blood pressure (a measure of hypertension) on the y-axis. Comparing the two conditions, we see that blood pressure steadily decreased in the intervention group but not in the control group, which supports the thesis that social networking can help reduce blood pressure and mitigate hypertension.

The graph shows that social networking appeared to reduce blood pressure, but it does not give any information about the possible mechanism. That's where Figure 2 comes in, which examines trends in self-esteem in parallel with changes in systolic blood pressure.

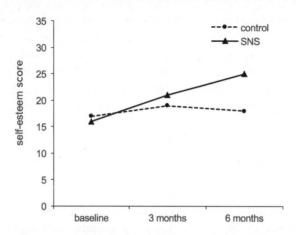

Figure 2. Self-esteem levels in SNS and control participants

According to this graph, it's clear that self-esteem levels rise in participants in the intervention group but are largely unaffected among controls. Integrating the information from Figures 1 and 2, an inverse relationship emerges between blood pressure and self-esteem changes in the intervention group. Several things could be going on here: perhaps a boost in self-esteem helps lower blood pressure, maybe reductions in blood pressure increase self-esteem (although this seems less probable), or possibly some other variable independently mediates both the drop in blood pressure and self-esteem boost. We can't really know for sure because correlation doesn't give us any information about causality.

The passage suggests that this might hint at the mechanism by which social networking alleviates hypertension. From this, we can infer that the researchers think social networking might reduce blood pressure in part by raising self-esteem. If this were true, then self-esteem would be a mediating variable that controls the effect of social networking on hypertension.

Next, the study examines how this response is affected by the age of participants. This next figure only refers to participants who were part of the intervention group, which is then categorized into three age groups.

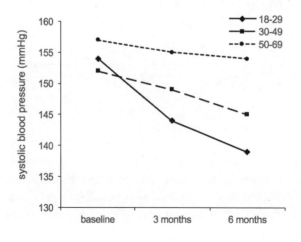

Figure 3. Systolic blood pressure among SNS participants with high and low self-esteem

We don't know what the researchers expected to find here, but what we observe is that younger participants experienced a more dramatic drop in blood pressure over the course of the study, as evidenced by the steepest downward slope for 18 to 29-year-olds. This more pronounced effect suggests that a younger age may have made participants more susceptible to the blood pressure-lowering effects of the intervention. Another way to look at it is that older age made participants more resistant to its effects. Why might this be the case? Well, maybe younger participants used the social networking site differently, or more frequently, or their response to the site interacted in complex ways with any number of age-related variables. Thus, age could be said to moderate the size of the effects that the intervention had on participants, making it an example of a moderating variable.

Mediating, moderating, and confounding variables are easy to confuse, so let's discuss what these might look like within this experiment. To review, **mediating variables** are those that provide a mechanistic link in the relationship between the independent and dependent variables. It might be that the intervention reduced blood pressure by raising self-esteem, or by spurring participants to engage in healthier behaviors, or by reducing anxiety or stress.

Moderating variables affect the strength of a relationship. Common examples of moderating variables are factors like age, gender, and socioeconomic class, as well as criteria like the amount of time participants were required to log into the social networking site, which we might expect to produce dose-dependent effects. The key distinction between mediating variables and moderating variables is that mediators help explain a relationship between two variables while moderators strengthen or weaken that relationship.

Finally, a **confounding variable** would be any external variable that affects both the independent variable, which is the intervention in this experiment, and the dependent variable, which is systolic blood pressure. By doing so, a confounding variable would obscure their true relationship. For example, suppose this experiment were poorly designed, and participants were allowed to choose their assignment to either the intervention or control group. Let's say that participants who were planning to start a regular exercise program, for whatever reason, were much more likely to sign up for the intervention. Then, perhaps to no surprise, we find that the intervention group experienced a much greater drop in blood pressure than control participants did. Is this due to the effect of the intervention or due to the confounding variable of exercise? We may never know! This tends to be a bigger problem with correlational studies than in well-designed experiments with proper randomization and controls. To reduce the risk of confounding effects, researchers can make statistical adjustments for variables like exercise that are expected to affect this relationship, and they should also report descriptive statistics to show that demographics and other important characteristics are similar across all groups.

Based on this analysis of the figures, we're well-positioned to answer any questions about the results, including ones that would require us to make hypothetical predictions.

Another category of questions about experimental design and results on the MCAT invites us to reflect on the strengths and weaknesses of a **study design**. As a well-designed experimental study, the results presented in this passage are strongly suggestive of a causal relationship between the independent and dependent variables, something that wouldn't have been possible if an observational design had been used or if the researchers had committed a grave blunder (like failing to randomize participants or not bothering to include a control group).

The results of a single experiment, like this one, certainly have the potential to be illuminating, and they can even permanently alter the course of a scientific field. But experiments can be flawed, and the results of many influential studies have proven difficult to reproduce. Therefore, a series of randomized controlled trials with similar results would provide even stronger evidence for these findings than one test ever could. So while this study is indeed interesting, we should be careful with how much credence we give it. A systematic review or meta-analysis combining the results of multiple randomized controlled trials would allow us to place more confidence in these findings. If asked for potential weaknesses of this study, other issues might include the small sample size, which might cause particular problems for the subgroup analyses in which participants are subdivided into age groups with no indication of how many belonged to each category. In any case, though, a solid understanding of experimental design allows us to quickly and efficiently hone in on what the results presented in a passage do and don't mean, with a direct payoff for questions dealing with those results.

3. MCAT Primary Research Passage Structure

Primary research passages focus on experiments or research studies. It can seem like there is enormous variation between research-based passages, which can make it tough to identify what these passages have in common and how you should approach them. After all, experiments in MCAT passages can relate to any science content tested on the exam.

More worrying still, **primary research passages** often focus on entirely unfamiliar content, like diseases, pathways, or processes that you never covered in your prep. This can be intimidating. It's easy to panic and think, "Oh my gosh, I must have forgotten to study this!" But in fact, you aren't supposed to recognize every process, disease, or acronym. Instead, the test-makers present unfamiliar material intentionally to assess whether you can stay calm, determine relationships from the text or figures, and apply the information you do know to get the correct answers.

In other words, primary research passages aren't about already recognizing and memorizing everything they describe. Instead, they require a combination of three things: understanding how science experiments work in general, using the stated or implied results to determine what happened in this particular experiment, and applying MCAT science content to understand certain aspects of the experimental design and make predictions. Only one-third of these skills actually involves content knowledge, but students often make the mistake of assuming that all or most questions can be answered from memorized information.

First, let's discuss the general structure of a primary research passage. In all three science sections, these passages tend to share the same basic structure, which includes four key parts: background information, the purpose or hypothesis, the methods and materials used, and the results. Let's break these parts down one-by-one.

The **background** is usually the first part of an experiment-focused passage, and it explains the context for the experiment. This background can be as short as a single sentence or as long as a paragraph or two, but the key idea is that it details why this experiment is relevant for society, modern science, or historical scientific advances. Something else to watch out for on the MCAT, though, is that the background can also give pieces of information that are vital to answering questions, such as numerical parameters of the molecules involved (like boiling points or K_m values) or clues to an enzyme's function.

The next part of a primary research passage is an indication of the researchers' **purpose** for the study. In other words, what are they trying to accomplish with this experiment? This differs from the background, which gives context without specifying the experimenters' intentions. For example, if researchers design a study to assess a new potential treatment for a disease, the background might give general information about the disease and its impact on society, while the purpose will actually specify the researchers' goals in analyzing this treatment, which could be determining whether it's successful or perhaps analyzing some side effect or aspect of the treatment to better understand how it works. In some passages, the purpose is stated as an actual hypothesis, which refers to a possible explanation for some observed phenomenon. Importantly, a hypothesis needs to be testable, meaning that we can design some experiment or procedure to confirm or reject it. In essence, then, the hypothesis introduces the idea that is being tested, and the rest of the passage proceeds to test it.

Where this gets tricky is that the MCAT may not give you a direct statement like "the researchers hypothesized that…". Instead, you might be required to infer the purpose of the experiment from other statements that might at first seem like random, informative phrases or sentences. Common examples are the phrases "it is thought," "it is believed," or similar variations. This wording indicates that scientists (either the researchers themselves or other scientists whose findings the researchers hope to confirm or prove wrong) *think* something happens a certain way but have not verified this with sufficient evidence. Guess what this experiment is almost certainly assessing: whether this process actually happens in this way!

The statement of an experimental purpose might also be much more subtle, or it could even be merged with a sentence that appears to describe the methods. For example, a passage might state, "To study X, the scientists built an elaborate booby trap," or even, "The scientists let all the rats in the lab loose to see what would happen." The parts of these sentences that might immediately jump out at you are "built an elaborate booby trap" or "let all the rats in the lab loose" because they're aspects of the methods. However, these sentences also contain a brief description of the experimental purpose too, in the phrases "to study X" and "to see what would happen." You might even see several related experiments described in a passage, and thus more than one purpose or hypothesis, although the experiments will generally make up a logically reasonable sequence aimed at answering a single larger-scale question. In such a passage, experiments presented later in the passage might be introduced very briefly, with something like, "To investigate Y, the scientists also did Z."

Let's look at a more realistic, specific example. Examining the effects of certain mutations is a major recurring theme in MCAT experimental design since what happens when a gene is mutated can tell us a great deal about the function of the unmutated, wild-type gene. So let's say you see this sentence in a Chemical and Physical Foundations passage: "The Asp346 residue of the ASIC3 protein is believed to play a key role in the protein's pH-sensing function." Ok, so why are they telling you this? It's not just a random factoid, and it probably isn't setting you up for a direct, factual-recall question. Instead, the test-makers are giving you a hint about what the researchers are probably testing. That is, the researchers are probably going to assess whether the aspartic acid residue at position 346 actually *is* important in sensing the pH of the protein's surroundings, and if so, they might also ask a question about the conditions or to what extent this occurs.

Now, how might they test this? It turns out that mutations can be incredibly helpful for exploring questions like this. The researchers could create a mutation with another amino acid substituted for the Asp residue at position 346, and then they could observe whether this missense mutation changes the protein's effectiveness at sensing pH. If the protein suddenly becomes much less sensitive to pH changes, and the only variable that they altered was the residue at position 346, then that residue must play an important role in pH sensation.

Now, consider that we started this example about the Asp346 residue with no direct textual statements about mutations. Based on our familiarity with MCAT science and the logic of how certain hypotheses tend to be investigated, we were already able to say to ourselves "oh, okay, if that's what the researchers are interested in, they'll probably use mutations to investigate this." Now, such predictions can never be 100% accurate, but at the same time, there are definitely some classic experimental strategies that recur on the MCAT and becoming familiar with them will improve your ability to read passages proactively.

Next, we have our third part of an MCAT experiment-focused passage: the **methods and materials**. This is where the passage tells us the sequence of steps in the experimental process, as well as any solutions, reagents, or lab equipment used. This part of the passage can be extremely detailed with lots of information about exact doses or volumes used or the pH or temperature at which each part of the experiment was conducted. It can also include information about how much time each step took or the criteria required of participants. Fortunately, most of these details are typically not terribly important to the questions asked, which tend to focus on results and conclusions rather than, say, the exact number of minutes a participant spent in a PET scanner. For this reason, don't get hung up on memorizing every detail of the methods. Instead, read through that section briskly, highlighting information that is relevant to MCAT content you've studied, like the names of amino acids, but not noting each concentration or number of minutes given.

Finally, we have the **experimental results**. Here, the outcome of the study is given, in the form of text, figures, or both. You should always examine the results with a clear idea of the hypothesis in mind. Very often, the results confirm the hypothesis, but in rare cases, they might contradict the hypothesis so the MCAT test writers can keep you on your toes. The findings might not even show a clear relationship where one was expected.

The structural components of primary research passages are very similar across all three science sections. However, three section-specific differences are worth noting so they don't throw you off when you encounter them.

First, in the Psychology/Sociology and occasionally in the Biological and Biochemical Foundations section, passages may consist of multiple experiments. Often you can spot these passages easily, especially if they contain some mention of "Study One" and "Study Two," or similar language. The first study is typically simpler or more general, or it may even replicate a historically familiar experiment. The second study or second experiment then either contrasts with or follows up on the first study. In the Biological and Biochemical Foundations section in particular, you might also see a pattern where the first experiment sets up the second by clarifying some preliminary point that must be established for the second experiment to make sense. It can also be the case that the experiments might work together to address a larger question. Regardless though, when reading these passages, it's important to identify the purpose of both studies and how they relate or contrast. If you have trouble determining the purpose of the second study, pay special attention to statements made at the end of the first study that describe things that are still unknown or follow-up experiments that still need to be done. Those unanswered questions most likely will be followed up in the second study.

Second, especially in the Psychology/Sociology section, an experimental design might have flaws in terms of lacking validity or reliability. The methods section is a good source of information about these limitations or flaws since it's usually where you'll find details about sample size, control group assignments, and other aspects of the design that could impact its validity. Third, in the Psychology/Sociology section, the experimental results are sometimes not given at all. Instead, you're required to infer what the results likely were from your content knowledge.

Nonetheless, across all three science sections, primary research passages have a similar architecture.

4. Details of Experimental Design

The structure of a primary research passage is a general framework that you can use to help orient yourself in a passage and make sense of the information it presents. The actual questions you'll encounter, though, are likely to have a more specific focus. In other words, to get points on questions dealing with experimental design, you'll usually need to look at the details of the specific experiment in the passage to understand why the researchers made certain decisions and what flaws might have been present in their chosen design.

First of all, understanding why the researchers made certain decisions can help you with any primary research passage. Sometimes this help is indirect, in that better understanding the passage will make you more confident in interpreting it. However, some MCAT questions do cut to the chase and directly ask why a certain decision was made by the experimenters. These questions fall into two categories: ones that can be answered solely using your science knowledge and ones that require some critical thought about the study design.

Here's an example of the first type: "A research design calls for the inclusion of a mutant strain in which the Gln36 residue has been mutated to Asn. Which of the following is the most likely reason for the researchers' use of Asn?"

We don't even need to see the answer choices here to predict what this question is probably getting at. This is a missense mutation, and Asn (or asparagine) and Gln (or glutamine) are highly structurally similar amino acids, so specifically, this is a conservative missense mutation. Our correct answer might mention conservative mutations directly, or it might indicate that we're trying to have a relatively minimal impact on the protein produced compared to the larger impact a nonconservative missense or a nonsense mutation would have had. Notice that we didn't need to know anything about the experimental design here. We could use our own science background to understand the researchers' choices.

The second type of question is a little bit more complex. These questions require some thought beyond your mental bank of science knowledge—specifically, about a certain experiment and its design, why the researchers did something a particular way, or if the scientists could have done something better. To answer these questions, remember the criteria of a good experiment: it should be valid and reliable. Any decisions the researchers made, then, most likely functioned to maintain one or both of these qualities.

Let's take a look at this example:

> Which of the following best explains why the researchers chose to measure levels of nitric oxide (NO) metabolites both before and after treatment?
>
> A. It allows for comparison between before-treatment and after-treatment values, with similarities between the values indicating reliability of the study design.
>
> B. The baseline measurement served to minimize confounding variables, improving the study's external validity.
>
> C. The earlier measurement established a baseline to which each participant could be compared, thus adding to the internal validity of the study.
>
> D. The baseline measurement of NO metabolite levels functions as an additional independent variable.

Now, the fact that baseline measurements should be included in a study design might seem kind of obvious, especially if you've designed or carried out experiments yourself during your studies. But even so, we can use this example as an exercise in asking why exactly, the researchers made this call. The first step is to clearly identify what decision the researchers made. Here, even though we weren't given any passage information, we can infer that the researchers chose to measure NO metabolite levels twice (before and after treatment) rather than just measuring once after treatment. Now that we understand what choice is being asked about, we should remind ourselves that the researchers likely made this decision for the benefit of the validity or reliability of the study design. There are many different kinds of validity and tons more factors that influence the validity of a study. So rather than blindly trying to predict the correct answer, let's move to the answer choices and use process of elimination.

We can start with choice A. This choice looks attractive because it starts off with a plausible-sounding statement about comparing before-treatment and after-treatment values, and it mentions reliability. However, a closer look shows us that it describes reliability as similarity between the before-treatment and the after-treatment measurements. This doesn't constitute reliability at all. In fact, our study could be enormously reliable and still have large differences between the before- and after-treatment data, because maybe the treatment worked! That is, it may have caused the after-treatment results to be reliably higher or lower than the baseline. So similarity between baseline and post-treatment values is not reliability. Instead, reliability exists if we can repeat the experiment over and over and see similar results for the difference between the before- and after-treatment values, assuming we're measuring that difference in the same way in every instance of the experiment.

Turning to choice B, although it may sound tempting because researchers definitely try to minimize the impact of confounding variables all the time, there are two issues here. First, it's not obvious that making baseline measurements necessarily accomplishes the goal of "minimizing confounding variables." That is, although making baseline measurements is a good idea, it's perfectly possible for confounding variables to exist nonetheless. Just the fact that we're taking an additional measurement wouldn't make them suddenly go away. It just gives us a consistent standard for comparison between groups. A second, and perhaps more clear, issue is that this answer choice says minimizing confounding variables increases external validity, which concerns the extent to which the results can be generalized to the larger population. In reality, minimizing the impact of confounding variables is associated with internal validity since the fewer and less impactful the confounding variables, the better able we'll be to draw causal conclusions, all else being equal. Both of these factors make choice B wrong.

Moving on, C looks like a solid option. The first part of this answer choice just describes the before-treatment measurement as a baseline, which is accurate and fits with the question stem. The second part mentions internal validity. This could absolutely be correct if the establishment of the baseline allowed us to infer a causal relationship more precisely, and in fact, that's exactly the point of making baseline measurements. The ability to infer causal relationships is related to the internal validity of the study. But before we choose C, we should take a look at D. Since we're measuring metabolite levels here, they serve as a dependent variable, not an independent one because the researchers didn't directly manipulate them. We can therefore safely eliminate D and pick C as our answer.

5. Experimental Flaws

Now so far, we've mostly been focusing on what makes a good experiment (in other words, a valid, reliable one) and what decisions made concerning its experimental design make it that way. However, the MCAT can also present flawed experiments, or ones where something about the study design is damaging to its validity or to the ability to repeat it reliably. The exact nature of the flaw depends on the particular study, but at its heart, virtually any legitimate flaw should undermine reliability and/or validity. Four key types of flaws are especially prevalent on the exam: a deficiency in internal validity, a deficiency in external validity, insufficient sample size, and errors in the choice or grouping of experimental participants.

Recall that **internal validity** describes the extent to which we can infer causal relationships. A major cause of deficiencies in internal validity is the presence of potential confounding variables. Biases, such as selection bias, can also interfere with internal validity, as can the choice of invalid or illogical measurements. For example, if we go back to the example in section 4, involving a nitric oxide study and the pre- and post-treatment measurements, the researchers made the wise decision to make baseline measurements. Not doing so would have damaged the internal validity of the study because, in the absence of baseline measurements, we would have no way to account for participants who improved very little from before- to after-treatment but who also just happened to come in with astronomically high baseline levels.

Alternatively, flaws might impact a study's **external validity**, or the generalizability of the results to a larger population. To understand why these flaws ever arise in studies designed by doctorate-level scientists, it's important to understand that experimental design often involves trade-offs, situations where an increase in one form of validity might result in a decrease in another. This makes it extremely difficult to create a perfect study design, meaning that some flaws are virtually inevitable. In particular, to increase a study's internal validity, it is helpful to eliminate confounding variables as best as possible. This often is accomplished by performing the study under very carefully controlled conditions. But the more "controlled-for" the study gets, the less it tends to resemble real life, which is very much not carefully controlled, as we all probably know from experience. And the less generalizable a study's conclusions are outside of that particular study, the lower its external validity. In this way, increases in internal validity can correspond to decreases in external validity.

The major remaining types of experimental flaws can impact validity too, but they are important enough to be reviewed separately. The third category is often the first one students think of, probably because it's perhaps the most commonly cited design flaw. This flaw is an insufficiently large **sample size**. Sample size is the number of participants in a given study. The larger the sample size, the less skewed the data will be by outlying data points, and the less likely it is that we'll erroneously see a relationship where none is present. Studies with small samples can be flawed, and their results may be both invalid (due to sampling bias) and unreliable (since repeating the experiment with a different sample may produce different results). You might be wondering, "How small is too small?" and the answer, unfortunately, is that there is no hard cut-off. Instead, the proper sample size for a procedure is specific to that procedure itself. For example, 200 participants may be plenty for an experiment on a rare neurological disease, while 2500 participants might be insufficient for a broad study intended to reflect the entire American population. This lack of a hard cut-off might seem frustrating, but this flaw is still easy to handle on the MCAT. Just pay attention to the sample size as you initially read the passage, and make a mental note to yourself if it seems unreasonably small given the procedure. If not, don't worry about it unless it comes up in a question. If you are still unsure and the question asks for experimental flaws, use the process of elimination to evaluate the other potential flaws. If all three can be eliminated, you know that sample size is the problem. But if one of the other flaws is both scientifically accurate and answers the question, that one is your answer.

The final category of experimental flaw relates not to sample size but to sample distribution. In other words, maybe the sample contains plenty of participants, but those participants were chosen or grouped in a way that could lead to biased results. Two major concepts can help us understand this flaw: sampling bias and random assignment. **Sampling bias** occurs when we're trying to study a certain population, but due to our sampling methods, some members of the population are more likely to be included than others. The result is that we end up with a different distribution of participants than we intended, and we might draw conclusions from that sampled group that aren't accurate for the entire population. For example, let's say we want to study the food preferences of the citizens of a certain country, and we want to do this by mailing out a survey and having our participants mail back their answers. But to mail it back, they need to put a stamp on the envelope, and in this particular country, a stamp costs $1000. Now the specifics here are ridiculous, but they make it easy to see how this would lead to a very biased sample. Only people who were both willing and able to spend $1000 on a stamp would answer our survey, and we'd end up with the food preferences of a very specific segment of that population. So much for getting every citizen in the country's opinion!

That simple example showed us how sampling bias makes it possible to obtain results that are not representative of what we're aiming to study. However, it can be even trickier when experiments involve multiple groups of participants that are treated differently, such as in a clinical trial where half of the participants are given an experimental medication and the other half receive a placebo. Here, we have to be careful to avoid grouping participants in a biased way, like putting all of the sickest patients in the placebo group. Doing that might make our experimental group look very healthy in comparison, even if our experimental treatment doesn't work. To avoid this, we can use **random assignment**, or the grouping of participants in a truly randomized way. Now, completely random assignment isn't necessary for all experiments, but it is a key way to prevent many of the participant grouping errors that appear constantly on the MCAT. By consciously avoiding sampling bias and using random assignment, researchers can make sure their experiment doesn't fall victim to this final category of error.

After all of this discussion of experimental flaws, it's worth mentioning what does *not* constitute a flaw, so you can avoid being lured toward an incorrect answer. On this note, by far the most important thing to remember is this: an experimental flaw is not simply something that the experimenters chose not to cover in the study design. For example, imagine that we're conducting an experiment that measures the effect of the number of books read by pregnant mothers in a two-week period on the likelihood that a child will grow up to be a New England Patriots fan. An answer choice might try to make you think that this experiment is flawed because it doesn't assess the number of books read by the fathers of these children. That seems like something we should be looking at, right? Some fathers are really into sports, and at least in some families, they might have more influence over their children's team preference than their mothers do. So is the fact that we didn't also study paternal book-reading a flaw? Nope, it's not. A good study tests exactly what it was designed to test, and no more. It's not a flaw that it doesn't test for everything else! If it were, every experiment would be required to test for every possible determining factor, and that's not the case. When trying to determine flaws, keep your thought process focused on validity, reliability, and classic flaws like insufficient sample size, and you'll avoid falling for a trap answer.

6. MCAT Experimental Design: Common Independent Variables

So far, we've talked in highly general terms about MCAT primary research passage structure, as well as aspects of experimental design. However, even though the content of passages can feel random, there are some common areas of focus and techniques that are worth familiarizing yourself with.

We'll start with commonly encountered independent variables and the outcomes of these experiments. Recall that independent variables are variables that are manipulated by the experimenter in order to study some resulting change in one or more dependent variables. When these variables are depicted graphically, the independent variable is typically on the x-axis, while the dependent variable is typically on the y-axis.

One important caveat is that technically, almost anything can be an independent variable. For example, if you're studying how your younger brother's mood is impacted by him being repeatedly pushed into the swimming pool, your independent variable might be "number of times he is pushed into the pool," while your dependent variable would be "his mood rated on a scale from one to ten." While this exact setup is somewhat unlikely to appear on the MCAT, something similar could appear on the Psychology/Sociology section, as well as thousands of other experimental variables. However, a much smaller set of classic variables appears with a much higher likelihood, and some of these have their own unique challenges and are described by their own unique notations. If you understand how to approach these variables, you can use the same skills to tackle any independent variables you happen to see on the exam.

More specifically, there are four independent variables that you'll see over and over again during your MCAT prep. These are time; concentration; the presence or absence of a certain molecule; and the presence or absence of a certain mutation, including genetic knockout models.

The first two of these variables (**time** and **concentration**) may seem very different, but they can actually be analyzed in similar ways. When time is the independent variable, it means that the experimenters were measuring the dependent variable repeatedly at regular intervals. These intervals might be on the order of seconds, minutes, hours, or even a weirder unit like nanoseconds, so be absolutely sure to verify these units using either the text of the passage, the x-axis, or the caption of an associated figure if one is given.

Take this figure from a biosignaling study, which looks at the effect of a treatment on plasma levels of three key signaling molecules.

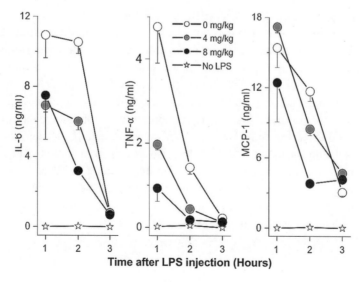

Figure 1. Cytokine response to LPS injection with EVK-203 pre-treatment

The x-axis shows time, which is a great indicator that time is an independent variable. Before going further, let's check the units, which are hours. But what starting point are these hours measured in relation to? In other words, are these the hours that have elapsed since the beginning of the experiment or since some other point of interest? This is relevant to this example because the figure tells us that two different events are occurring near the beginning of the study. First, the mice are "pre-treated" with a compound called EVK-203, and second, they are injected with lipopolysaccharide, or LPS. So, is time being measured from the time of treatment with EVK? Or from the time of LPS injection? Here, the x-axis gives us our answer. It states "time after LPS injection," meaning that the timer started when the mice were injected with a dose of LPS. Of course, on the MCAT, this figure would be associated with a passage, where more information about this study would certainly be given! But we don't even need that information to see that the "1 hour" mark on the x-axis refers to an hour after LPS injection, not one hour after EVK-203 treatment or anything else. From here, we can draw conclusions about the dependent variable, which here is the plasma levels of these signaling molecules.

Our second "standard" independent variable is **concentration**, and it tends to be even more straightforward than time. This can be the concentration of a drug, a biological molecule, hydrogen ions, or any other substance. Imagine a variation on the same cytokine experiment, except we measure cytokine levels only at the two hour mark, thereby eliminating time as an independent variable since it doesn't vary.

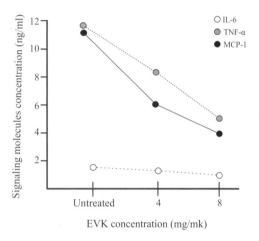

Figure 2. Signaling molecule concentration in response to EVK-203 pre-treatment at different conditions

Now, the only variable manipulated by the experimenters is concentration of the EVK treatment. As we did before, we should check our units first (mg/kg). But here, we don't need to worry about our starting point. Instead, our x-axis ranges from the simple values of 0 mg/kg (no treatment) to 8 mg/kg (the highest dose). We can therefore jump right into analyzing the relationships shown by the graph, where we see that the higher the EVK dosage, the lower the levels of cytokine biosignaling molecules in the plasma. Therefore, here, our steps were to determine that concentration is our independent variable, check the axes for units, and then move directly into drawing conclusions.

However, it's also common for the presence of a drug or molecule to be given by a simple, binary "yes" or "no" distinction. This brings us to our third key variable: the **presence or absence of something**. In other words, the experimental data distinguishes between "yes, the treatment or molecule was present" and "no, it was not present." This is commonly shown using a plus sign to denote "yes, present" and a minus sign to denote "no, not present." When dealing with experiments that involve this distinction, it's very helpful to compare two trials that differ only in that the molecule is present in one and absent in the other. If those two trials result in very different levels of the dependent variable, the molecule must have had an effect on that variable, while if the two trials have similar results, the molecule might not have had an impact on what is being studied.

The fourth variable is the presence or absence of a certain genetic **mutation**, which is important enough to be covered in a section of its own below.

7. MCAT Experimental Design: Mutations as Independent Variables

One particularly important independent variable in MCAT experimental design involves **mutations**, specifically, whether a cell or protein is the wild-type (or unmutated) version or whether it's a mutant. Typically, the wild-type is compared to one or more mutants with respect to physical or biochemical properties, such as denaturation temperature or catalytic efficiency. Just like you've learned in your content review, don't assume that all mutations are deleterious! In other words, don't jump to the conclusion that all mutant strains will be worse than the wild-type in whatever parameter is being measured. Instead, always use the actual data given to make a comparison.

You might think that this doesn't seem too hard, as we just have to compare wild-type or mutant variants to each other to see which of them are higher, lower, or at similar levels of the dependent variable. This is simple enough from a conceptual standpoint, but the MCAT tends to compound the difficulty of these experiments by using certain forms of notation to describe mutations. If you aren't familiar with the code, you'll likely miss the question, regardless of how well you understand the underlying content.

The first notation in this code is used to describe substitution mutations, specifically missense mutations. It consists of a letter, a number, and a second letter, in that exact order. Both letters are single-letter amino acid abbreviations, while the number is the position of the amino acid in question in the peptide sequence. By convention, the amino acid that is present in the wild-type protein is the first single-letter abbreviation, while the amino acid that replaces it in the mutant is the second letter abbreviation. For example, you might see the abbreviation "N375K" in an MCAT passage. The first letter is N denotes asparagine. This, coupled with the number "375," tells us that asparagine must be the residue in the 375th position in the wild-type protein. The wild-type is unmutated, so that "N375" is how things "should" be! In this case, however, we have a letter "K" after the number, so the amino acid lysine must replace asparagine in the mutant protein. The mutant, then, has lysine at position 375 instead of asparagine.

This is important, so let's work through another example:

> Researchers identify several variants of a mammalian DNA polymerase. They discover that these mutant proteins differ in the rate at which they introduce errors during DNA replication. These rates are shown below for both the wild-type polymerase and the mutant enzymes.

Variant	Error rate (errors per base pair)
WT	2.8×10^{-9}
K482E	3.6×10^{-10}
D85A	4.9×10^{-6}
L201V	2.7×10^{-9}

Given this data, which of the following changes in the wild-type is most deleterious?

A. A substitution in which the lysine residue at position 482 is replaced by glutamic acid

B. A substitution in which the glutamic acid residue at position 482 is replaced by lysine

C. A substitution in which the aspartic acid residue at position 85 is replaced by alanine

D. A substitution in which the alanine residue at position 85 is replaced by aspartic acid

Alright, so researchers are looking at the effect of certain mutations on the accuracy of DNA replication. The question wants us to find which mutation is most deleterious, or harmful. Since all of the information required to answer this question is found in the table, we should look there first. The wild-type polymerase is denoted by WT, and it has an error rate of 2.8×10^{-9} errors per base pair. That's a pretty tiny error rate. It's somewhere close to an error every billion nucleotides or so. Let's see if any of the variants have a HIGHER error rate since a deleterious mutation would correspond to more errors being introduced. Does K482E? No, it has a more negative exponent, which corresponds to a smaller or lower error rate. L201V also has a lower error rate since 2.7 is lower than 2.8. The only variant with a higher rate is D85A, which has a less negative exponent (10^{-6}) and therefore a larger value for its error rate.

At this point, we know our answer, but we could still get the question incorrect if we misinterpret the notation! D85A means that the original amino acid in position 85 was aspartic acid, but the new amino acid in the mutant enzyme is alanine. This corresponds to answer choice C, but notice how similar C and D are. We know from correctly deciphering the notation that we want a substitution in which the aspartic acid residue at position 85 is replaced by alanine. But we need to be careful not to get this backwards, like in answer choice D!

You should be aware of an additional convention used to describe mutations. This convention is the use of the delta (Δ) symbol to describe when something is missing, and that something is usually a gene or part of a gene. For example, let's say we're dealing with the human carcinoma cell line Hep G2. First of all, you don't need to know anything about Hep G2 (in fact, the MCAT will use the names of cell lines and signaling molecules that you don't know all the time, so it's important to get accustomed to it). Let's say that the passage or question tells us that a mutant strain of these cells is missing the *CASR* gene, which codes for a calcium receptor. We could describe these cells as Hep G2$^{\Delta CASR}$. Alternatively, if a genetic deletion causes a person to lack the *CASR* gene on both copies of the chromosome, we could describe that person as *CASR*$^{\Delta/\Delta}$. The notation rule here simply indicates whatever is associated with the Δ is missing. Here, we see *CASR* listed along with the Δ, so the *CASR* gene must be missing.

Researchers can learn a lot from genetic knockouts, or models where all or part of a gene is inactivated or totally eliminated. But they can sometimes investigate even further by trying to re-introduce the missing gene into those mutant cells to see if this restores or "rescues" its function. For example, if we wanted to rescue our poor Hep G2 cells, which are struggling through their *CASR* deficiency, we'd basically need to add the *CASR* gene back in again. This would be described using notation like: Hep G2$^{\Delta CASR}$ + *CASR*. This means the cell line was missing *CASR* but it was added back again, and we might expect these cells to more resemble wild-type cells in whatever we happen to be measuring.

Sometimes the fact that a gene is knocked out is not denoted by a Δ but rather by a simple minus sign. As we'd expect, minus means "not present," while plus means present. Someone with a genotype of *CASR*$^{+/-}$, then, has one copy of *CASR* but lacks a second. In other words, they're a heterozygote. If you see this in a graph or figure, don't be alarmed, even if the figure looks complicated like the one below with four different things being shown on the x-axis.

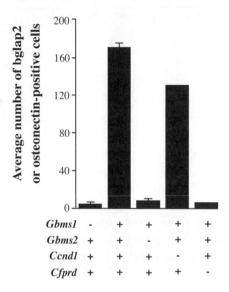

Figure 3. Relationship between genotypes and bglap2

Just remember that plus means present and minus means absent. In the leftmost column, then, *Gbms1* has been knocked out while the other three transcription factors are present.

8. MCAT Experimental Design: Common Outcomes Measured

Independent variables are a vitally important aspect of experimental design, but no study can exist with independent variables alone. Instead, experiments need at least one dependent variable, which simply put, is a thing that we are measuring or an "outcome" of the study. Let's take a look at some commonly-investigated outcomes. Our goal with these is not only learning about their specifics but also understanding the general ideas that connect dependent variables on the MCAT as a whole.

Common dependent variables on the MCAT can be broadly divided into three categories: changes in some physical or chemical property, biological measurements, and biochemical measurements. None of these categories include psychology or sociology, which is because the Psychology/Sociology section has considerably more variation in the content of its experiments. Dependent variables could be anything from the number of words remembered from a list to the number of aggressive behaviors displayed after watching a video to the extent of activation of a certain region of the brain. For this reason, it's best to evaluate each Psychology/Sociology passage individually and clearly focus on what the experimenters aim to study. Therefore, in this section, we'll take a deeper look at the Chemical and Physical Foundations and Biological and Biochemical Foundations sections, where clearer patterns in dependent variables do emerge.

Let's first consider physical or chemical dependent variables. These can include things like changes in pressure or boiling points. The data for these experiments are typically straightforward, and associated questions often require an understanding of the underlying science more than anything else. That is to say, if boiling point is the dependent variable, you can expect MCAT questions to focus on factors that you should know impact boiling point more than they do on the experimental setup.

One thing to be careful about, however, is exactly how the results are depicted. Are they directly-measured values, like a blood pressure of 135 mmHg? Are they measured relative to another value, like if we had a 1.65 ratio of systolic to diastolic blood pressure? Or are they measured as a change from a previous value? Consider the following example:

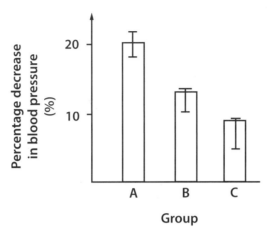

Figure 4. Blood pressure in groups A, B, and C

Here, for example, if we read hastily, we might be tempted to think that column A corresponds to a 20-fold change in blood pressure, or even that, since it's a higher bar, it denotes a higher blood pressure than what are shown in columns B and C. In fact, a few extra seconds spent looking at the axis would tell us that this value represents a percent decrease. In other words, column A represents a 20% drop from some original or reference value. If our original blood pressure were 100 mmHg, then the new blood pressure for this group would be 80 mmHg. This idea of potentially interpreting experimental results backwards, or at least incorrectly, is common across very different studies. For example, another dependent variable often measured in MCAT experiments is protein folding or unfolding. Don't be the person who misses a question just because you misread an axis and mistook 90% folded for 90% unfolded! Incorrect answer choices on the MCAT like to take advantage of how easy it is to misinterpret a graph in this way, so we can't emphasize enough the importance of reading carefully.

Turning to biological outcomes, by far the most common are growth and gene expression. **Growth** is as simple as it sounds. It is the extent to which a cell or an entire organism increases in mass or volume. A related concept is the increase (or decrease) in the number of cells, which is also a common dependent variable on the MCAT. When dealing with growth or changes in cell number, we run into the same issue that we did for the physical parameters earlier: if we don't identify exactly what is being measured, we risk drawing incorrect conclusions. For example, imagine a study where the independent variable is the plasma concentration of a certain signaling molecule that is thought to promote apoptosis in cancer cells. We might think that "level of apoptosis" is our dependent variable, but what if instead, the variable measured by the researchers is tumor volume? Tumor volume is an inverse measure of apoptosis, which means the more apoptosis going on, the smaller we'd expect the tumor volume to be. If a question asked us about the most effective pro-apoptotic concentration of the signaling molecule, then we'd want to look for the trial showing the lowest tumor volume.

Like growth, gene expression is an extremely common experimental outcome on the MCAT. **Gene expression** simply refers to the extent to which a gene is used to form a gene product, which we usually quantify as the amount of mRNA transcribed from that gene or, more indirectly, as the amount of protein translated from that mRNA. Higher levels of gene expression correspond to more transcription and thus more mRNA produced. Often, we aren't particularly concerned with the absolute level of gene transcription (when's the last time you saw something like "3×10^6 transcripts were produced in this cell"?). Instead, we care about relative gene expression, or the level of transcription compared to some reference, often a wild-type control group. In these cases, the researchers set the reference level of transcription at a certain value, often 1, and all other values are scaled in comparison. This adjustment relative to a reference value is called normalization. The MCAT will indicate when data have been normalized, but it is important to notice and interpret that information. Consider, for example, the figure below:

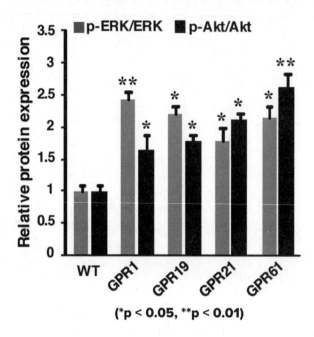

Figure 5. Relative gene expression

Here, the protein expression of the wild-type variant has been set at one, and the expression of four GPCR mutant variants has been normalized to that value. Looking at the GPR1 column, we can say that p-ERK/ERK expression for that variant is almost 2.5 times the level of expression for the wild-type. However, if you wanted to know the absolute quantity of transcripts produced, you'd be out of luck! This graph only tells us these values relative to each other.

Another classic biological dependent variable is **binding affinity**. Several measurements reflect the binding affinity of a biochemical molecule, such as K_M, the Michaelis-Menten constant, or K_a, the affinity constant. Often, however, MCAT experimental results do not directly provide the measured values for these constants. Instead, this is another place where experimental results may be presented as relative values. For example, a study might give its results as a ratio of K_a to some original K value, where K_a gives the affinity constant under the experimental condition and K gives the original affinity constant for the untreated, or wild-type control. A K_a/K ratio of one means that K_a and K are equal, while a K_a/K ratio near zero means that Ka is smaller than K or that the experimental condition has reduced the binding affinity. In this way, we see that the greater the effect of the experimental condition on K_a, the farther K_a/K will be from one, and vice versa.

All of these dependent variables have their own quirks, especially in the ways that data can be presented. While understanding these quirks is extremely helpful in knowing what to expect and recognizing what's going on in a passage, at heart, how we approach these variables should be largely the same. First, clearly identify what is being measured and understand how the results of this measurement are displayed, and then try to draw conclusions from that information. That's all there is to it!

9. MCAT Experimental Methods: Cell Culture Basics

In previous sections in this chapter, we've discussed high-level aspects of experimental design, and then zoomed in to look more closely at common choices of independent and dependent variables. Now it's time to get even more specific. Let's look at some common aspects of experimental methods with a particular focus on the Biological and

Biochemical Foundations section. This is not to say that all primary research passages draw on these methods, but they're common enough that familiarizing yourself with them will pay off.

The first set of methods we'll discuss relates to **cell culture**. In such experiments, some cells or biological samples are isolated or cultured, and they're treated with biological, chemical, or physical agents or exposed to some other experimental conditions. Then they undergo some sort of procedure (either before or after treatment) to prepare the sample, and finally some outcome is measured and presented as data. Let's talk about each of these steps in more depth:

First, there will usually be some kind of starting biological sample. This might be tissues or cells harvested from patients, in some cases patients with genetic disorders or some other condition. There might be an animal model, typically mice or rats. In fact, if you see a word ending in "-ine," like "murine" or "canine," this refers to an animal model, where "murine" refers to mice, "canine" to dogs, "porcine" to pigs, and so on.

More frequently, the biological sample will be derived from a cell culture, meaning cells that are "cultured" (or grown) in a Petri dish. Over the years, research labs have developed and shared what are called cell lines, which are permanently established, immortal cell cultures derived from a single starting cell, so all cells in a given cell line theoretically all have the same or at least a very similar genetic makeup. The HeLa cell line is one such example. This line was derived from cervical cancer cells taken (controversially) from a patient named Henrietta Lacks, hence the name "HeLa." The advantage of a cell line is that cells from a given line in one lab theoretically should behave very similarly to cells from the same line in any other lab around the world.

You're certainly not expected to memorize or even recognize specific cell lines. In fact, try not to get too bogged down by the terminology. Whether you're dealing with HeLa cells or LNCaP cells or ATCC cells or something else, the key is to identify the important, big-picture details and move on. Ask yourself how connected the cell type is to the purpose of the experiment. For example: What's special about the cells used? Are macrophages being used to study phagocytosis? Are cancer cells being used to study metastasis? Are the cells genetically altered or engineered to express (or lack) a certain gene or protein? Are two cell types being incubated together in the same culture to see how those cell types communicate and how their secretions affect each other? Focusing on the big picture will help you better understand the data and, by extension, your answer choices.

If we're working with a cell culture, there's a good chance you'll be told how the cells are grown in the lab. There are a few synonyms for this in the scientific literature ("grown," "cultured," "incubated," "maintained," "nourished"), but they all pretty much mean the same thing. Basically, just like cells in our body, cells grown in the lab need water and nutrients to survive. For that reason, cells are cultured in a fluid known as a culture medium, which contains the necessary glucose, nutrients, and survival factors that the particular cell type likes. This medium might have a fancy name for it, like Dulbecco's modified eagle's medium or enriched medium, but again, don't get too tied up in the details. You might even come across something called "conditioned medium," which is essentially medium taken from one cell culture and then transferred over to another cell culture. This isn't just some budget-friendly recycling scheme to cut down on lab costs. The idea is that, after a few hours or days, this conditioned medium is rich in all the metabolites and growth factors secreted by the first culture, and transferring it over to the second culture allows scientists to study how those secretions affect the behavior of the latter cell culture.

Cells are usually grown on plates or flasks in the lab, which provide a solid surface for cells to anchor and immobilize themselves to. The size of the well or plate may vary from that of a 96-well microplate to a 75 centimeter-squared culture flask, but they all serve essentially the same purpose: allowing cells to thrive so we can perform interesting experiments on them.

When reading a primary research article dealing with cell culture, it's important to identify the **treatment groups**. For example, maybe we start with two different cell types, like wild type versus a genetically engineered cell type lacking the p53 gene. Then perhaps each is divided further into two conditions: a control and an experimental group exposed to, say, UV radiation. Afterwards, maybe each is divided again, with half receiving treatment with a cell cycle inhibitor and half receiving a control treatment. In this example, the control treatment might just be the solvent that the cell cycle inhibitor was dissolved in to control for the effects of adding that volume to the culture.

Treatment conditions pose three challenges. The first is understanding the methodology itself. Is the sample being treated with a biological molecule, a chemical, or a physical agent like radiation? Is a gene being introduced into the sample, maybe via a plasmid or virus? Are the cells being treated with an agonist or an inhibitor?

The second challenge is connecting the method to its purpose. At the end of the day, research methods are simply the means to answering questions about broader scientific phenomena. UV radiation might have been used to model induced DNA damage, and cell cycle inhibitors could have been used to evaluate how each cell type would respond to various chemotherapies. As you go, be sure to interpret each step in light of the question the researchers are pursuing.

The last key challenge is keeping track of all the different treatment conditions and acronyms. It's not reasonable to expect yourself to remember every detail and acronym perfectly without ever referring back to earlier parts of the passage. Instead, the trick is to create a tracking system that allows you to refer back in an efficient manner. One tactic is highlighting each acronym the first time it appears, and you might even consider jotting it down on your wet-erase board with a symbol that helps you recall its identity. For example, you might draw a symbol to represent the cell cycle with an inhibition arrow next to "INK4" to help you remember it's a cell cycle inhibitor. Anytime you see "INK4" in the passage, replacing this in your mind with "cell cycle inhibitor" or "drug that blocks cell division" will help you make sense of the experimental findings. Another highlighting tactic that we endorse is highlighting the familiar parts of long names or descriptions that are unfamiliar overall. For example, if a passage describes the "release of an array of cytotoxic granule proteins, one of which is ECP, or eosinophil cationic protein," the description of this process overall might not ring a bell. However, it can help immensely to highlight the words "cytotoxic" and "cationic" since we are supposed to know what those mean and they're relatively more likely to come into play in the questions.

Before or after treatments are applied, the sample will likely undergo auxiliary procedures like DNA extraction or centrifugation in preparation of obtaining results from the sample. The passage may expect you to infer the purpose of these steps, and questions may even ask you about them, so it's important to practice recognizing them, drawing connections to your content knowledge, and learning the terminology used to describe specific techniques.

Now, let's say a passage rattles off a list of procedures, using the following wording:

> A buccal swab sample was obtained from each patient and suspended in an isotonic buffer containing a nonionic detergent. The samples were homogenized by blender and centrifuged at $1200 \times g$. The supernatant was then removed, and samples were stored at 4°C.

In essence, a tissue sample is taken from a patient, and an isotonic buffer is added that contains detergent. Then the sample is homogenized and centrifuged, the supernatant is removed, and the sample is cooled. Don't get too lost in the methods, and instead, focus on the essentials, like the actual treatment groups. But if you are asked about any one of these steps, the good news is you can (and should) lean on your content knowledge to decipher its purpose, even if it's a technique you've never encountered before. For example, why would an isotonic buffer be added to the sample? Well, based on our understanding of tonicity, if you place the sample in a hypertonic buffer, the cells would lose water and shrink, and if you use a hypotonic buffer, the cells would swell up and possibly burst. Therefore, an isotonic buffer will least disturb fluid homeostasis. What about a detergent? Recall that detergents have both hydrophobic and hydrophilic components, so that allows them to disrupt and lyse cell membranes, which is useful if we want to extract organelles or proteins or DNA or some other intracellular component from our sample. If we really want to lyse those membranes, we can facilitate this process using mechanical disruption, or homogenization. Moving on, centrifugation separates particles in solution by their size and density, so if we spin a sample in a centrifuge and then isolate the supernatant, we've essentially left behind a pellet of cell debris and larger membrane fragments and organelles. Finally, why might we want to keep our sample cool? We know that temperature is linked to enzyme function, so if we lower the temperature, we might be able to limit the activity of DNAses and proteolytic enzymes that would otherwise degrade biomolecules in the sample.

Let's quickly mention a few other steps that you might come across on the MCAT. Sometimes a cell culture will be treated with an enzyme like trypsin or endopeptidase in order to cleave proteins. This may simply be used to help cells detach from the plate or to cleave proteins in a specific or nonspecific matter. It really depends on the purpose of the experiment, so read carefully! Furthermore, there will often be a wash or rinse step in which the culture medium is temporarily replaced by a buffer. This removes treatment molecules, metabolites, and impurities from the culture. There might even be an extraction step used to isolate DNA, protein, or some other biomolecule from the sample, and the details of that extraction shouldn't concern you so much as what exactly is being extracted and why.

If we're interested in studying cell or chromosome behavior at a specific point in the cell cycle, certain drugs can be added to arrest proliferating cells in one stage of the cycle, which can be helpful for karyotype analysis, among other things. Cultured cells might even be grown in a Petri dish before being injected into a study animal, as will often be done with cancer cells to observe the rate of tumor growth in an organism. And finally, flow cytometry (or cell sorting) is a technique that may be used to physically sort and separate cells in a heterogeneous sample based on certain characteristics, such as their protein expression.

We mention these techniques as a quick heads-up, so they don't catch you off guard if you see them on your exam. The goal of this overview is not to teach you everything about them. In fact, flow cytometry is a great example of a methodological procedure that the MCAT might present without expecting you to know all the details. If a new technique does show up on your MCAT, however, don't allow yourself to be weighed down by unfamiliar terms or by a belief that you have to know absolutely everything about flow cytometry (or whatever new technique is presented) to be successful. Your content knowledge, the information you're given, and strong reasoning skills are all you need.

10. MCAT Experimental Methods: PCR and Sequencing

Polymerase chain reaction, or **PCR**, is a molecular technique used to amplify genetic material. In research labs, PCR is commonly used to create molecular clones and sequence genes, and it's also used to identify pathogens responsible for new outbreaks of infectious disease, in DNA fingerprinting to identify criminals (and exonerate the innocent), and in molecular paternity tests. You may already know that it's used to genotype DNA, such as if you've ever undergone any kind of DNA or ancestry testing. Therefore, PCR can show up in diverse contexts on the MCAT.

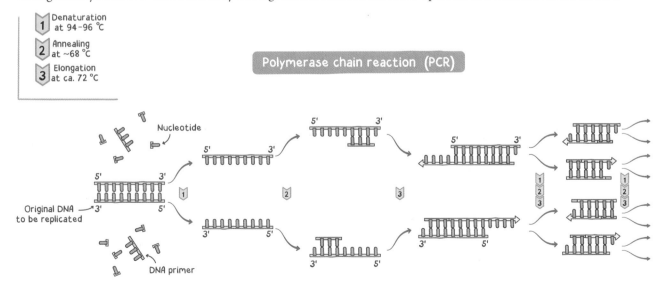

Figure 6. PCR cycles

In a nutshell, PCR uses repeated cycles of heating and cooling to amplify even very small amounts of DNA. So even if a passage doesn't explicitly mention PCR, the word "amplification" should clue you in that this is the method being used. There are a few things to keep in mind when reading about PCR in a passage. First of all, what is the starting material? DNA is used as the starting sample for genotyping or sequencing DNA, of course, but in other situations, we might alternatively want to use RNA, such as if we were interested in studying the mRNA expression of various genes. When RNA is used as the starting sample, it first has to be converted into DNA because PCR exploits cellular replication machinery that replicates DNA, not RNA. Plus, RNA is far less stable than DNA and more difficult to work with. So when RNA is used as the starting sample, the enzyme reverse transcriptase is used to reverse transcribe RNA into DNA before amplification occurs, and this is referred to as reverse transcription PCR, or RT-PCR.

Now, the next question on our minds is: what genes are being studied? PCR is only used to amplify select segments of the genome, typically fragments between 100 and 10,000 base pairs, which means we need forward and reverse primers flanking our genes of interest. Pay attention to the genes being analyzed and the functions or roles of those genes as described in the passage.

Questions like these tie back into the most important question you should be asking yourself: how do these methods facilitate the goals of the experiment? If we're using RT-PCR, we're probably interested in gene expression, so there's a good chance our results will take the form of an electrophoresis gel. You may also see these results depicted in a table representing the presence or absence of specific genes, sometimes with relative expression levels indicated by one or more asterisks or plus signs, as in Figure 6. Additionally, the intensity of the bands on the gel could be quantified as proxy markers of expression levels. In fact, there's even a form of PCR designed expressly for this kind of quantitative analysis, and fittingly, it's called "quantitative PCR."

If we're interested in gene expression on a larger scale, a microarray might come into play. A microarray is essentially a small glass slide or membrane filter spotted with hundreds or thousands of unique DNA fragments that's used to analyze the expression of up to tens of thousands of genes at a time. To prepare a microarray, a sample's mRNA content is isolated and reverse-transcribed into complementary DNA (or cDNA). PCR is then sometimes used to amplify those sequences prior to hybridization on the microarray. Again, this is a place where the passage might describe a sample's genetic material being "amplified" without explicitly mentioning PCR. As with RT-PCR, the results might be presented as raw data in the form of a photograph of the microarray, or the results might be quantified and presented in a table or bar graph. To analyze these results, note that the goal of a microarray is to compare the relative expression of genes between a reference and an experimental sample. In a microarray image, then, red spots indicate genes that are more strongly expressed in the experimental sample, and green spots indicate genes that are more strongly expressed in the control. Relative fluorescence can also be displayed in the form of a table or bar graph, which will often highlight a select number of genes of interest with marked differential expression between the two groups. In fact, sometimes the result is simply the identification of those genes, which is essentially as simple as "these two (or three, or five) genes are expressed more strongly in the experimental sample." Results of this nature might then give way to a follow-up experiment to investigate those genes more thoroughly.

If DNA is used as the starting material for an experiment using PCR, we're not so much interested in the expression of these genes as we are in what those genes actually look like at the nucleotide level. This almost always means one of two experimental outcomes: genotyping or sequencing. Both aim to determine the precise nucleotides that make up genetic material, but they differ in scope. While DNA sequencing looks at the sequence of a stretch of DNA up to the entire genome, genotyping has a narrower focus of looking for specific features of a DNA sequence, like the presence of single nucleotide polymorphisms, variable number tandem repeats, introns, point mutations, and so on.

These days, genotyping is routinely performed using microarrays, in which target sequences hybridize to their complementary sequences on a microarray chip. Alternatively, **sequencing** can be used to genotype DNA. Recall that in Sanger sequencing, after labeled dideoxynucleotides are incorporated into the DNA, the DNA fragments are subjected to gel electrophoresis, which separates the fragments by size such that the shortest fragments migrate farthest through the gel. It's quite possible that you will be presented with a schematic of such a gel and asked to reconstruct the sequence of the DNA segment. Truthfully, this is only a challenging task if it's something you've never done before. If you've done it once or twice, it makes for easy points on the MCAT. All you have to do is start with the shortest fragment, whose label corresponds to the identity of the first nucleotide in the DNA sequence. Then work your way up the gel, with successively longer fragments providing the identity of the next nucleotide in sequence.

As you can imagine, this task would be quite laborious for a thousands-of-nucleotides-long DNA sequence, so these days, the electrophoresis results are typically illuminated by a laser and read by a camera. Those results are generally presented in a fluorescent peak trace chromatograph, which is a little easier to read. All you have to do is read the colored peaks in order from left to right, as each peak corresponds to one position along the length of the DNA sequence, with each color corresponding to one of the 4 nucleotides.

11. MCAT Experimental Methods: Electrophoresis and Blotting

As you already know, **electrophoresis** is a technique that separates charged particles in an electric field. What's more, you can think of an electrophoresis gel as a circuit itself. Since current is the movement of electrically charged particles, you can think of the large, charged molecules in an electrophoresis gel as carrying part of that current through the gel, with buffer solution providing varying levels of resistance.

This points to the interdisciplinary nature of electrophoresis, which bridges physics, chemistry, and biology. Therefore, let's explore the reasoning that underlying how you interact with gel electrophoresis on the MCAT, regardless of the specific context in which it appears. Let's start by talking about the methods and variations on gel electrophoresis that you might encounter in a passage. The first question you should be asking yourself is, what exactly is being electrophoresed? Prior to electrophoresis, the sample is prepared in a specific manner depending on the source material and the purpose of the experiment, so pay attention to what kind of biomolecule we're working with and what questions the experiment intends to answer.

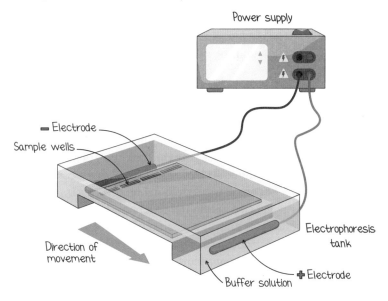

Figure 7. Gel electrophoresis experimental setup

There are a few important methodological considerations at hand. For instance, the type of electrophoresis gel that's used serves a specific function. Your standard gel is composed of an agarose or polyacrylamide matrix, although the exact makeup of the gel is not all that important. Instead, what you should be paying attention to is charge. In a typical gel, negatively charged species will migrate toward the anode of the gel when exposed to an electric field. For this reason, electrophoresis gels normally have a basic pH so that the biomolecules in the sample will carry a negative charge and migrate toward the anode pole of the gel. Thus, if we don't alter the charges of the sample molecules further, their degree of migration down the gel will be affected by their mass, shape, and charge. This is called native gel electrophoresis, and you won't see it very often for protein analysis because it's hard to precisely identify proteins of interest when there are so many factors affecting their movement through the gel. More common is SDS-PAGE, or sodium dodecyl sulfate-polyacrylamide gel electrophoresis, in which the detergent SDS linearizes and applies a uniform, negative charge to all proteins such that their migration is differentially affected by mass alone.

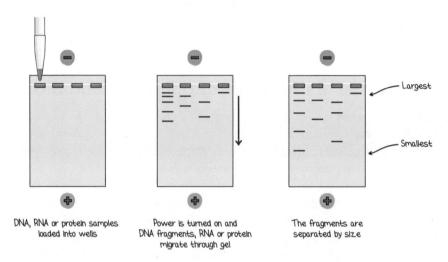

Figure 8. Separation of macromolecules by size in gel electrophoresis

In isoelectric focusing, in contrast, the entire point is to separate molecules by charge. Therefore, we use a gel with a pH gradient that separates compounds by their charge, or, more specifically, by their isoelectric point. If we want even more information about the compounds in our sample, we can combine SDS-PAGE and isoelectric focusing in 2D gel electrophoresis, which separates compounds by size in the first dimension and then by charge in the second dimension.

In some cases, electrophoresis is a procedural step used to separate and isolate biomolecules for the purposes of subsequent cloning or sequencing, for example, but in other cases, the experimental results can be interpreted from the migration patterns on the electrophoresis gel itself. However, since we're unable to see bands on the gel with the naked eye, we might have to take another step to visualize the molecules of interest. The simpler version of this involves staining DNA or protein with a dye, illuminating with UV light, or exposing radiolabeled samples in the gel to X-ray film. A more complex version, known as **western blotting**, involves transfer (or "blotting") of the gel onto another membrane, and then applying labeled antibodies that bind specifically to the proteins of interest on the gel. You're probably familiar with western blotting as a technique used to detect and analyze proteins, most commonly to analyze protein expression. Analogous terms for protein expression like gene expression, protein levels, and transcriptional activity may also hint at the use of a blotting method, but be careful to distinguish between mRNA expression and protein expression. mRNA expression is routinely analyzed using reverse transcription PCR, microarrays, or northern blotting, whereas western blots are used to analyze protein expression.

Regardless of the method of visualization, interpreting the results of an electrophoresis gel involves the same general steps. Reading gels is a skill that takes practice, so let's discuss a few things you should be looking for when analyzing a gel. First, consider the sample under study. Are we looking at a Southern blot for DNA samples, a western blot for protein samples, the results of Sanger sequencing, or something else? Then ask yourself what factors affected the migration pattern: mass, shape, and/or charge? In SDS-PAGE, for example, we'd add the detergent SDS to equalize charge across all proteins, whereas in isoelectric focusing, we wouldn't want to neutralize the effects of charge since differences in charge are the whole point. Another possibility is that a reducing agent like beta-mercaptoethanol was added to the sample to disrupt tertiary and quaternary protein structure to help linearize proteins in the sample.

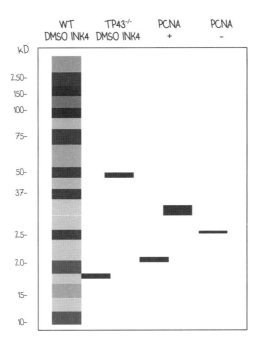

Figure 9. Results of gel electrophoresis of DNA, with ladder

You'll also want to look for a ladder, typically on the leftmost lane of the gel, with known size markers that you can use to estimate the size of sample proteins in adjacent lanes. Also, note the nonlinear relationship between migration distance and size, such that a 50-kDa protein is going to be located closer to the 100-kDa marker than to the 10-kDa marker. The units here hint at the methods: the units of this ladder are shown in kilodaltons, a unit of atomic mass. So there's a good chance these are the results of SDS-PAGE, as the ladder suggests we should be able to distinguish between bands based on mass alone.

Since each lane of the gel normally corresponds to a unique sample, next we want to identify what condition each lane represents. This can sometimes be the trickiest part if there are multiple conditions and acronyms and symbols all over the place. Don't be afraid to refer back to earlier parts of the passage so you know exactly what each acronym refers to and, more importantly, the scientific concept it's meant to represent. One or more lanes may be reserved for positive or negative controls.

There's another kind of control that's commonly used in western blotting, and that's when in addition to the protein of interest, a protein that is expected to be present in approximately equal amounts across samples is also detected on the membrane. A commonly used example is GAPDH, glyceraldehyde 3-phosphate dehydrogenase, a critical housekeeping enzyme that is expressed fairly equally across cells. This controls for the proper loading of samples, such that if levels of GAPDH vary widely across samples, that indicates that perhaps unequal volumes of the various samples were added to the gel or something else is going on that we didn't intend. For this reason, it's not uncommon to standardize or "normalize" expression of the protein of interest to the control protein to account for that source of variation.

In terms of analyzing the bands themselves, your approach is going to depend on the goal of the experiment. If the question is whether or not a given gene or protein is expressed at all, the presence or absence of the expected band in each lane should answer that question. This can also be displayed in the form of a table with plus and minus symbols indicating the presence or absence of each protein. Note that gels aren't always perfectly clean, so a very, very faint band might be treated as a negligible expression level, but the MCAT will not leave this up to personal discretion. On the other hand, if the experiment intends to compare or quantify expression levels, then you'll want to evaluate the intensity of the bands present. On a gel, this will be a relatively subjective, qualitative kind of evaluation, but quantitative analysis is possible if a photograph of the gel is taken and analyzed by densitometry, which quantifies the optical density of each band. Such results can then be presented in a bar graph and evaluated statistically.

How might all this information show up in an MCAT question? As you might expect, you'll definitely be expected to analyze and interpret the significance of electrophoresis results, so the ability to read a gel, identify controls and treatment conditions, and connect the results to the experimental hypothesis will absolutely benefit you. The other way this may show up is in the form of a question that asks about methodology and experimental flaws. For example, suppose you're asked why a single protein with an expected molecular weight of 100 kilodaltons shows up as two distinct bands at 20 and 60 kilodaltons in SDS-PAGE analysis. To answer this question, you should use reverse-engineering and trace back the steps of SDS-PAGE to determine the most logical explanation. In this case, recall that a reducing agent is often used in SDS-PAGE to disrupt quaternary protein structure, breaking apart subunits, which could certainly explain how a 100-kilodalton protein might disassemble into more than one distinct subunit. However, 60 and 20 don't quite add up to 100 kilodaltons. But if the 100-kDa protein disassembles into one 60-kDa subunit and two 20-kDa subunits, that would suffice to explain why it appears as just two bands. Even if you weren't able to make that leap, if you can draw the connection to the use of a reducing agent like beta-mercaptoethanol, you may be able to look at the answer choices to identify an explanation that's reasonable and fits in with your understanding of the science of electrophoresis.

12. MCAT Experimental Methods: Genetic Nomenclature

Imagine growing up using your favorite computer program for years, and then one day, you're given access to the code and allowed to tinker with it, swapping out one element at a time to figure out how it works and make it work even better. That's analogous to the series of breakthroughs scientists had when they first started to develop DNA cloning methods in the 1970s and later sequenced the entire human genome in the early 2000s. With the genome mapped down to the last nucleotide and tools at our hands to silence, swap out, and mutate any gene we want, the possibilities for genetic engineering are almost endless.

A prerequisite to understanding these experiments is mastery of the relevant nomenclature. You're certainly not expected to memorize all the nuances of genetic naming conventions, but familiarity with them can help you decipher complex gene names and relate them back to the experimental methodology. Starting with vertebrates, human genes are given a 3-8-character identifier that is both italicized and in all-caps, and this is the same identifier used for mRNA and cDNA. Proteins use the same identifier, but without italicization, so italics are the key differentiator between genes and proteins. In other vertebrates, the gene may not necessarily be all-capitalized, but the gene will always be italicized and the protein non-italicized. However, there are a few exceptions to these conventions in which an unofficial name is commonly used in place of the official identifier for a protein. For example, the TP53 tumor suppressor protein is more commonly called the p53 protein in the literature, but in any case, the gene name remains italicized and the protein in normal font.

In bacteria, genes are designated by three lowercase letters representing the relevant biological pathway followed by a single capital letter for the actual gene and possibly an allele number. Take the rpoA gene codes for the alpha subunit of RNA polymerase, for example. You'll often see three-letter gene abbreviations for amino acids and metabolic compounds you might recognize, like ala for alanine, and lac for lactose, particularly in the context of the lac operon. When a bacterium is engineered with a gene conferring antibiotic resistance, an abbreviation for the antibiotic is used, followed by the superscript R, as in ampR for ampicillin-resistant bacteria. Like vertebrates, the gene is italicized, but the protein is not.

What it means

CTLA4+/+	Mouse carrying two wild-type alleles of CTLA4 gene (homozygous WT)
CTLA4+/-	Mouse carrying one wild-type and one mutant allele of CTLA4 gene (heterozygous)
CTLA4-/-	Mouse carrying two mutant alleles of CTLA4 gene (homozygous mutant)
thrC	bacterial threonine synthase (italicized for gene, regular for protein)
ΔdnaK	deletion of bacterial dnaK, a chaperone protein
ΔdnaK::thrC	dnaK replaced with threonine synthase gene in bacterial genome

Figure 10. Genetic nomenclature

Where things get more complicated is nomenclature for genetic modifications. When a gene or protein is genetically altered, one way of expressing this is to use superscripts that describe the alteration. For example, "WT" is often used as a superscript to denote wildtype, and something like G172R might be used to denote the replacement of glycine with arginine at the position 172 on the mutant protein. In bacteria, a superscript + symbol will denote wildtype, and a superscript (symbol or no symbol at all) generally denotes the mutant genotype. In *Drosophila*, much of this nomenclature follows similar rules, but you'll also see X-linked mutations given as superscripts to the letter X.

In gene knockout experiments, recall that + and − symbols are used to indicate which gene copies are present for a given gene. For example, *CTLA4*+/+ mice are the wild type, containing normal copies of both alleles of the *CTLA4* gene; *CTLA4*+/- mice are heterozygous mutants, containing only one copy of the wildtype gene; and *CTLA4*-/- mice are homozygous mutants, in which both alleles have been knocked out. If you had previously wondered how such heterozygous and homozygous mutants lost their alleles, gene knockout is the answer! When this nomenclature isn't used, other descriptions of gene knockouts might be used, such as "*CTLA4* knockout mice," "mice heterozygous for or lacking the *CTLA4* gene," "mice in which the *CTLA4* gene was deleted," or "mice engineered to no longer express the *CTLA4* gene." Additionally, you might also see the delta symbol used to indicate a gene deletion, sometimes followed by a double colon and the replacement gene.

13. MCAT Experimental Methods: Genetic Techniques

Now that we've got basic nomenclature out of the way, we're ready to explore the genetic techniques you're most likely to see on the MCAT. Let's start with plasmid-based research models because these methods are notorious for generating confusion on the MCAT. It's less important to know extensive details about plasmids as it is to understand what they allow researchers to do. In short, a **plasmid** is composed of an insert placed into a vector. The insert contains the gene or genes of interest, and the vector contains sequences that enable the construct to do noteworthy things, like confer resistance to an antibiotic or regulate gene expression under specific conditions. Understanding the basic insert-vector anatomy of a plasmid will go a lot farther than getting into the weeds trying to decipher a plasmid description like: "a pREB126 *E. coli* plasmid containing a 2-kb segment of the pVR1 replicon with a pUC19 origin of replication, T7 promoter, a multiple cloning site, a TEV-site, an ampicillin resistance cassette, and an origin of transfer allowing transfer via bacterial conjugation." Most of the time you should avoid getting too bogged down by alphabet soup like this. Instead, focus on any notable features that you recognize, like that ampicillin resistance cassette, the origin of replication, and the promoter.

Among the important landmarks on a plasmid are the restriction sites that flank the insert and vector. When digested by the appropriate restriction enzymes, these sites on the insert and vector become complementary and, if all goes well, will ligate together. One way this might be tested on the MCAT would be if you were asked to identify the appropriate restriction enzymes to use for a cloning experiment. In such a case, you would want to choose two different restriction enzymes that flank both the insert and vector without excising any critical components.

After a restriction digest, the DNA fragments then undergo electrophoresis so that the insert and vector can be isolated from the gel while leaving behind any excess DNA trimmings. This combination of a restriction digest followed by electrophoresis is specifically known as restriction fragment length polymorphism or RFLP analysis, which for a long time formed the basis of DNA fingerprinting before sequencing became more widely available. In essence, this technique identifies unique polymorphisms based on which restriction sites or how many variable number tandem repeats (VNTRs) are present in someone's DNA. For example, suppose you're shown a gel with several DNA samples that have undergone RFLP analysis using the EcoRI restriction enzyme. From a control sample, let's say three bands appear on the gel, and in a disease state, only two bands appear. This suggests that DNA in the disease state lacks one of the restriction sites present on the control DNA, which might be the result of a mutation or deletion. As you might imagine, sequencing provides more granular information about the specific nucleotides in a DNA sequencing, taking out a lot of the guesswork, but unfortunately, this is still a method you should be prepared to see on the MCAT.

There are several synonyms for plasmids and their components to be aware of. In addition to plasmid, insert, and vector, be on the look-out for the terms construct, clone, and transgene. The term "construct," as in a "DNA construct," refers to the same thing as a plasmid, and the term "clone" is sometimes used to refer to a plasmid and at other times used to refer to a group of genetically identical cells derived from a parent cell that incorporated a gene of interest from a plasmid. The term "transgene" refers to the gene of interest on the insert, which might be a novel or mutant gene or a gene from one organism introduced into another organism or species. So when you see these terms, start thinking plasmids.

Plasmids are delivered to cells in one of several ways, which brings us to the three T's of plasmid biology: transformation, transfection, and transduction. Transformation is the uptake of DNA by prokaryotic cells from the environment, and it's a really popular way of mass-producing a specific protein for subsequent protein purification. Transfection refers to the transfer of DNA into eukaryotic cells. Eukaryotic cells are a bit more stubborn and require a reagent that permeabilizes the plasma membrane to promote uptake of external DNA. Researchers then can select for clones that have successfully been transfected and incorporated the gene of interest into their genomes. Finally, transduction refers to the infection of eukaryotic cells using a viral vector. This is another common approach that essentially has the same outcome as transfection but by using a different method of DNA transfer.

So if you see any of these terms, you're likely working with some kind of plasmid. Plasmids can do all sorts of interesting things. They're frequently used in cell culture research, but they're also used in animal models and even in human clinical trials. Essentially, they're used any time there is interest in introducing or modifying a target gene. The easiest scenario to imagine is the introduction of a new gene into a genetically engineered cell line or animal.

However, plasmids can also be used to delete genes in what's known as a gene knockout model. If you really want to get rid of a cell's *STAT3* gene and see what happens, one way to do this is to introduce a plasmid that lacks (but is complementary to) the gene of interest. During DNA replication, the hope is that the host genome will undergo homologous recombination with the DNA construct and replace the target gene with the decoy plasmid DNA. Hopefully, all future daughter cells will also lack this gene. A heterozygous knockout is one in which just one allele copy is deleted, and more commonly, a homozygous knockout is one in which both allele copies are deleted. It's also possible to have double knockouts in which two genes are deleted, triple knockouts in which three genes are deleted, and so on, depending on the complexity of the experiment.

Gene knockouts are a highly powerful technique, but they pose some practical challenges. For one, gene knockouts can be quite expensive and require tremendous resources, especially in animal models. Furthermore, depending on the target gene, a knockout animal model might not be viable. Therefore, in some cases it can be useful to use gene silencing as a non-permanent approach. Gene silencing takes advantage of RNA interference by introducing small interfering RNA or short hairpin RNA that binds to and inactivates complementary mRNA, thereby suppressing the expression of target genes for as long as the interfering RNA is present. These kinds of experimental set-ups are ripe for questions about identifying complementary nucleic acid sequences, and they're ripe for interpreting the effects of the loss of a gene product.

The key aspect of analyzing gene knockout and gene silencing studies is understanding that a gene or two is deleted or silenced, at which point all sorts of follow-up questions are possible: What do the cells' gene expression profiles look like? What are their survival rates? How responsive are they to various treatments? Interpreting the results of such experiments might at first be counterintuitive because we're used to thinking in terms of adding a gene or treatment and then measuring its effects. Instead, in gene knockout and gene silencing studies, we're examining how the loss of a gene affects cellular behavior, which requires us to use careful logic.

In the absence of a gene, if the result is the complete loss of some effect or the elimination of some biological outcome, then we can conclude that the gene in question must be essential for that biological process. For example, if deletion of the *STAT3* gene results in phosphorylation of Akt proteins being completely eliminated, we can conclude that the STAT3 protein is required for Akt phosphorylation. Now, if deletion of this gene results in a diminished effect, like reduced Akt phosphorylation, then we could conclude that STAT3 plays some kind of important role but that other factors allow for some Akt phosphorylation in the absence of STAT3. In fact, it might be the case that deleting *STAT3* alone doesn't completely eradicate Akt phosphorylation, and deleting some other gene doesn't completely eradicate it either, but together they abolish Akt phosphorylation when deleted. This indicates that one can compensate for the loss of the other to some extent, but at least one is required for this biological process. And finally, if gene deletion results in an enhanced effect, such as if *STAT3* deletion results in greater Akt phosphorylation, then we can conclude that STAT3 plays some kind of inhibitory or otherwise regulatory role when present. We could further support these conclusions if we re-introduced the STAT3 protein and show that Akt phosphorylation was recovered or restored to normal levels. Consider mapping this out on your wet-erase board if needed: if the absence of X gene results in Y outcome, the presence of that gene should result in the reciprocal outcome.

14. Must-Knows

> Some especially key points about study design (see Psychology and Sociology Chapter 1 for more details):
  - Study design: choice depends largely on nature of phenomenon under investigation.
  - Experimental study design: manipulate independent variable and measure dependent variable.
  - Observational study design: observe what happens without direct intervention.
  - Forms of bias may be a concern (e.g., sampling bias from non-random population inclusion).
  - Moderating variables affect the strength of a relationship; mediating variables explain a relationship by providing a mechanism, confounding variables affect both sides of a relationship.
> Primary research passages tend to present background, purpose/hypothesis, methods/materials, and results, often in order.
> Some potential flaws to be on the lookout for:
  - Internal validity (ability to infer causal relationships) can be impeded by confounding variables, bias, and poor design.
  - External validity (or generalizability) can be impeded by highly controlled design, insufficient sample size, sampling bias, non-random assignment.
> Common independent variables:
  - Time and concentration: often on x-axis of line graphs or bar graphs.
  - Presence or absence of some condition.
  - Mutations (presence/absence).
> Common outcomes measured:
  - Changes in physical/chemical properties, like pressure, boiling point: generally straightforward, but watch out for direct measurements vs. ratios.
  - Biological outcomes: growth, gene expression, binding affinity; again, care is needed to analyze details of how information is presented properly.
> Common methods to familiarize yourself with:
  - Cell culture: key is to focus on treatment groups and outcomes, abstract away from details.
  - PCR: be sure to understand which genes are being amplified and why; what is relationship to goal of the experiment?
  - Sequencing: how does that relate to experimental question?
  - Electrophoresis and blotting: note conditions of electrophoresis (e.g., native, reducing, etc.) and nature of biomolecule being analyzed (protein [western blotting], DNA [Southern blotting], RNA [northern blotting]).
  - Genetic techniques: review terminology in Sections 12-13, especially related to mutations and plasmids; again, focus on purpose/goals of experiment.

Applied Practice

The best MCAT practice is realistic, with detailed analytics to help you assess where things went wrong. For those reasons, we recommend completing practice questions in an online setting that simulates the real MCAT interface, and using the analytics provided to help you decide how to best move your studies forward.

CARS does not require knowledge of specific subject areas, but it does require development of strong test-taking skills. To ensure you are honing those skills as you work through this book, we suggest you go online after wrapping up each chapter and generate a Qbank Practice Set of 2-3 CARS passages to practice and review. While not every chapter of this book is directly applicable to CARS, regular CARS practice is key to test day success.

As a further supplement, given the importance of active learning for effective studying, we also suggest that you consult the Must-Knows at the end of each chapter of this Reasoning text as a basis for creating a study sheet. This is not a sheet to memorize in the more traditional sense of content memorization, but rather a quick reference of the most important strategies for you to refer to during and after practice in your early prep. Frequently revisiting the most important strategies for the MCAT - in both CARS and the Sciences - will help you continue to improve your performance.

This page left intentionally blank.

Answering Science Questions

0. Introduction

We all know that the killer MCAT score you're looking for depends entirely upon your ability to get questions correct in the time allowed. This is definitely easier said than done, though. Even relatively straightforward questions on the MCAT require an understanding of both how the question is worded and the science itself. More complex questions might require you to integrate or apply that science to contexts you've never seen before. The goal of this chapter is to give you a framework for tackling science questions.

As an important methodological point before we get started, our strategy here is not to make you read this chapter once and absorb every point within the chapter. Instead, practice is essential. Answering questions isn't an all-or-nothing process. Finding the correct answer often requires multiple steps, and it's possible to miss a question even if you did some of those steps correctly. Focusing on taking a question one step at a time both helps you parse out exactly where you're falling prey to question traps and gives you discrete, manageable goals to work toward. The goal of this chapter, therefore, is to provide strategies that will give you the tools (and confidence) to handle any question thrown your way.

1. Getting Started

As a broad overview, there are four steps to tackling MCAT questions:

> Interpreting the question
> Getting the information you need to answer the question
> Making a generalized prediction
> Evaluating the answer choices

The first step, interpreting the question, means understanding exactly what you're being asked. This may seem straightforward, but it's especially important for questions that are confusing or easy to misinterpret. In such cases, interpreting the question is simply a matter of taking a moment to paraphrase the question in a way that makes sense to you.

Here's a prime example of a long-winded psych/soc question:

> Jane is part of a large group of friends wishing Alice a happy birthday. As the group sings "Happy Birthday," Jane gets distracted, checks her phone, and winds up singing along very quietly, missing some lines. What concept from group psychology best explains this behavior?
>
> A. Peer pressure
>
> B. Socialization
>
> C. Social loafing
>
> D. Bystander effect

It's a common pattern for MCAT science questions to present an example or analogy of some scientific concept, where these questions naturally run on the longer side. Our job is to trim away the details to reveal what the question is asking. In this case, we can conceptualize this question stem as describing an individual who doesn't fully participate and exerts less effort in a group setting. It's only after we understand the question that we can begin evaluating our answer choices, which is a process we'll be examining later in the chapter. For now, the point is that we need to paraphrase the question stem into a shorter summary that better captures its main idea.

In addition to paraphrasing, another useful strategy is to highlight the words that express the basic idea of a long or multi-part question stem. However, if you do so, remember to keep the highlighting to a minimum. Paraphrasing and highlighting can come in handy in special circumstances, such as NOT, EXCEPT, or LEAST questions, for which it may be useful to highlight these words in the question stem and rephrase the question in positive words.

Don't get too bogged down if you encounter unfamiliar terms in a question stem (whether that's an acronym from the passage, or the name of an unfamiliar chemical, or a new technique you've never heard of before). For such questions, it can be useful to substitute each term with a placeholder when paraphrasing. These placeholders can be general, or, if the passage gave some information about the unfamiliar term, they can be more specific. For instance, the question, "Flow cytometry was used to analyze pre-pro-opiomelanocortin in the AtT20 cell line for what purpose?" can be made a little more manageable by rephrasing it as "Why was this particular cell sorting technique used to study the precursor to ACTH in a pituitary cell line?"

If you're still puzzled by the question stem, it may be best to move on to the answer choices, as reading through them may shed new light on the question and can aid in your interpretation.

For passage-based questions, interpreting the question stem also involves determining whether a question stem truly requires passage information, or is a **pseudodiscrete**," a term that we use for questions that do not require the passage to correctly answer, even though they are tied to a specific passage. In other words, what we're assessing here is the degree to which the question requires passage information, outside science knowledge, or both.

Most questions associated with a passage will require some passage information, but the amount varies. Some may simply require you to recognize a fact, like the idea that pre-pro-opiomelanocortin is a peptide hormone precursor, while others require you to analyze or synthesize multiple facts. Others might require you to examine and draw conclusions from a figure. You can be more confident that a question requires passage information if it directly refers back to a specific paragraph or figure, or if it refers to a technique, perspective, or term from the passage. You might not remember every term and technique mentioned in the passage after your initial read-through, so if a term is unfamiliar, that may be a signal that it comes from the passage. If the answer choices refer back to terms or concepts from the passage, that is also a signal that the question draws upon passage information.

To establish whether a question is a pseudodiscrete, pretend you don't have the associated passage directly in front of you. Does the question stand on its own? Does it test concepts that are exclusively covered by the MCAT curriculum? For instance, a passage about how the circulatory system could be modeled from a biophysics perspective might just throw in a question that draws only on your knowledge about fluids. If you encounter a question like this, and you understand what it's asking and how to answer it, go for it! Where it gets tricky is that sometimes you might sense that a question could be a pseudodiscrete, in that it draws on concepts that are covered in the content sections of the MCAT curriculum, but you personally might not feel very confident about your knowledge. In this case, there's nothing wrong with briefly skimming the passage, as it may contain some useful clues.

Even if a question is entirely answerable using outside content knowledge, the passage may reiterate some of background information in the introduction or present hints elsewhere. In particular, this can happen for questions drawing on content knowledge at the fringes of what the MCAT tests. The point is not that you should go back to the passage for every pseudodiscrete question, but if you're completely stuck on what you think is a pseudodiscrete question, you have nothing to lose by doing a quick skim of the passage for related topics. That said, the converse danger—of trying to integrate passage information for literally everything—can also be very real. Some pseudodiscrete questions are quite simple if you've studied the relevant materials, and if feel that you've understood what the question is asking and why the correct choice is correct, don't psych yourself out by thinking that every single question must draw on the passage in some non-obvious way.

To reiterate, the first step in our process is to understand what the question is asking, and what science and passage information are needed to answer it. With this in mind, let's move on to discuss the remaining steps to tackling science questions.

2. Working Through the Question

The second step in answering a question is gathering all the information you need to answer the question. You may or may not need to return to the passage. There's not a one-size-fits-all trick about when to return to the passage, as all people vary in what they remember. However, the only cost associated with going back to the passage is time, so if you think there's a chance the passage could help you, you should return to the passage. If a question tests the main idea or a major theme that requires an entire re-reading of the passage, you may instead want to rely on your memory and comprehension of the passage as a whole.

If you return to the passage, it's in your best interest to do so strategically and efficiently. Your ability to do this will be supported by reading the passage thoroughly on the first pass and highlighting in such a way that creates a passage map, so you can quickly identify the relevant parts to return to. Once you've identified where to look—either based on where the question tells you to look, or key ideas or terms referenced in the question stem—then you're in the right neighborhood as the information you need is almost always in the vicinity — if not within the same sentence, or flanking sentences and same paragraph.

In some cases, you may need more than one piece of information from the passage. This tends to occur for questions that require information from a figure, table, equation, or constant in addition to other textual information that provides the necessary context. If you're ever stumped, a quick, 10-second skim of your highlighting should help remind you of any related concepts discussed in the passage. There will also be cases for which you'll need to return to the passage for each answer choice. This usually occurs with relatively open-ended question stems that have four answer choices that refer back to four different parts of the passage. Your best bet is to evaluate each option one by one, and if you're running low on time, it's okay to stop and move on once you're confident that you've identified the correct answer.

You'll also need to determine what outside science information is necessary, if any. This decision is inherently linked to your ability to paraphrase the question stem in an effective manner. For example, suppose we're asked: *What work is performed on a 3000-kg SUV accelerating from 0 to 30 m/s?*

Of course, there are many different equations for work. Knowing which one to use requires us to examine the information we're given, and draw connections to the broader scientific concepts tested by the question. Here, we're given information about the vehicle's mass and velocity at its initial and final states, and, most importantly, we're asked for the amount of work performed as it accelerates. If this were a passage-associated question, there may be more information in the passage we'd need to consider, but fortunately this appears to be a fairly straightforward discrete question. Now, you might recognize that the SUV's mass and velocity give us all the information we need to calculate its kinetic energy, or more specifically, its change in kinetic energy as it accelerates.

Therefore, we might initially paraphrase this question as, "What equation can we use for work knowing a moving object's mass and initial and final velocity?" Then, hopefully, as you draw the connections between work and kinetic energy, this will crystallize in your mind as a work-energy theorem problem that can be solved using the equation that equates work with the change in kinetic energy.

After gathering the information we need from the passage and from our arsenal of scientific knowledge, it's now time to make a prediction, by making a general conceptualization of what you're looking for in the right answer and what you're trying to avoid in the wrong answers. Predictions can save you time by helping you focus in on the correct answer in an efficient manner, and they also help you avoid tempting or distracting wrong answer choices. They can be especially helpful on questions that require you to start with a broad, generalized principle and then find a specific example or analogy among the answer choices that is the best fit.

An example of how predictions could play out in the Chemical and Physical Foundations section might include a question about which element has the smallest radius. Based on general scientific knowledge, you can predict that this will be an element located near the top right of the periodic table. Then you can review the answer choices and pick the one with the smallest atomic radius on that basis. In the Biological and Biochemical Foundations section, you might be asked about amino acids that tend to be found in the interior of proteins in an aqueous solution. In such a case, correctly predicting that such amino acids are likely to be hydrophobic will help you immediately concentrate on finding a hydrophobic amino acid without being distracted by the other answer choices. In the Psychology and Sociology section, it's common to be presented with a psychology or sociology concept in the question stem (e.g. the bystander effect) and then be asked to select the example or analogy that best demonstrates this concept among the answer choices.

Of course, predictions won't be necessary or even helpful for every question. For example, an open-ended question like "Which of the following interpretations is best supported by the results presented in the passage?" does not lend itself well to predictions. We might get some benefit by briefly reviewing the logic of an experiment and its major findings, but ultimately, we're not going to be able to get very far without examining the answer choices.

But for those questions that do benefit from making a prediction, once we have that prediction in mind, our last step—and the most crucial—is to evaluate the answer choices. Identifying and eliminating wrong answers in the science sections is covered elsewhere in this chapter. As a brief note, however, evaluating the answer choices generally involves a combination of identifying the characteristics of correct answer choices and identifying reasons to eliminate wrong answer choices. If approaching a question from one direction (by looking for the right answer) isn't working, approaching it from the other direction (by eliminating the wrong answers) may yield better results.

3. Science Questions in Practice

No matter how robust your reasoning toolkit is, odds are good that you'll get stumped from time to time. When this happens, half the battle is avoiding getting stuck in your head. Sometimes all you need is a fresh perspective. So, once you realize you're not making progress on a question, first try re-reading the question stem. Ask yourself if there might be a clue from the passage or some other science concept you haven't taken into consideration yet. Give yourself a limit so you're not spending minutes on the question, which is counterproductive, and then give it your best guess, flag the question, and move on, with the understanding that you'll have an opportunity to come back to it later if time permits.

A common question is: *What questions should I be flagging?* It's tempting to think you should flag every question where you aren't certain of the correct answer. However, uncertainty is a very broad. Odds are that you'll only feel absolutely confident of your answer selection on a subset of questions. Therefore, it's very difficult to establish a certainty threshold for which questions to flag. What's more, thinking about things in terms of certainty isn't the most helpful from the cold, rational perspective of maximizing your score. Instead, you should try to flag the questions that stand the most to gain from additional time or a fresh perspective, including ones where something hasn't quite "clicked" just yet, questions that started to frustrate you and caused you to lose focus, or those involving time-consuming calculations that you'd like to try again or check your work on. Try to limit flagged questions to under 25% of questions in a section so you can be strategic about the use of your review time.

When you've reached the end of the section, you'll see three options for reviewing questions at the bottom of your review screen: Review All, Review Incomplete, and Review Flagged. Make sure you haven't left any questions incomplete or unseen, and address those questions first. Then, clicking "Review Flagged" will allow you to revisit just your flagged questions. This extra time during the review period may afford you the second wind you need to focus exclusively on difficult or time-consuming questions, without the added stress of seven incomplete passages ahead of you. You may also return to these questions with a fresh perspective, having answered the other questions associated with that passage if it's a passage-based question, or perhaps after being reminded of a related science concept on a subsequent question. This is your chance to take a deeper dive on complex questions and seek that "Aha!" moment.

Fortunately, however, getting stuck is something you can prepare for. The first thing you can do is diagnose patterns in your performance in terms of the types of questions that tend to leave you stumped. Throughout your MCAT prep, periodically take a look at your recent score performance, and ask yourself questions like:

> Do you tend to flag questions associated with content areas you haven't studied yet?
> Are your flagged questions more likely to ask about figures, involve multi-step calculations, or have Roman numerals?
> Do you tend to answer these questions incorrectly, or do you change your answer from incorrect to correct when you have a chance to review them?

Based on these patterns, set actionable goals for yourself. If you appear to be missing questions based on content deficiencies, you have several options for reviewing scientific content. If you notice that a particular question type tends to trip you up, pay special attention to these question types in practice and work on identifying what you could do differently to answer them correctly on your real MCAT. If your flagging strategy isn't working for you (maybe you're over-flagging or missing lots of unflagged questions), that's certainly something you can work on during your next Full Length practice test. If your major issue is not having sufficient time to review, we suggest reviewing the timing and pacing strategies we discussed elsewhere in this book.

4. Special Question Types: Part 1

Although the MCAT does test a very broad range of scientific knowledge and skills, the specific questions tend to follow some general trends, and being aware of those patterns will help you take the test more effectively. In this section, we'll discuss some examples of commonly occurring question types in the science sections, namely: Analogy, Roman numeral, Two-Part, Ranking, Quantitative, and Figure questions.

Analogy questions present a scientific concept in the question stem and then ask for an example, or analogy, to that concept. Alternatively, they can present an analogy to a scientific concept in the question stem, and ask you to identify that concept among the answer choices. This question type is especially prevalent in the Psychology/Sociology section. In fact, the question that we previously used to discuss how to paraphrase is an Analogy question:

> Jane is part of a large group of friends wishing Alice a happy birthday. As the group sings "Happy Birthday," Jane gets distracted, checks her phone, and winds up singing along very quietly, missing some lines. What concept from group psychology best explains this behavior?
>
> A. Peer pressure
>
> B. Socialization
>
> C. Social loafing
>
> D. Bystander effect

Notice how the question stem presents a descriptive example of an individual's behavior, or what you can almost think of as a case study for some psychological or sociological phenomenon. Our job is to recognize the basic pattern represented in this question and match it to the correct term among the answer choices. As discussed above, we could paraphrase this as a scenario in which an individual participates less fully or exerts less effort in a group setting. Now, all we have to do is tap into our psychology and sociology knowledge and pull out the correct term.

Fortunately, we only need to choose between four answer choices, so we can first eliminate peer pressure and socialization, which have to do with how people conform to or acquire norms. Jane's not really acquiring norms, so much as side-stepping her duties as a friend because her other friends are carrying the load. The bystander effect is related to the presence of others, but it more so has to do with how likely observers are to intervene in a situation in which someone requires help when others are present. The best fit is choice C, social loafing, which describes the tendency for people to participate less intensely in a group setting because other members of the group are pulling the majority of the weight. In this analogy, we can think of Jane as loafing around while her friends as busy singing their hearts out for their dear friend Alice.

The reciprocal example of an Analogy question would be if the question stem introduced a Psych/Soc concept, and then required us to identify an appropriate example. For example, we might be asked "Which of the following is an example of social loafing?" followed by four answer choices, each of which describes an individual or group's circumstances and behaviors. This is where making a prediction comes in handy, as having a general idea of what to look for will help us focus in on the correct answer without being distracted by tempting wrong choices. Therefore, if we go into such a question thinking, "Hmm, which of these best exemplifies someone who's slacking off while expecting the rest of the group to do the bulk of the work?" This should guide us to the right answer.

Analogy questions are common in the Psychology and Sociology section, so on your next full length, see if you can start recognizing these patterns. **Roman numeral questions**, by contrast, appear in all sections of the test. Here's an example:

In military training, an intense sense of group belonging coexists with extensive formal rules and regulations. Which of the following group psychology concepts likely apply in this situation?

I. Formal social control
II. Informal social control
III. Peer pressure

A. I only

B. I and II

C. II and III

D. I. II, and III

Our approach to Roman numeral questions is to first evaluate the numeral that appears in exactly two answer choices. If this choice is true, we can eliminate any answer choices that lack this Roman numeral, and if it's false, then we can eliminate any answer choices that contain it. Thus, let's begin with Roman numeral III since it appears in both choices C and D. Numeral III is peer pressure. Even those of us who haven't undergone military training can understand how peer pressure may reinforce certain social expectations, especially when those pressures come from an "intense sense of group belonging." Based on this, we can eliminate choices A and B because they do not contain Roman numeral III. From here, we need only evaluate Roman numeral I to decide between choices C and D. Numeral I is formal social control. Formal rules and regulations certainly fall under the definition of formal social control, so we can confidently choose choice D. For the sake of completeness, numeral II reads informal social control. This term refers to the reactions by individuals that enforce community and social standards, and includes peer pressure. Numeral II is definitely true, but notice that, by using our strategy, we really didn't even need to evaluate II. This is precious time we saved!

Elimination is also a suitable strategy for our next category of questions: **Two-Part questions**. Consider the following example:

In which of the following ways does an inclined plane differ from a lever?

A. An inclined plane should never have a mechanical advantage less than 1, while a lever can.

B. A lever should never have a mechanical advantage less than 1, while an inclined plane can.

C. Inclined planes and levers should never have a mechanical advantage less than 1.

D. Both inclined planes and levers may have a mechanical advantage less than 1.

Note how each answer choice has two parts that you must evaluate separately. In this way, two-part questions are similar to Roman numeral questions in that you must make determinations on multiple pieces of information, and for this reason, elimination also makes for a useful strategy. With these question types, the structure of the answer choices shows us which decisions we have to make. In this case, we have to decide (1) whether an inclined plane's mechanical advantage can drop below 1, and (2) whether a lever's mechanical advantage can drop below 1.

Let's evaluate each independently. What do we know about an inclined plane's mechanical advantage? Well, the mechanical advantage of an inclined plane is equal to the ratio of its length to its height, but the height can never exceed its length. It's mathematically impossible. The implication of this is the mechanical advantage must never be less than 1. This allows us to eliminate choices B and D. Next, what about levers? It is possible for levers to have a mechanical advantage less than 1, if the output distance is greater than its input distance. The forearm is actually a great example of this. In the human body, the elbow acts as a fulcrum as the muscles of the forearm contract to lift whatever the hand is holding. This actually requires more effort relative to the load, so you could call it a mechanical disadvantage. Where the physiological advantage comes in is that this is compensated by a large movement of the forearm (over a greater output distance) produced by just a small muscle contraction. Therefore, levers can have a mechanical advantage of less than 1, while inclined planes cannot. Thus, choice A must be correct.

Many two-part questions will be like this one, with two relatively independent parts to each answer choice. An analogous example would be if a question asked you to predict the direction of a temperature change and the direction of a pH change needed to increase the reaction rate for some chemical process.

In other cases, the two parts may be closely intertwined, such as in questions where the first part provides a short one- or two-word answer, followed by its rationale. For example, we might be asked if a particular conclusion is supported from a passage, and each answer choice might begin with the word "Yes" or "No," followed by a reason for that conclusion. In this case, the order of investigating each of the two parts does matter, as typically you'll want to arrive at the correct conclusion first, and then match your reasoning to the explanation provided. However, if you're stuck on the first part, you can eliminate answer choices by ruling out their explanations. But when you're making your answer selection, make sure that the explanation provides solid justification for the initial conclusion. The second part to the answer choice might be a true or scientifically accurate statement, but if it doesn't answer the question or explain the first part of the answer choice, then it's not correct.

Next, **Ranking questions** most often occur in the Chemical and Physical Foundations section. Generally speaking, Ranking questions won't literally ask you to rank choices in increasing or decreasing order, but they will ask you to identify the choice that has the greatest or least value of some scientific property. Examples might include questions that ask you to identify the element with the largest atomic radius, or the organic molecule with the lowest boiling point. However, the question might not directly tell you what property they're testing. For instance, a question about atomic radius might be disguised as a question about chemical reactivity, while another question might ask you what compound would distill first from a vacuum distillation apparatus when it's really asking you which compound has the lowest boiling point. The key to answering these questions, is to first identify it as a Ranking question, and then determine the scientific property in question. Next, figure out what factors you can use to differentiate between the answer choices that relate to the property in question. If you aren't sure which answer choice fits the bill, try eliminating any intermediate choices or those with any disqualifying factors so that you at least have a 50/50 shot between the extremes when selecting your final answer.

5. Special Question Types: Part 2

In this section, we'll discuss **Quantitative questions**, which include all math, calculation, formula, and Figure questions. Quantitative questions can be quite diverse. You might be asked to utilize a new formula, recall a formula from your content knowledge, or perform math without any formula at all. Moreover, you may be expected to make a broad estimation, calculate a precise value, or simply evaluate the relationships between multiple variables.

Let's return to a question that came up earlier in our discussion: *What is the work performed on a 3000-kg SUV accelerating from 0 to 30 m/s?* Once we establish that we're looking for the work performed on a vehicle as it accelerates based on its mass and initial and final velocities, we next need to ask: What MCAT concepts are at play here? Perhaps more importantly, what MCAT formulas are needed?

If you aren't sure what formula to use, it may be helpful to consider all the variables that we need to account for, and it may even be beneficial to jot them all down on your wet-erase board. Here we need an equation that involves some combination of work, mass, initial velocity, and/or final velocity. Kinetic energy is defined as $\frac{1}{2}mv^2$, so if kinetic energy comes to mind, you're on the right track! In fact, since we have both the initial and final velocities, we can solve for the change in kinetic energy from the initial to final state. We also know that work is closely related to energy, as they both share the units of joules. By now we've hopefully drawn a connection to the work-energy theorem, specifically the definition of work as the change in kinetic energy. So now we can set up our equation, as $W = KE_f - KE_i$ and plug in our values, which can be done on your wet-erase board, using the following steps:

$$W = KE_f - KE_i$$

$$W = \tfrac{1}{2}mv^2_f - \tfrac{1}{2}mv^2_i$$

$$W = \tfrac{1}{2}(3000\text{kg})(30\text{m/s})^2 - \tfrac{1}{2}(3000\text{kg})(0\text{m/s})^2$$

$$W = 1{,}350{,}000 \text{ J}$$

We do have to be careful when performing calculations. Just because you've calculated a value that matches one of the answer choices doesn't mean you've identified the correct answer. More often than not, wrong answer choices will be carefully selected based on predicted problem-solving errors or common miscalculations, such as choices involving the wrong units or order of magnitude. Because the AAMC is tricky, be sure to check your work!

Furthermore, you won't have a calculator on your exam. Therefore, it's important both to be careful and to become familiar with estimation. A helpful trick is to be sure to check that your units work out to be equal on both sides of the equation before you start solving. This often comes up in thermodynamics problems where you might be given an enthalpy or heat value that uses kilojoules, and a specific heat or entropy value that uses joules, and there may be a trap answer choice lying in wait for the student who forgets to convert from one to the other.

Note that we didn't stop to make a prediction before solving the question, as you won't get very far by trying to predict specific numeric values. However, there is value in comparing your answer choice to what might be a reasonable prediction for the question at hand. For example, would it be reasonable to expect negative work to have been performed on the SUV? No, because the SUV's kinetic energy increases, so work must have been performed on the vehicle, and it should be a positive value. If our calculation tells us otherwise, we might've reversed the initial and final kinetic energy terms in our equation. Would it be reasonable to expect something very small, like 1 joule of work, to have been performed on the SUV? No, because 1 joule doesn't correspond to very much energy. That's enough energy to power a 100-watt light bulb for one one-hundredth of a second.

In this problem, we only had one equation to consider. But what if we were told the SUV's acceleration occurred over an interval of 10 seconds, and we were asked to calculate the power? In this case, we'd need the equation that states that power equals work over time ($P = \frac{W}{t}$). In such cases, it can be helpful to work backwards. In other words, start by identifying what you're asked to calculate and any equations you can use to do so. Then, identify what equations we need for those variables. Logically, we can represent the process as follows:

$$P = \frac{W}{t}$$

$$P = \frac{\Delta KE}{\Delta t}$$

$$P = \frac{(KE_f - KE_i)}{\Delta t}$$

$$P = \frac{(\frac{1}{2}mv_f^2 - \frac{1}{2}mv_i^2)}{\Delta t}$$

That said, it's entirely up to you whether you prefer to write out a single complicated equation, like $P = (\frac{1}{2}mv_f^2 - \frac{1}{2}mv_i^2)/t$, or to calculate work in a separate step and then substitute that into the equation $P = \frac{W}{t}$. As you work through practice materials, try to identify which approach is more intuitive to you, and, crucially, try to determine which way allows you to check your work more effectively.

Science questions that involve figures are also common. This includes everything from molecular structures, to experimental set-ups, to figures with data. That last category includes things like graphs and tables, which are commonly used to present experimental data in primary research passages or even reference data in informational, textbook-style passages. You may not be told when or which or how many figures to refer back to, which underscores the importance of thoroughly reading the passage and coming away with a general sense of the story each figure tells, before you even get to the questions. In particular, if you're asked something broad and open-ended like, "What conclusions can be drawn based on Figure 1?," you'll have a head start if you know what experimental question it's designed to address, and any larger patterns or trends you noticed on the graph.

When you encounter a Figure question, the first thing to determine is whether the question refers to information presented in passage figures that you should return to. Is the question open-ended, and asks for general conclusions based on data, or does it ask something more specific about one or more figures? Next, go back to the figure. Even if it's just a basic force diagram you could recreate, we don't want to leave any room for error. That figure is there for a reason. Then, try to come to your own conclusions based on the figure and make a prediction. Consider whether you need any more information to answer the question, either from elsewhere in the passage or from outside science knowledge. Finally, evaluate the answer choices as you normally would.

If you encounter a more open-ended question with multiple possible conclusions that could be drawn based on passage figures, it'll be worth your while to investigate each possibility fully so you aren't enticed by alluring, but misleading, answer choices before finding the best fit. Along those same lines, it's important to avoid assuming that a given question must refer to a particular figure, especially when that question doesn't reference the figure specifically. This often happens with passages that contain a single graph, especially when that graph looks complex or difficult to interpret - it's easy to assume that your answer will be found in that graph. But in reality, it's possible that the question isn't asking about that figure at all and that the answer can be found elsewhere in the passage. To avoid falling for traps here, first make sure that the experimental question the graph was designed to address is aligned with what the question is asking. Second, if you do return to the graph, but simply can't figure out the answer no matter how hard you try, ask yourself whether you may have jumped to conclusions and went back to the wrong part of the passage.

6. Identifying the Correct Answer

Just like there are only so many ways you can ask a question about the power of a lens or the index of refraction, there are only so many tricky ways to write a clever or tempting wrong answer choice. Understanding these patterns should give you a better idea of what to expect and allow you to recognize wrong answers when you see them, which will hopefully make this whole experience less daunting. Breaking down the anatomy of a science question and understanding its logic is kind of like revealing the man behind the curtain, stripping away its mystique so we can dissect it part by part.

In the broadest sense, science answers can only be wrong for one of three reasons:

> Being scientifically wrong
> Being wrong based on the information in the passage or question prompt
> Containing a reasoning flaw, even if they technically don't violate any science or passage information (for example, if an answer choice doesn't actually address what the question is asking)

Therefore, in order to answer a question correctly, you must first get your science knowledge in order, and then you must make sure you're interpreting new information correctly, and finally you have to make sure you're using air-tight logic.

Let's try working through an example. Consider this passage on optics:

Light typically propagates through a medium in a linear fashion. However, if light moves into a different medium or hits a curved lens, it will change direction. The refractive index of the medium will determine the angle of these changes. Positive lenses have a focal length greater than zero, while negative lenses scatter incoming light beams and have a negative focal length. Figure 1 shows typical shapes of a positive and negative lens, where R is the radius of curvature for each lens.

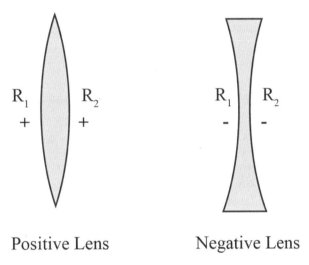

Figure 1. Positive (L) and negative (R) lenses

Figure 2 is an optical representation of the human eye, which is a transparent, biconvex structure with a focal length approximately equal to the distance from the lens to the retina. These dimensions ensure that incoming light is refracted such that it will be focused on the retina.

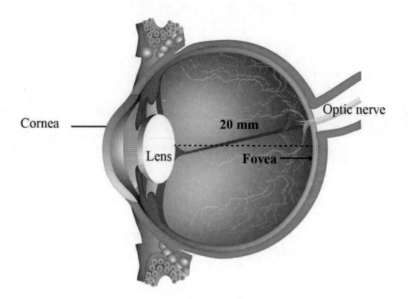

Figure 2. Human eye

True lenses have a non-negligible thickness. This causes the lens to have two radii of curvature, one at the front and another at the rear. The approximate equation relating focal length and radii of curvature for these lenses is given by the following equation:

$$\frac{1}{f} = (n - 1)[\frac{1}{R_1} - \frac{1}{R_2}]$$

where f is the focal length, n is the refractive index of the lens material, and R_1 and R_2 are the front and back radii of curvature, respectively.

The human fovea is where most of the rods and cones are concentrated. These receptors are stimulated by the light coming through the eyes and are responsible for visual perception. The cornea has its own lens with a fixed radius of curvature while the focal length of the eye lens is under muscular control. When relaxed, the radius of curvature is at its largest. The relationship between a source of light, the focal length of a lens, and the distance to the image created by the lens is given by:

$$\frac{1}{f} = \frac{1}{i} + \frac{1}{o}$$

where o is the distance from the object to the lens, and i is the distance from the lens to the image (i.e., the distance at which the image will be clear).

Let's assume that the first question we encounter for this passage is:

Which of the following best explains why older people have a hard time focusing on nearby objects?

A. Muscle weakness around the eye lens inhibits shortening of the radius of curvature.

B. Muscle weakness around the eye lens inhibits lengthening of the radius of curvature.

C. Muscle paralysis around the eye lens inhibits shortening of the radius of curvature.

D. All of the parts of the eye naturally become stiffer and weaker with age.

This question asks us about the biological structures and functions that allow us to focus on nearby objects, as well as how those structures are affected by aging. Let's see what the passage has to say about this. Paragraph 2 reminds us that the human eye is basically a fancy lens. So if the eye is a lens, what does that have to do with viewing up-close objects? From a physics standpoint, the distance of the object from the lens (or "o") decreases. From a biological standpoint, what parameters would have to change to accommodate a reduced object distance?

Equation 2 indicates that object distance is related to both the focal length of the lens and the distance between the lens and the image formed, so one or both of these parameters are going to have to change. Based on the structure of the human eye, the image distance is unlikely to change, as the distance between the lens and retina is fixed. What about focal length? The last paragraph indicates that the "focal length of the eye is under muscular control." Okay, now we're getting somewhere! In order to focus our gaze on an up-close object, the eye's focal length must change, and that requires muscular involvement. We know that focal length is determined by the radius of curvature of the lens, and specifically we know it's equal to half the radius of curvature, so we can imagine the muscles of the eye contracting and relaxing to change the shape of the lens, allowing it to focus on objects at various distances.

Therefore, we have a robust prediction of what the correct answer choice will look like. We'll want something about muscles or radius of curvature. So let's at look at the answer choices! First, let's consider choices A and B, which make opposite predictions about the effects of muscle weakness: choice A says that muscle weakness around the eye lens inhibits shortening of the radius of curvature, and the other says that muscle weakness inhibits lengthening. Although we don't always get two answer choices that are exact opposites, when we do, there's a strong chance that one of them is right.

Distinguishing between choices A and B requires us to determine the direction in which the radius of curvature may change. This requires some math. Let's take a look at the relationship between the relevant variables from Equation 2. Since the radius of curvature is just twice the focal length, let's focus on these two variables. Image distance must remain constant, so let's get rid of that term altogether. By doing so, we can see that as object distance decreases, the focal length must also decrease. Consequently, so must the radius of curvature. Therefore, choice A seems very tempting. Plus, we know that muscle atrophy and weakness is certainly part of the aging process, so this answer choice makes a lot of sense! In fact, it does turn out that A is the correct answer.

Thus, choice B was incorrect because it muddled the appropriate mathematical relationships. However, let's look more closely at reasons why we might have been tempted to select this wrong answer choice. For example, this answer choice could be tempting if we put all the pieces together correctly, like if we knew muscle weakness and radius of curvature were related, but we didn't know in which direction. Maybe we made assumptions about how we'd expect muscle weakness to affect the radius of curvature, but we didn't draw the right connection to image distance or realize that we should rely on Equation 2. We might have also been tripped up by the language here: "inhibits shortening" sounds kind of like a double negative, so maybe our gut told us to choose the answer choice that said "inhibits lengthening" instead. Make sure your reasoning for choosing the right answer is grounded in scientific logic. If you're not confident in your answer selection, consider whether you've made all the necessary connections.

In this case, we built up a strong prediction before we got to our answer choices, but that's not always absolutely necessary. Sometimes you might not be 100% sure how to get started on a question, but the answer choices may get our cognitive gears turning. Thus, having a solid framework for tackling science questions will certainly give you a head start, but knowing how to critically examine answer choices is also an important skill.

7. Science Wrong Answer Patterns

In the previous section, we evaluated the following passage-based question: "Which of the following best explains why older people have a hard time focusing on nearby objects?" The correct answer was "muscle weakness around the eye lens inhibits shortening the radius of curvature," but let's also look at some ways the answer choices might have gone wrong. For instance, choice C read "Muscle paralysis around the eye lens inhibits shortening of the radius of curvature." The mention of paralysis is a red flag, because that would imply only being able to focus on objects at a single length, which completely violates common sense. Thus, an answer choice like this is too extreme in the sense that we shouldn't expect the eye lens to be completely fixed with aging. Keep your eye out for extreme, or appealing-sounding but unrealistic, answer choices because an answer choice that is so close to being spot on, but then takes it a little too far, is every MCAT writer's favorite trick.

You'll often see words like "always," "never," and "only" in extreme answer choices, but also be on the lookout for less obvious variations on extremes, such as when two things are described as the "same" or "identical," or when something is called the "ideal" or absolute "best," or when something can only be "exactly" or "precisely" one thing. Moderating terms, like "may," "might," or "often," are more flexible and thus harder to invalidate, making for better answer choices. Notice how "muscle weakness may inhibit shortening of the radius of curvature" has softer language than something like "muscle weakness always completely prevents shortening of the radius of curvature," and that sort of flexibility or generality is something you're going to want to look out for in correct answer choices. That said, context matters, too. Muscle paralysis is extreme for this question, but it might not be for a question about botulinum toxin, which literally does paralyze muscles.

There are, of course, other reasons why an answer choice might be a poor fit. For example, we want to avoid answer choices that are too broad or too narrow. An answer choice that's too broad might suggest that all of the parts of the eye naturally get stiffer and weaker as we age, like choice D, which isn't quite as specific as an answer choice that focuses on the muscles controlling the shape of the lens. An answer choice that's too narrow might just focus on the stiffness of the lens itself, while discounting the role of the eye muscles that are at least partly responsible for this stiffness. So, by having a prediction in mind, we'll be better equipped to identify the answer choice that truly is the best fit for the question.

Let's now imagine another answer choice, which attributes this age-related process to the refractive index of the vitreous humor changing. First, let's consider whether that possibility is scientifically plausible from a physics standpoint. If the refractive index of the vitreous humor changes, that will affect how light refracts between the lens and the vitreous humor, and where that light hits the retina. Thus, the lens would have to overcompensate or undercompensate to refract the light onto the retina, and it's hard to say whether that would have a disproportionate effect on visualizing close-up objects. Now, what is the likelihood that the refractive index of the vitreous humor would change? The refractive index of a material only changes if its density changes. Theoretically, the amount or type of protein secreted into the vitreous humor could change with aging, although the extent to which that would have a significant effect on its refractive index is dubious. At best, this explanation is maybe plausible, or at least possible, but we have absolutely no information to support it. There's nothing in the passage or from required MCAT knowledge that suggests this, so we'd really be going out too far on a limb to select this answer choice. There are also too many question marks and missing links, too many places where this could go wrong. Instead, you should select answer choices with at least some direct support, either in the passage or in your reserve of MCAT-specific content knowledge.

Let's examine two more possible wrong answer choices, one that claims that the shape of the cornea flattens with age, and one that claims the shape of the eye lens flattens with age, scattering incoming light less effectively. Although scientifically speaking, the cornea and the overall shape of the eye might flatten with age, and that would certainly affect refraction of light onto the retina, such changes would affect both near and far vision, so they fail to provide an explanation specific to near vision. Instead, we need to look for something that would focus on the lens failing to do its job focusing on up-close objects.

Additionally, it's worth noting that the latter choice, which says this "scatters incoming light less effectively," echoes the part of the passage that says "negative lenses scatter incoming light beams." Keyword matching like this doesn't automatically invalidate an answer choice, but it's a warning sign because keyword matching patterns are a trick that writers can use to make incorrect answer choices superficially tempting. The basic flaw with this answer choice is that it refers to the wrong part of the passage - specifically, it refers to negative lenses. Based on Figures 1 and 2, it's pretty clear that the lens of the human eye is a positive lens, meaning that this answer choice flat-out contradicts the passage. However, this remains a tempting answer choice for students for two reasons. For one, the use of passage keywords can automatically tempt test-takers. Second, if we like the first half of this answer choice, confirmation bias might tempt us to nod along with its second half and ignore what's otherwise a subtle error. Instead, we must remember to be critical of every part of an answer choice: if an answer choice is even 1% incorrect, then it's 100% incorrect.

Let's take a look at another wrong answer choice. This one states that a reduction in photoreceptor density in the retina impairs visual perception during aging. Technically this is scientifically legitimate, right? A loss of photoreceptors is something that could, and does, occur with aging. So what's the problem? The problem is that it doesn't really answer the question, which is: *What best explains why older people have a hard time focusing on nearby objects?* Photoreceptors have nothing to do with the optics of focusing light on the retina. For this reason, it's essential not to lose sight of what we're really being asked, and it almost never hurts to refer back to the question stem. Additionally, this answer choice does keyword matching itself, by referring to the rod and cone receptors "responsible for visual perception" in the last paragraph. Again, this refers to a different idea from the passage that is not relevant to the immediate question at hand. Be wary of answer choices that are out-of-scope or irrelevant to the topic of the question.

A final important wrong answer pattern involves errors in causality. The question we've been exploring is exactly the kind that might contain answer choices with causal errors, precisely because it asks for the cause or explanation for something. You might see this when asked for a putative explanation for some scientific phenomenon, or when you're asked to explain the results of an experiment. Suppose an answer choice suggested, for example, that straining of the eye to see nearby objects as we age causes the muscles controlling the lens of the eye to weaken. That proposal may or may not be true, perpetuating some kind of positive feedback loop, but it fails to explain why our eyes strain to see nearby objects as we age in the first place. Be careful to avoid reversing the causal variables, as happened here, and also to make sure you've correctly identified the causal variables at play. Furthermore, be careful not to confuse correlation with causation. Lots of changes happen as we age—our bones become more fragile, our hearing ability diminishes, short-term memory starts to decay—but none of these sufficiently explains the cause of the visual impairment described in the question stem.

8. Process of Elimination

Now let's integrate our knowledge about how to tackle MCAT science questions from top to bottom, and how to identify wrong answer patterns, by discussing how exactly to evaluate and eliminate answer choices.

Process of elimination is a legitimate strategy for any question you encounter. If you can latch onto the correct answer right away, fantastic! Then you can move right along. But most of the time, answering science questions won't be quite as straightforward. Elimination isn't just a backup strategy: it's a key tool you'll use to triage answer choices based on how likely they are to be correct. Even eliminating just one incorrect choice increases your likelihood of getting the question right on chance alone up to one-third, and eliminating two boosts your chance of answering correctly up to 50:50.

When eliminating answer choices, we suggest literally striking out each answer choice that's no longer in the running. There are two benefits to this. First of all, if you choose to flag this question and review it later, you can pick up right where you left off. Second, visually narrowing down your options has psychological benefits, reducing distractors so you can dedicate all your focus only on the most likely contenders.

To play devil's advocate, there is one significant risk with being overzealous with the strikethrough tool: accidentally striking out the correct answer choice. This is very common, and the first step in coping with it is to carefully review your practice material to determine whether you should eliminate answer choices more cautiously. If so, you can put this into practice in two ways. First, up your threshold for striking through an answer choice. Make sure you've vetted it thoroughly and feel confident about removing it as an option. Evaluate your reasons for eliminating that answer choice rather than getting rid of it on impulse or for flawed reasons. Second, if you've eliminated one or more answer choices but feel stuck on the question, re-evaluate those choices in case you've eliminated one in error. This is particularly true when returning to review flagged questions, as your perspective on a question may evolve with time, perhaps casting the answer choices in a different light. Third, unless you're seriously crunched for time, make sure to check all the answer choices before selecting the best answer. And finally, be sure to flag questions when you feel like you've hit a dead-end so you can come back to them later.

A few question types are particularly well-suited to the process of elimination, including Roman numeral questions. Here's an example:

> Consider the following pipe, which is closed at x = 0 and open at x = L, and which contains a standing wave. Which of the following statements are accurate?

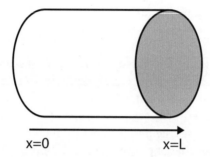

x=0   x=L

> I. The velocity of air molecules is zero at x = 0.
> II. The velocity of air molecules is zero at x = L.
> III. The velocity of air molecules is constant throughout the pipe.

> A. I only

> B. III only

> C. I and II only

> D. I and III only

With these questions, if we can eliminate any one of these Roman numerals, we may be able to knock out more than one answer choice. Let's start with numeral III since it occurs in exactly two choices. At x=0, the pipe we're shown is closed. This means there is a node at this point, and the velocity of air molecules here must be zero. However, at x = L, the pipe is open. This means that this point represents an antinode, or point of maximum amplitude. Numeral III is false, so we can eliminate choices B and D. At this point, we need only evaluate numeral II to choose an answer. However, notice that we've actually already addressed both numerals I and II in thinking through numeral III. Numeral I must be true and II is false. We can confidently choose A and move on.

A similar procedure can be used for Two-Part questions. For example, suppose this same basic question were posed, but in a different form:

> Consider the following pipe, which is closed at x = 0 and open at x = L, and which contains a standing wave.

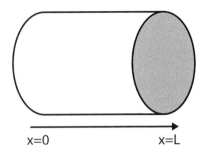

Which of the following statements are accurate?

A. The velocity of air molecules is zero at x = 0 and zero at x = L.

B. The velocity of air molecules is zero at x = 0 and nonzero at x = L.

C. The velocity of air molecules is nonzero at x = 0 and zero at x = L.

D. The velocity of air molecules is nonzero at x = 0 and nonzero at x = L.

Based on these answer choices, we have two decisions to make. First, what is the velocity of air molecules at x = 0, and what is the velocity of air molecules at x = L? If we know that the velocity is zero at x = 0, we can eliminate any answer choices that say otherwise, and then look for an answer choice that gives a non-zero velocity at x = L.

Elimination is also a good strategy for questions that contain the words NOT, EXCEPT, or LEAST and require you to select the answer choice that's unlike the rest. For this example, suppose this same question was instead posed in such a way:

Consider the following pipe, which is closed at x = 0 and open at x = L, and which contains a standing wave.

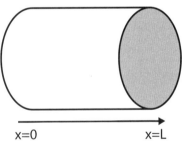

Which of the following statements is NOT accurate?

A. The velocity of air molecules is zero at x = 0.

B. The velocity of air molecules is nonzero at x = L.

C. The velocity of air molecules is constant throughout the pipe.

D. The velocity of air molecules varies throughout the pipe.

One way to approach such a question is to simply identify the one we know to be false. An equally legitimate approach is to eliminate all the ones we know to be true. As you do so, be mindful to strike through the true statements so we're left with one that's false.

The final category of questions particularly well-suited for elimination strategies are Ranking questions that ask you to identify the answer with the greatest or least value of some property. For example, suppose we were asked:

When white light moves from a vacuum to a glass prism, the component color that bends the most is:

A. blue light.

B. yellow light.

C. green light.

D. All colors of light bend the same when changing from one medium to another.

Before we even start evaluating the answer choices, let's make a prediction. We know that when light travels from a vacuum into glass, it bends toward the normal at an angle based on the index of refraction. The key to answering this question is realizing that different colors of light have different refractive indices in glass. First, we can eliminate choice D. It won't always work to immediately eliminate the "none of the above" option right off the bat, but in this case, we know this answer choice is scientifically invalid, so let's get rid of it. Now we're left with three colors to choose between. The refractive index of different colors in glass ultimately boils down to their wavelength, with shorter wavelengths having larger indices of refraction and bending the most. So even if we don't know yet which color to pick, the correct answer to a Ranking question is most likely going to be one of the extreme choices on a spectrum, meaning eliminating intermediate choices is a relatively safe bet. On the visible spectrum, yellow falls in between green and blue, so it's unlikely to have the shortest wavelength, and we can eliminate it. At this point, you might recall that red is the color with the longest wavelength, and violet light has the shortest wavelength. Since blue is closest to violet on the visible spectrum, it's going to have the shortest wavelength among these answer choices and bend the most in a glass prism.

Finally, you should also use this method to eliminate obviously absurd or flawed answer choices. If one of the answer choices gives you a number that's orders of magnitudes out of the ballpark, uses the wrong units, introduces an unrelated term, or is unreasonable or illogical for some other reason, go ahead and strike it out.

9. Must-Knows

> Four basic steps to answering MCAT questions:
  - Interpreting the question.
  - Getting the information you need to answer the question.
  - Making a generalized prediction.
  - Evaluating the answer choices.
> Interpreting the question seems obvious, but can be a source of a surprising amount of difficulty:
  - Questions may present an example or analogy of some concept, so we must trim away the details by paraphrasing.
  - Unfamiliar terms may be distracting. When paraphrasing, try to figure out what they represent.
  - Analyzing the answer choices may help figure out what a question is getting at.
> Working through the question:
  - You may or may not have to go back to the passage. "Pseudodiscretes" can be answered with minimal, or no, passage information.
  - If it is necessary to return to the passage, do so strategically and efficiently.
  - Make a prediction (i.e., a general conceptualization of what you're looking for in the right answer).
> Special question types:
  - Analogy questions present a scientific concept and ask for an example or analogous concept, or present an example and ask what scientific concept applies.
  - Roman numeral questions: key is to work systematically through the Roman numeral options and then eliminate answer choices.
  - Two-part questions: use logic to break up the answer choices and evaluate one component at a time.
  - Ranking questions: figure out what parameter they're trying to test, focus on extreme examples (i.e., ends of the spectrum).
  - Quantitative (calculation-based questions): think carefully about how to solve the problem before writing down equations, write calculations legibly, and don't rush too much.
  - Figure questions: use figure caption to determine what the figure is getting at, then read the figure carefully to make sure the information you're taking actually answers the question.
> Science answers can be wrong for three basic reasons:
  - Being scientifically wrong.
  - Being wrong based on the information in the passage or question prompt.
  - Containing a reasoning flaw, even if they technically don't violate any science or passage information (for example, if an answer choice doesn't actually address what the question is asking).
> Process of elimination: can be very useful. Watch out for specific flaws (errors in causality, answers that are too extreme, etc.). Reasoning skills developed in CARS practice can pay off here too.

Applied Practice

The best MCAT practice is realistic, with detailed analytics to help you assess where things went wrong. For those reasons, we recommend completing practice questions in an online setting that simulates the real MCAT interface, and using the analytics provided to help you decide how to best move your studies forward.

CARS does not require knowledge of specific subject areas, but it does require development of strong test-taking skills. To ensure you are honing those skills as you work through this book, we suggest you go online after wrapping up each chapter and generate a Qbank Practice Set of 2-3 CARS passages to practice and review. While not every chapter of this book is directly applicable to CARS, regular CARS practice is key to test day success.

As a further supplement, given the importance of active learning for effective studying, we also suggest that you consult the Must-Knows at the end of each chapter of this Reasoning text as a basis for creating a study sheet. This is not a sheet to memorize in the more traditional sense of content memorization, but rather a quick reference of the most important strategies for you to refer to during and after practice in your early prep. Frequently revisiting the most important strategies for the MCAT - in both CARS and the Sciences - will help you continue to improve your performance.

This page left intentionally blank.

This page left intentionally blank.

INDEX